# HOMOCYSTEINE AND VASCULAR DISEASE

# Developments in Cardiovascular Medicine

VOLUME 230

# Homocysteine and Vascular Disease

*edited by*

## KILLIAN ROBINSON

*Department of Cardiology,*
*The Cleveland Clinic Foundation,*
*Cleveland, Ohio, U.S.A.*

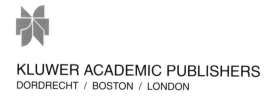

KLUWER ACADEMIC PUBLISHERS
DORDRECHT / BOSTON / LONDON

A C.I.P. Catalogue record for this book is available from the Library of Congress.

ISBN 0-7923-6248-9

Published by Kluwer Academic Publishers,
P.O. Box 17, 3300 AA Dordrecht, The Netherlands.

Sold and distributed in North, Central and South America
by Kluwer Academic Publishers,
101 Philip Drive, Norwell, MA 02061, U.S.A.

In all other countries, sold and distributed
by Kluwer Academic Publishers,
P.O. Box 322, 3300 AH Dordrecht, The Netherlands.

*Printed on acid-free paper*

# TABLE OF CONTENTS

# FOREWORD

This is an important and timely volume. The history of research in homocysteine metabolism can be divided into three periods. The first phase was the exploration of the individual reactions and metabolites that characterize the transmethylation and transsulfuration sequences. The former originated with his description of the biosynthesis of methylpyridine and culminated in the work of Cantoni and Axelrod. Similarly the finding that insulin contained cystine was a potent catalyst for the metabolic and nutritional studies of Rose and du Vigneaud.

The description and the definition of homocystinuria, a rare inherited metabolic disorder, marked the beginning of the second historical period. Where previously there had been few laboratories located largely in the United States soon there were numerous research groups representing many nationalities. The more intense focus led to major advances, both in the laboratory and in the clinics. Studies of afflicted individuals, when combined with investigations in experimental animals, provided the basis for a concept of methionine metabolism that encompassed both transmethylation and transsulfuration. The central role of homocysteine was apparent.

Conversely, the early clinical observations of these patients opened a new area for investigation - the relationship between biochemical abnormalities and several significant pathologies. Researchers sought explanations for the mental retardation, skeletal abnormalities and thrombovascular disorders. Although the first two areas remain relatively unexplored, studies of vascular dysfunction have proliferated following the suggestion that disordered homocysteine metabolism might explain vascular diseases in a population broader than those with the rare genetic defects. Thus it remains for the next generation of investigators to tell us whether lower levels of hyperhomocysteinemia, have the same vascular toxicity that occurs at the much higher levels found in homocystinuria. Furthermore they must define the pathochemical mechanisms. Lastly, we must know whether reduction of plasma homocysteine concentrations halts and/or reverses the vascular pathology.

Thus this volume rests comfortably on the border between the second and third periods of homocysteine study. It will prove to be an invaluable road map - providing a comprehensive review of the earlier work while offering us an outline for future expectations.

James D. Finkelstein, M.D.
February 1999

## EDITOR'S HISTORICAL PREFACE

In 1959, Claude Field, a pediatrician at Belfast City Hospital, was referred a 6 year old girl for evaluation of convulsive episodes for which no cause could be found. Patricia, aged 6 years, was a first child, and the mother had had two previous miscarriages. Patricia had a younger sister of almost identical appearance. She was a premature infant of 1023 gms, due to pre-eclamptic toxemia. She sat up at 10 months and walked at 18 months. At three years she was thought to be quite fit, although still slow to develop mentally. Talking began at five years. She was placid, plump and obviously mentally backward. She was at the 50th percentile for height and 75th percentile for weight. She had fine, dry, sparse blond hair and blue eyes showing iridodonesis due to bilateral posterior dislocation of the lenses. Her complexion was fair with bright pink patches of colour on each cheek. Her skin elsewhere was covered with erythematous blotches resembling the pattern of erythema ab igne. She had genu valgum and pes cavus. Her liver was enlarged. The Babinski responses were equivocal on the right side and extensor on the left. She had about a dozen words of speech. She was cooperative and could obey simple commands. Later that month, her sister Pauline was brought to hospital by request. She was four years old, birth had been normal, she had walked at 15 months and had not yet started to speak. She had a major motor seizure in July 1959 lasting two hours. Her height and weight were at the 3rd and the 25th percentiles respectively. Her liver was not enlarged.

Extensive investigations, including chromosome analysis, were performed but revealed nothing untoward. Samples of urine were sent to Nina Carson and Desmond Neill at the Royal Victoria Hospital, Belfast, who were studing metabolic abnormalities in the mentally handicapped. The cyanide nitroprusside test for cystine was positive and amino acid screening showed a spot in the cystine position. However, as this was not accompanied by the other amino acids found in cystinuria, further urine specimens were sent to Professor Charles Dent at University College Hospital, London. In his laboratory, amino acid chromatography on these, and subsequent 24 hour specimens, appeared to show that the amino acid was not cystine but homocystine.

Simultanously, another group had been working in Wisconsin, in the United States. At that time, development of amino acid analysis in physiological fluids had reached the stage where, in different laboratories all over the world, qualitative information was obtained by (2-dimensional) paper chromatography and/or electrophoresis, and quantitative data by ion-exchange column chromatography. Thus, essential amino acids and other ninhydrin-positive compounds acting as intermediates in different metabolic pathways could be analysed.

These compounds were often undetectable in urine or blood of healthy normals, but were found to be present in the urine (and often plasma) of pediatric patients with congenital anomalies. In 1962, this group discovered an infant with congenital anomalies, mental retardation and failure to thrive and provided the first definitive chemical proof of homocystine excretion in the urine of which they gave qualitative data. They also mentioned the increased urinary excretion of methionine.

Claude Field presented the results of their work at the 10th International Congress on Paediatrics in Lisbon, Portugal in September 1962 (1). That year, Gerritsen et al published the findings on their patient (2) and, also that year, Carson and Neill published a fuller description of the two cases as part of their survey of mentally backward children (3). In this manner, Drs Carson, Field, Gerritsen and Waisman were collectively responsible for the initial clinical descriptions of homocystinuria and for the correct initial identification of homocystine in the urine of the first cases. Their seminal observations were followed by the mapping of the underlying genetic and metabolic abnormalities by Finkelstein and Mudd (4). Later, McCully (5) would raise the homocysteine hypothesis of vascular disease and Wilcken and Wilcken (6) would apply all these principles to the coronary disease population. The rest, as they say, is history. Although the two little sisters are now dead, the descriptions of them by all these earlier investigators have now become a burgeoning research area, intimately connected with vascular diseases, molecular biology, vitamin nutrition and clinical trials.

It is rare privilege for an editor to have had the opportunity to work with the founders of a field some of whom have contributed to this volume. I am deeply grateful to Drs Carson, Field and Gerritsen, all now retired, who provided personal notes and background information. Special thanks go to both Professor Alun Evans at Queens University, Belfast and Dr Godfried Boers Academisch Ziekenhuis, Nijmegen who facilitated this process.

## REFERENCES

1.  Field CMB, Carson NAJ, Cusworth DC, Dent CE, Neill DW. Homocystinuria: a new disorder of metabolism. Annales Nestle 1962;9:73 (Xth International Congress on Paediatrics, Lisbon, Portugal).
2.  Gerritsen T, Vaughn JG, Waisman HA. The identification of homocystine in the urine. Biochem Biophys Res Commun 1962;9:493-6.
3.  Carson NAJ, Neill DW. Metabolic abnormalities detected in a survey of mentally backward individuals in Northern Ireland. Arch Dis Childh 1962;37:505-13.
4.  Laster L, Mudd SH, Finkelstein JD, Irreverre F. Homocystinuria due to cystathionine synthase deficiency: the metabolism of L-methionine. J Clin Invest 1965;44:1708-19.

5.  McCully KS. Vascular pathology of homocysteinemia: implications for the pathogenesis of arteriosclerosis. Am J Pathol 1969; 56:111-28.

6.  Wilcken DEL, Wilcken B. The pathogenesis of coronary artery disease. A possible role for methionine metabolism. J Clin Invest 1976; 57:1079-82.

# LIST OF CONTRIBUTORS

Professor Generoso ANDRIA, Dipartmamento di Pediatric, Federico II University, Via S. Pansini 5, I-80131 Naples, Italy

Dr Ruma BANERJEE, Biochemistry Department, University of Nebraska, N 133 Beadle Center, Lincoln, NE 68588-0664, U.S.A.

Dr Henk BLOM, Laboratory of Pediatrics and Neurology, University Hospital Nijmegen, P.O. Box 9101, 6500 HB Nijmegen, The Netherlands

Dr Godfried BOERS, Department of Endocrinology, Katholieke Universiteit Nijmegen, Postbus 9101, 6055 HB Nijmegen, The Netherlands

Dr Robert CLARKE, Clinical Trial Service Unit, Nuffield Department of Clinical Medicine, Harkness Building, Radcliffe Infirmary, Oxford 0X2 6HE, UK

P. Barton DUELL, M.D., Division of Endocrinology, Diabetes, and Clinical Nutrition, Oregon Health Sciences University, L465, 3181 SW Sam Jackson Park Road, Portland, OR 97201-3098, U.S.A.

Professor Ian GRAHAM, Cardiology Department, Charlemont Clinic, Charlemont Mall, Dublin 2, Ireland

Dr J. Ralph GREEN, Department of Pathology, University of Davis Medical Center, 2315 Stockton Boulevard, Sacramento, CA 95817, U.S.A.

Dr Brian FOWLER, Kinderspital Basel, Univ. Child. Hospital, Romergasse 8, Postfach, CH-4058 Basel, Switzerland

Dr Martin den HEIJER, Department of Internal Medicine, University Hospital Nijmegen, P.O. Box 9101, 6500 HB Nijmegen, The Netherlands

Dr Donald W. JACOBSEN, Department of Cell Biology, The Cleveland Clinic Foundation, Desk FF40, 9500 Euclid Avenue, Clevelanad OH 44195, U.S.A.

Dr Warren KRUGER, The Fox Chase Cancer Center, 7701 Burholme Avenue, Philadelphia, PA 19111, U.S.A.

Dr Joseph LOSCALZO, Whitaker Cardiovascular Institute, Boston University School of Medicine, 715 Albany Street, W507, Boston, MA 02118, U.S.A.

Dr M. Rene MALINOW, Laboratory of Cardiovascular Diseases, Oregon Regional Primate Research Center, 505 NW 185th Avenue, Beaverton, OR 97006-3499, U.S.A.

Dr Kilmer McCULLY, Pathology and Laboratory Medicine Service, Department of Veterans Affair, Medical Center, Providence, RI 02908-4799, U.S.A.

Dr Arno MOTULSKY, Department of Medicine, Division of Medical Genetics, University of Washington, Box 356423, Seattle, WA 98195-6423, U.S.A.

Professor Ivan PERRY, Department of Epidemiology, Univesity College Cork, Cork, Ireland

Professor Helga REFSUM, Department of Pharmacology & Toxicology, University of Bergen, Haukeland Hospital, Armauer Hansen Hus, N-5021 Bergen, Norway

Dr Killian ROBINSON, Department of Cardiology, The Cleveland Clinic Foundation, Desk F15, 9500 Euclid Avenue, Cleveland, OH 44195, U.S.A.

Dr Rima ROZEN, Department of Human Genetics, McGill University, 4060 St. Catherine W. #242, Momtreal, Quebec, Canada H3Z 2Z3, Canada

Dr Barry SHANE, 6465 Swainland Road, Oakland, CA , U.S.A.

Professor Lloyd TAYLOR, Department of Surgery, Division of Vascular Surgery, Oregon Health Sciences University, 3181 SW Sam Jackson Park Road, Portland, OH 97201-3098, U.S.A.

Dr Johan B. UBBINK, Department of Chemical Pathology, University of Pretoria, Faculty of Medicine, P.O. Box 2034, 0001 Pretoria, South Africa

Dr Per Magne UELAND, Clinical Pharmacology Unit, University of Bergen, Central Laboratory Haukeland Hospital, Armauer Hansens hus, N-5021 Bergen, Norway

Dr Petra VERHOEF, Wageningen Centre for Foord Sciences, and Wageningen University, Division of Human Nutrition and Epidemiology, 6703 HD Wageningen, The Netherlands

Professor David WILCKEN, Department of Cardiovascular Medicine, Prince of Wales Hospital, Blacket Building, South Avoca Street, Randwick, 2031 New WALES, Australia

Dr Peter WILSON, The Framingham Heart Study, Five Thurber Street, Framingham, MA 01701, U.S.A.

NOTE ON NOMENCLATURE

Specifically, the term homocysteine refers to the free reduced form of this amino acid. Other circulating forms include homocysteine-cysteine mixed disulfide, homocysteine-homocysteine (homocystine) and protein-bound homocysteine. Total homocysteine is defined as the sum of reduced and oxidized forms of homocysteine in plasma. Homocysteine thiolactone is another form which may exist in small amounts in human plasma. Different options for nomenclature are used by various authorities in the field. In this text, for simplicity, unless specifically qualified, the term homocysteine is used generically to refer either to total homocysteine or to one of the above species. The term homocysteinemia and the spelling hyperhomocyst(e)inemia have both been deliberately avoided as they may be confusing to the non-specialist. If the precise details of the exact biochemical form of homocysteine which was used in any particular study are required the reader should consult the original references.

To Jackie Yew Ming, Síofra, Ríoghnach, Liam, Kathleen, Orna, Ferga and Dara. And Séamus.

# 1. INTRODUCTION

This is the first text specifically devoted to homocysteine and its relationship to vascular diseases. This amino acid, which plays a central role in folate and methionine metabolism, is now regarded by many as a potentially major risk factor for cardiovascular diseases and venous thrombosis. It is also a risk factor for the vascular complications of other systemic disorders such as end stage renal disease and systemic lupus erythematosus. There has been an exponential increase in the scientific output in this field in the last ten years. As with all risk factors for vascular disease, investigations have been undertaken in many fields including epidemiology, the basic sciences and clinical medicine. This text brings together many of the workers in these fields including some of those responsible for the original clinical and pathological reports which made the initial connection between homocysteine and vascular disease over twenty years ago. The reader will therefore see that this field is by no means new but it has certainly received a renewed and increased interest in the last decade.

Atherosclerotic vascular disease, particularly coronary heart disease, is a leading cause of death world-wide and, with the decline in communicable diseases, will become even more important over the next 20 years. While age specific death rates have declined substantially in many developed countries, total mortality has changed less, because of a transference of cases from younger to older age groups. Furthermore, death rates are rising in developing countries. At a population level, atherosclerotic vascular disease appears to be primarily environmental, although individual susceptibility may be genetically determined. Of more than 200 putative risk factors for coronary heart disease, a high fat diet with consequent hyperlipidemia, cigarette smoking and hypertension consistently emerge as powerful, graded and independent causal risk factors. These risk factors may be modified by both genetic and environmental factors; for example hyperlipidemia may be genetically determined, but also relates strongly to a high saturated fat diet.

The observation that a raised plasma homocysteine level might be a new and powerful risk factor is comparatively recent, starting with the description

1

K. Robinson (ed.), Homocysteine and Vascular Disease, 1-4.
© 2000 Kluwer Academic Publishers. Printed in the Netherlands.

of homocystinuria in 1962. Such subjects, with genetically determined severely raised plasma homocysteine levels and the excretion of the dimer homocystine in the urine have a high risk of premature atherothrombotic events. By 1964, the most frequent enzyme defect responsible for homocystinuria was described, followed by the description of the vascular pathology and the formulation of the homocysteine theory of arteriosclerosis. In formulating this theory, McCully noted that hyperhomocysteinemia arising from different metabolic defects was associated with premature arteriosclerosis. These observations set the scene for clinical and epidemiologic studies which examined whether milder elevations of plasma homocysteine might also be associated with vascular disease.

As reviewed by Jacobsen, plasma homocysteine levels are controlled by the interplay between genetically determined enzyme activity and nutritional factors, notably vitamins $B_6$ and $B_{12}$ as co-factors and folate as a co-substrate. S-adenosylmethionine modulates these interactions. Ubbink presents reference ranges for homocysteine concentrations. As with a number of other risk factors, statistically defined reference ranges of total plasma homocysteine of, for example, 5-15 µmol/L may not reflect normal, defined as desirable for health. In one large case-control study, a fasting total plasma homocysteine of 12 µmol/L or more was associated with a doubling of risk of cardiovascular disease and it may be that risk rises in a graded manner from considerably lower levels.

Refsum, Ueland and Schneede explore further the relationships between genetic and environmental causes of an increased plasma homocysteine level, and note that suboptimal vitamin intake is a primary determinant. Smoking, physical inactivity, coffee, certain drugs and diseases such as renal failure may all contribute, substantially so in the case of renal disease. Wilson notes that 20 to 30% of the US population may have insufficient folate intake and that recently introduced food fortification may reduce the prevalence of hyperhomocysteinemia in the adult population.

Homocysteine may be damaging to the vascular tree, through direct toxicity, interaction with other risk factors, impairment of endothelial function, or the promotion of the proliferation of vascular tissues. A precise mechanism, however, is still not clear and much of the basic research requires replication and extension. Whatever the mechanism, the association with vascular disease is beyond doubt. In observational epidemiological studies, the risk appears to be stronger in case-control than prospective studies. That said, the suggestion that a raised plasma homocysteine is a cause rather than effect of vascular disease is not well founded, particularly in view of the aggressive disease experienced in genetic cases. It is possible that the risk is stronger for the recurrence rather than for the first occurrence of a vascular event. Between them, the Naples group, Taylor, Duell and Malinow, den Heijer and Perry indicate that a raised plasma homocysteine is associated with increased risk of all form of atherosclerotic vascular disease, including coronary heart disease and venous thrombosis.

The relationship of homocysteine to other risk factors is described in the sections on vascular diseases and in the appropriate basic science section. Two areas have been given special attention. As homocysteine requires a number of enzymes for normal metabolism and several disorders have been described in which high levels of the amino acid may be produced by a genetic abnormality it is not surprising that hyperhomocysteinemia may be familial, and the studies in this area have been reviewed separately by Genest. It is also important to note that many of the studies of patients with vascular disease have been performed on men only and a separate chapter has therefore been written by Verhoef to address the published data on homocysteine as a risk factor for vascular disease in women.

For reasons which remain unclear, a high plasma homocysteine concentration is often found in patients with renal failure. Proposed mechanisms for the hyperhomocysteinemia include reduced elimination by either renal or non-renal routes and inhibition of essential vitamin-related reactions in the uremic environment. Studies using both case control-type and prospective designs have now established that hyperhomocysteinemia is an independent risk factor for vascular complications in dialyzed patients with en-stage renal disease. Trials are now are underway to evaluate the effects, if any, of homocysteine reduction on vascular risk in patients with renal failure.

The molecular biology of the enzymes controlling homocysteine levels has been the subject of intense and elegant research. These aspects are reviewed by Rozen, Banerjee and Kruger. Initially, interest focused on cystathionine β-synthase, (CBS), the enzyme responsible for the irreversible degradation of homocysteine. While homozygous deficiency of CBS is associated with homocystinuria and aggressive vascular disease, it is still unclear if heterozygotes for this enzyme defect are at increased risk or not. This mutation does not appear to be a major contributor to the burden of risk associated with modestly raised homocysteine levels. Recently, much interest has focused on the thermolabile variant of methylenetetrahydrofolate reductase. Subjects with this mutation have modestly elevated homocysteine levels, particularly if folate deplete, but the association with risk, if any, is modest. To date, rather less attention has been paid to methionine synthase in relation to cardiovascular disease.

Homocysteine interacts with conventional risk factors, particularly hypertension and smoking to powerfully increase risk. It may also interact with cholesterol but Blom finds little evidence that this is mediated through promotion of the oxidation of low density lipoprotein cholesterol. It would be expected that homocysteine might react with hemostatic factors and this is explored by Green. The explosive interest in vascular endothelial function extends to studies of homocysteine effects and this topical area is dealt with by Loscalzo.

Homocysteine is a very sensitive marker of folate, $B_{12}$ and $B_6$ status. Homocysteine levels start to rise as plasma concentrations of plasma folate or vitamin $B_{12}$ fall below the mean value and long before overt deficiency is present. Supplementation with these factors, particularly folate, can reduce homocysteine levels by perhaps 30% in most subjects. Thus, cheap, apparently risk free therapy to lower plasma homocysteine levels is available. There has, however, been little financial incentive to explore such therapy and randomized control trials of homocysteine lowering with folate and other nutrients are only now being undertaken. As both Rubba and Clarke point out, it does appear that homocysteine reduction by the use of vitamins in subjects with severe genetic hyperhomocysteinemia does indeed delay or prevent the occurrence of vascular disease.

Does a raised plasma homocysteine cause vascular disease? The relationship is strong, graded, consistent, independent and has biological plausibility. Although it has been suggested that vascular disease might itself cause a raised plasma homocysteine level this is not consistent with the observation that subjects with genetic hyperhomocysteinemia develop premature vascular disease. However, causality cannot be implied beyond reasonable doubt unless it can be shown lowering homocysteine levels with therapy such as folate reduces cardiovascular risk. This lends both clinical and public health importance to the randomized controlled trials reviewed by Clarke.

Fortmann, Motulsky and Shane point to the directions of future research through randomized control trials of therapy and suggestions for further research into putative mechanisms whereby homocysteine may be atherothrombotic. They also note that vitamin therapy may affect other aspects of methyl group homeostasis than homocysteine levels alone.

As far as possible, the chapters in this book have been presented for non-workers in the different areas and a summary has been provided at the beginning of each chapter to facilitate a rapid perusal of the state of each field at present. It is hoped that this book will serve as a useful reference source for the results of the major clinical and basic studies which have been performed to date and should also be a useful resource to anyone wishing to become fully familiar with the scope of this rapidly expanding field. This may include not only those who are already actively involved in any one area outlined in this book but also clinicians, nurses, nutritionists, epidemiologists, scientists, and others interested in risk factors and prevention of vascular disorders.

Ian Graham, Dublin, Ireland
Killian Robinson, Cleveland, USA

## 2. HISTORICAL ASPECTS OF THE RELATIONSHIP BETWEEN HOMO-CYSTEINE AND VASCULAR DISEASE

## SUMMARY

The possibility that modest elevations of circulating homocysteine (hyperhomocysteinemia) could contribute to cardiovascular risk arose from investigation of patients with greatly increased plasma homocysteine due to the rare inborn error of metabolism, cystathionine β-synthase deficiency. Such patients often had thromboembolic events before the age of 30 years. Because the established cardiovascular risk factors could only partly account for the occurrence and severity of vascular disease in the general population, other risk factors had to exist, and modest homocysteine elevation seemed a possible candidate.

Australian case-controlled studies to explore this hypothesis identified an association between mild homocysteine elevation and early-onset coronary disease; and in separate studies of patients with chronic renal failure, a patient group with a high prevalence of unexplained vascular disease, it was shown that they too had elevated homocysteine. It was also demonstrated that the modest homocysteine elevations in vascular patients could usually be normalized by daily oral folic acid (1 - 5mg) whilst in the patients with chronic renal insufficiency 5mg of folic acid daily markedly reduced the increased concentrations.

These initial observations have been confirmed by many investigators and biologically plausible mechanisms for homocysteine-induced vascular dysfunction, and particularly endothelial dysfunction, have been identified. Ho-

*K. Robinson (ed.), Homocysteine and Vascular Disease, 5-14.*
© 2000 *Kluwer Academic Publishers. Printed in the Netherlands.*

wever associations between hyperhomocysteinemia and other risk factors, eg smoking and hypertension, have also been documented and need to be controlled for when assessing any increase in risk that mild homocysteine elevation may independently confer. Whilst we have established that lowering the greatly elevated levels found in homocystinuria unquestionably reduces cardiovascular risk, it remains to be determined whether or not this is true for the normalising of the mild homocysteine elevation common in vascular disease patients in the general population. Trials to test this have been initiated and others planned.

## INTRODUCTION

Recognition of an association between the sulfur-containing amino acid homocysteine and vascular disease had its origin in the 1960s. It followed the identification of a new inborn error of metabolism in which a large quantity of homocysteine was excreted in the urine[1] and shown to be associated with precocious vascular disease[2]. It was soon established that the disorder was due to cystathionine β-synthase deficiency[3]. Several years elapsed before it became evident that among the complex metabolic changes identified in this inborn error it was the markedly elevated level of homocysteine itself which was the likely mediator of the vascular changes[4]. Some years later the possibility that modest homocysteine elevation might also interact with established risk factors and enhance cardiovascular risk was considered[5]. Further evidence for the hypothesis was obtained with the demonstration of increased homocysteine in chronic renal insufficiency and the suggestion that homocysteine elevation was a significant contributor to the well-documented greatly increased risk of vascular disease in patients with varying degrees of renal failure[6-9].

The many studies that followed have, in general, been supportive of a role for small increases in homocysteine in enhancing cardiovascular risk. However, the recent results of genetic, prospective, case control and population studies of mild homocysteine elevation have cast doubt on the validity of some aspects of the hypothesis. It is therefore an appropriate time to have a reflective assessment of homocysteine in relation to cardiovascular risk. There are several recent authoritative reviews of methionine metabolism and the relevance of homocysteine to vascular disease[10,11]. Thus this chapter must of necessity be selective and it seems appropriate for it to have some emphasis on the work which has emanated from our group.

## EVOLUTION OF THE CONCEPT OF HOMOCYSTEINE-INDUCED VASCULAR DISEASE

The st[1]ory begins with the publication in 1962 of the results of a search for metabolic abnormalities as causes of mental retardation and the identification by Carson and colleagues of a subset of patients who excreted large amounts of homocystine in the urine[1]. A new disorder of methionine metabolism was, in this way, uncovered and referred to as homocystinuria. The identification of other cases soon followed and in 1964 there was the first documentation of the pathological findings in homocystinuria and the description of widespread vascular changes and thrombosis[2]. It was also in 1964 that Mudd and colleagues identified the enzyme defect in the disorder showing that absence of, or diminished activity of, cystathionine β-synthase was responsible for the abnormality in the metabolism of the essential sulfur-containing amino acid methionine[3].

From the pathway shown in Fig. 1 it was therefore logical that the enzyme defect would result in a marked elevation of circulating methionine and homocysteine and a decrease in cysteine. These are the characteristic amino acid changes resulting from cystathionine β-synthase deficiency. Circulating homocysteine is almost entirely oxidized to homocystine and on the amino acid analyser it is measured as homocystine together with the mixed disulfide of homocysteine and cysteine; and in the urine it is measured as homocystine. It has become customary to refer to all measured circulating homocysteine moieties as homocysteine* to include twice the molar concentration of homocystine plus the molar concentration of cysteine-homocysteine. However, it was not until 1969 that it was first suggested that among the complex metabolic changes occurring in cystathionine β-synthase deficiency the factor mediating the vascular changes was a greatly elevated concentration of homocysteine. This was the result of two separate studies undertaken in the same patient.

The patient was an infant who died at the age of 7½ weeks. Biochemical studies undertaken by Mudd, Levy and Abeles established that the infant's urine and plasma contained markedly elevated levels of homocysteine and of cystathionine but that, unlike the findings in cystathionine β-synthase deficiency, methionine was extremely low in plasma and undetectable in urine[12]. In the detailed studies that followed they established that the elevated homocysteine was due to a disorder of remethylation of homocysteine to methionine and, as there was also methylmalonic aciduria and a normal concentration of vitamin $B_{12}$ in the patient's liver, they concluded that abnormal metabolism of vitamin

---

* See Note on Nomenclature p. xix

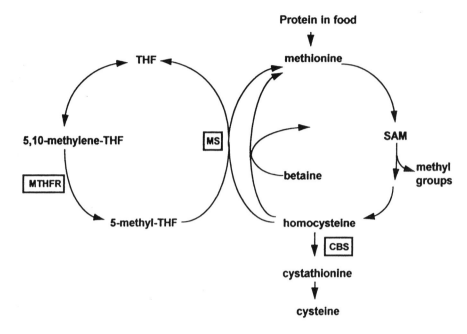

*Figure 1. The methionine degradation pathway. Methionine is metabolized via S-adenosyl me-thionine (SAM) and S-adenosyl-homocysteine to homocysteine in the course of producing methyl groups for use in synthetic processes. On a normal diet about 50% of the homocysteine formed is metabolized via the transsulfuration pathway (see text). The first step involves the enzyme cystathionine synthase (CBS) for which pyridoxine (B$_6$) is the co-factor and deficiences of this enzyme result in the usual form of homocystinuria. The remaining 50% of formed homocysteine is remethylated to methionine and requires 5, 10-methyltetrahydrofolate as substrate, and me-thylcobalamin as a co-factor. Remethylation by trimethylglycine (betaine) may also occur via a separate pathway.*

*MS = Methionine synthase*
*MTHFR = 5, 10 Methylenetetrahydrofolate Reductase*
*THF = Tetrahydrofolate*
*CBS = Cystathionine β-synthase*
*SAM = S-adenosyl methionine*

B$_{12}$ was the most likely explanation[12]. The remethylation of homocysteine to methionine is mediated by reactions which
depend upon both folate and vitamin B$_{12}$ (Fig 1) and the measured concentrations of folate in serum and tissues were not abnormal.

When McCully undertook the autopsy in this infant he documented the presence of widespread vascular changes and thromboses[4]. Thus there was evidence for early-onset vascular disease in a remethylating disorder associated with low circulating methionine as well as in a transsulfuration disorder due to cystathionine β-synthase deficiency and associated with elevated methionine. The common biochemical factor in the two disorders was the elevated homocysteine. McCully therefore suggested that elevated homocysteine was the likely mediator of the precocious vascular changes[4].

## CONFIRMATION OF A ROLE FOR ELEVATED HOMOCYSTEINE IN THE PRODUCTION OF VASCULAR DISEASE

Confirmation of the homocysteine hypothesis depended upon firstly a demonstration that a lowering or normalization of markedly elevated homocysteine reduced cardiovascular risk and secondly on the identification of biologically plausible mechanisms by which an elevated homocysteine might mediate changes in vessels leading to vascular disease. Resolution of both these issues in relation to the greatly increased homocysteine levels found in homocystinuria is now beyond doubt. The first of these depended upon the development of treatment regimens which would effectively lower increased circulating homocysteine. As the treatment of homocystinuria will be considered in a later chapter this will be referred to only briefly here.

The development of effective treatment regimens for cystathionine β-synthase deficiency began with the observations of Barber and Spaeth in 1969[13]. They showed that in some patients with cystathionine β-synthase deficiency high oral doses of pyridoxine (250 - 500mg daily) lowered greatly the elevated circulating and urinary homocysteine and methionine. It was shown in later studies that 100mg daily of pyridoxine was usually an effective dose, and that approximately 50% of cystathionine β-synthase patients were responsive to pyridoxine[12]. It was also established that patterns of responsiveness were consistent within families[12] and that for an optimal response there was also an important need for additional folate to maintain and enhance the remethylation of homocysteine to methionine[14]. As can be seen from Fig. 1, in pyridoxine-responsive patients, ie in those patients with defects associated with some residual cystathionine β-synthase activity, the activity of the enzyme could be increased by a therapeutic dose of pyridoxine to permit enhanced flow through the transsulfuration pathway. And as can also be seen from Fig. 1, the availability of adequate folate (and vitamin $B_{12}$) to maintain or increase remethylation of homocysteine to methionine would contribute to a further decrease in the elevated homocysteine.

In pyridoxine non-responsive patients the later studies of Smolin and colleagues[15] and our own[16] established that the addition of oral betaine lowered homocysteine effectively long-term, and that this was usually associated with a further increase in the already elevated methionine because of enhanced re-methylation of homocysteine to methionine (Fig 1). With regard to clinical outcomes, the crucial observations were that effective lowering of elevated homocysteine resulted in greatly reduced cardiovascular risk in both pyridoxi-ne responsive[17,18] and pyridoxine non-responsive patients[18]. Together, these studies provide powerful evidence for the relevance of markedly elevated ho-mocysteine to vascular disease and establish that high methionine concentra-tions persisting over long periods - more than sixteen years in our patients[18] - are not harmful.

There are now biologically plausible mechanisms whereby the very high homocysteine levels found in untreated homocystinuric patients might increase cardiovascular risk. Evidence for a potentially damaging effect on endotheli-um, for increased risk of thrombogenesis and for homocysteine-induced en-hanced smooth muscle cell proliferation has been carefully documented and summarized in two recent extensive reviews[10,11]. The pathology of the vascular changes in homocystinuria will be discussed in a further chapter but in our own patients we have shown that in children with untreated homocystinuria there is intimal thickening and reduplication of the internal elastic lamina re-sulting in luminal obstruction; the lesions are essentially fibrous and without evidence of lipid accumulation[19]. However, in older patients, there may also be lipid accumulation as a result of complicating standard risk factors, and the lesions may then appear more characteristically atherosclerotic[19]. But the un-derlying process as seen in children before the advent of effective therapy was in the nature of a "non-lipid" model for arteriosclerosis and an important one for the understanding of the pathogenesis of vascular disease.

## MILD HOMOCYSTEINE ELEVATION (HYPERHOMOCYSTEINEMIA) AND CARDIOVASCULAR RISK

Whereas there is no doubt about the pathological effects of the high homocysteine concentrations found in untreated cystathionine β-synthase deficiency it is a contentious issue as to whether or not the hyper-homocysteinemia in which circulating homocysteine levels are $1/20^{th}$ or less of those in patients with untreated homocystinuria contributes independently to increased cardiovascular risk. It is an issue of much current interest.

In our original study we measured concentrations of plasma cysteine-homocysteine mixed disulfide after a standardized oral methionine load in men aged 50 years or less with angiographically documented coronary artery di-sease and in age- and sex-matched controls. The patients had significantly higher levels[5]. In a subsequent study we measured total free homocysteine in 20 patients with premature coronary artery disease and found increased fasting and post-load homocysteine concentrations in 2 patients, identical twins; and in these the increased levels and abnormal methionine loads were normalized by oral folic acid[20]. Numerous subsequent studies, including our own[21] have confirmed these early results and established that some 20 - 30% of patients with coronary, cerebrovascular, and peripheral vascular disease have mild homocysteine elevation, either after an overnight fast or following the challenge of a standardized methionine load - see recent reviews[10,11]. However the question that has to be asked is whether or not these modest elevations simply represent an "epiphenomenon" and are "fellow travellers" occurring as a consequence of other risk factors. The reasons are as follows.

In a very extensive Scandinavian study[22] it was demonstrated that hyperhomocysteinemia is associated with many of the standard risk factors for vascular disease; these include smoking, lack of exercise, increased age, hypertension and, as we originally showed[23], with male sex. Thus there is a need to control for these factors in assessing any risk that homocysteine might independently confer; and control for these factors has not been adequate in some of the earlier studies.

The other important recent finding which is very relevant to this issue is a lack of any association between the methylenetetrahydrofolate reductase (MTHFR) C677T mutation and vascular disease even although in subjects with serum folate levels below the population median there is a significant association between the mutation and modest homocysteine elevation. This issue has been examined comprehensively recently, most notably in a meta-analysis of over 6,000 patients and their controls genotyped for the mutation[24]. The findings confirm the absence of an association between the mutation and vascular disease. Thus unless the mutation is in some other way protective against the development of vascular disease it is difficult to reconcile these findings with the notion that modest homocysteine elevation independently enhances cardiovascular risk even although there is evidence for reduced endothelial dependent vasodilatation in patients with only modest homocysteine elevation[25]. The answers must await the results of controlled clinical trials of the effects of homocysteine lowering with folic acid. Some are in progress and others planned.

## HOMOCYSTEINE AND RENAL DISEASE

In chronic renal failure there is a 20-fold increase in cardiovascular risk, often for unexplained reasons[26]. This has been long recognized. Because of the contribution of the kidney to the metabolism of homocysteine and the excretion of sulfur-containing metabolites we measured homocysteine levels in patients with varying degrees of chronic renal failure and in renal transplant recipient patients who had only modest impairment of renal function. The homocysteine levels were significantly elevated[6-9] and to a level considerably above the levels commonly found in vascular disease patients with hyperhomocysteinemia.

For a mean serum creatinine level of 0.56mmol/L the mean total free plasma homocysteine after an overnight fast in the renal patients we studied was 12.9µmol/L ie the equivalent of approximately 50µmol/L of free plus bound (total) homocysteine - a level likely to interact with other risk factors and contribute to the enhanced vascular risk seen in these patients[9]. Furthermore, in chronic renal insufficiency both cysteine and homocysteine are also elevated[9] and so too is lipoprotein(a), itself a significant risk factor when elevated[27]. Since increased levels of both cysteine and homocysteine enhance the binding of lipoprotein(a) to fibrin with the effect of reducing fibrinolysis[28], these interactive effects are likely to be important contributors to the development of vascular disease in chronic renal insufficiency by promoting antifibrinolytic changes in the vessel wall.

It is noteworthy that in patients with renal disease the elevated homocysteine levels are strikingly reduced by oral folic acid in the absence of overt folate deficiency and without altering methionine or cysteine levels[9]. We showed that the extent of the decline in total free homocysteine after folate was linearly related to the initial plasma concentration, findings which have clear implications for the importance of adding folic acid to treatment regimens in chronic renal insufficiency. Interrelations between homocysteine, vascular disease and renal insufficiency are the subject of a later chapter.


CONCLUDING COMMENTS

Lessons from the recessively inherited inborn error of metabolism, cystathionine β-synthase deficiency, have provided us with a homocysteine-induced non-lipid model of vascular disease and it is clear that the changes produced by elevated homocysteine will interact with other established risk factors to increase further cardiovascular risk. Biologically plausible mechanisms through which elevated homocysteine may result in vascular damage have been identified, although not entirely clarified; and effective treatment to lower elevated homocysteine unquestionably reduces cardiovascular risk in both pyridoxine-responsive and non-responsive homocystinuric patients. However the post treatment homocysteine levels, particularly in pyridoxine non-responsive patients, remain well above those found in the some 20 - 30% of patients with usual forms of commonly occurring vascular disease. In these vascular patients there are also associations between the mildly elevated homocysteine and other risk factors and it remains to be established in these patients whether or not normalising homocysteine concentrations with folic acid reduces cardiovascular risk. However in renal disease there appears to be stronger evidence for the relevance to vascular disease of the higher homocysteine levels found in chronic renal insufficiency. Together with the associated increases in cysteine and lipoproteina, these elevated levels could contribute importantly to the pathogenesis of vascular disease in this high risk patient group.

## REFERENCES

1.  Carson NAJ, Neill DW. Metabolic abnormalities detected in a survey of mentally backward individuals in Northern Ireland. *Arch Dis Child.* 1962;37:505-513.
2.  Gibson JB, Carson NA, Neill DW. Pathological findings in homocystinuria. *J Clin Path.* 1964;17:427-437.
3.  Mudd SH, Finkelstein JD, Irreverre F, Laster L. Homocystinuria: An enzymatic defect. *Science.* 1964;143:1443-1445.
4.  McCully KS. Vascular pathology of homocysteinemia: Implications for the pathogenesis of arteriosclerosis. *Am J Pathol.* 1969;56:111-128.
5.  Wilcken DEL, Wilcken B. The pathogenesis of coronary artery disease: A possible role for methionine metabolism. *J Clin Invest.* 1976;57:1079-1082.
6.  Wilcken DEL, Gupta VJ. Sulfur containing amino acids in chronic renal failure with particular reference to homocystine and cysteine-homocysteine mixed disulphide. *European Journal of Clinical Investigation.* 1979;9:301-307.
7.  Wilcken DEL, Gupta VJ, Reddy SG. Accumulation of sulfur-containing amino acids including cysteine-homocysteine in patients on maintenance haemodialysis. *Clinical Science.* 1980;58:427-430.
8.  Wilcken DEL, Gupta VJ, Betts AK. Homocysteine in the plasma of renal transplant recipients: Effects of cofactors for methionine metabolism. *Clin Sci.* 1981;61:743-749.
9.  Wilcken DEL, Dudman NPB, Tyrrell PA, Robertson MR. Folic acid lowers elevated plasma homocyst(e)ine in chronic renal insufficiency: Possible implications for prevention of vascular disease. *Metabolism* 1988;37:697-701.
10. Mudd SH, Levy HL, Skovby F. Disorders of transsulfuration. In: Scriver GR, Beaudet AL, Sly WS, Valle D, (eds): *The Metabolic and Molecular Basis of Inherited Disease.* 7th ed. New York, NY: McGraw-Hill; 1995:1279-1327.
11. Refsum H, Ueland PM, Nygård O, Vollset SE. Homocysteine and Cardiovascular Disease. *Annual Review of Medicine.* 1998;49:31-62.
12. Mudd SH, Levy HL, Abeles RH. A Derangement in $B_{12}$ Metabolism Leading to Homocystinemia; Cystathioninemia and Methylmalonic aciduria. *Biochemical and Biophysical Research Communications.* 1969;35:121-126.

13. Barber GW, Spaeth GL. The successful treatment of homocystinuria with pyridoxine. *Journal of Pediatrics*. 1969;75:463-478.

14. Wilcken B, Turner B. Homocystinuria: Reduced folate levels during pyridoxine treatment. *Archives of Disease in Childhood*. 1973;48:58-62.

15. Smolin LA, Benevenga NJ, Berlow S. The use of betaine for the treatment of homocystinuria. *J Pediatr*. 1981;99:467-472.

16. Wilcken DEL, Wilcken B, Dudman NPB, Tyrrell PA. Homocystinuria—The effects of betaine in the treatment of patients not responsive to pyridoxine. *N Engl J Med*. 1983;309:448-453.

17. Mudd SH, Skovby F, Levy HL, Pettigrew KD, Wilcken B, Pyeritz RE, Andria G, Boers GHJ, Bromberg IL, Cerone R, Fowler B, Grobe H, Schmidt H, Schweitzer L. The natural history of homocystinuria due to cystathionine β-synthase deficiency. *Am J Hum Genet*. 1985;37:1-31.

18. Wilcken DEL, Wilcken B. The natural history of vascular Disease in homocystinuria and the effects of treatment. *J Inher Metab Dis*. 1997;20:295-300.

19. Wilcken DEL. Novel risk factors for vascular disease: the homocysteine hypothesis of cardiovascular disease. *Journal of Cardiovascular Risk*. 1998;:217-221.

20. Wilcken DEL, Reddy SG, Gupta VJ. Homocysteinemia, Ischaemic Heart Disease, and the Carrier State for Homocystinuria. *Metabolism*. 1983;32:363-370.

21. Dudman NPB, Wilcken DEL, Wang J, Lynch JF, Macey D, Lundberg P. Disordered Methionine/Homocysteine metabolism in Premature Vascular Disease. The Occurrence, Cofactor Therapy, and Enzymology. *Arterioscler Thromb*. 1993;13:1253-1260.

22. Nygård O, Vollset SE, Refsum H, Stensvold I, Tverdazl A, Nordrehaug J, Ueland P, Kvale G. Total plasma homocysteine and cardiovascular risk factor profile. The Hordaland Homocysteine Study. *JAMA*. 1995;274:1526-1533.

23. Wilcken DEL, Gupta VJ. Cysteine-Homocysteine mixed disulphide: differing plasma concentrations in normal men and women. *Clin Sci*. 1979;57:211-215.

24. Brattström L, Wilcken DEL, Öhrvick J, Brudin L. The common Methylenetetrahydrofolate reductase Gene Mutation leads to hyperhomocysteinemia but not to vascular disease - The result of a meta analysis. *Circulation*. 1998;98:2520-2526.

25. Tawakol A, Omland T, Gerhard M, Wu JT, Creager MA. Hyperhomocysteinemia is associated with impaired endothelium-dependent vasodilatation in humans. *Circulation*. 1997;95:119-1121.

26. Wheeler DC. Cardiovascular disease in patients with chronic renal failure. *Lancet*. 1996;348:1673-1674.

27. Black IW, Wilcken DEL. Decreases in apolipoprotein(a) after Renal Transplantation: Implications for lipoprotein(a) metabolism. *Clin Chem*. 1992;38:353-357.

28. Harpel PC, Chang VT, Borth W. Homocysteine and other sulfhydryl compounds enhance the binding of lipoprotein(a) to fibrin: A potential link between thrombosis, atherogenesis and sulfhydryl compound metabolism. *Proc Natl Acad Sci*. USA. 1992;89:10193-10197.

# 3. BIOCHEMISTRY AND METABOLISM

DONALD W. JACOBSEN

## SUMMARY

Homocysteine, a metabolite of the methionine cycle, is a strong independent risk factor for cardiovascular disease. Although the methionine in dietary protein can transiently affect levels of total plasma homocysteine, the B complex vitamins folic acid, $B_{12}$, $B_6$, and $B_2$, which drive homocysteine metabolism, are essential for maintaining homocysteine homeostasis. To prevent cytotoxic accumulations of homocysteine, cells can export homocysteine to the circulation, or they can convert homocysteine to non-cytotoxic metabolites. Two pathways are available for homocysteine metabolism- remethylation and transsulfuration. Most cells in the body can remethylate homocysteine back to methionine using $B_{12}$-dependent methionine synthase. In a limited number of organs, homocysteine can be catabolized through the transsulfuration pathway. This pathway is initiated by $B_6$-dependent cystathionine β-synthase. The remethylation and transsulfuration pathways are regulated by S-adenosylmethionine. When methionine is abundant, the intracellular concentration of S-adenosylmethionine increases and more homocysteine is converted to cysteine through the transsulfuration pathway. S-Adenosylmethionine is a negative allosteric effector for the remethylation pathway and a positive allosteric effector for the transsulfuration pathway. It appears that even under conditions of optimal vitamin sufficiency and metabolism for homocysteine, a finite amount is exported to the circulation. Here, homocysteine can undergo autooxidation or participate in thiol/disulfide exchange reactions to form homocystine, a mixed disulfide with

*K. Robinson (ed.), Homocysteine and Vascular Disease, 15-39.*
© 2000 *Kluwer Academic Publishers. Printed in the Netherlands.*

cysteine and mixed disulfides with protein. Less than 2% of total plasma homocysteine remains as free reduced homocysteine.

## INTRODUCTION

Homocysteine, a metabolite of the methionine cycle, is a strong independent risk factor for cardiovascular disease [1,2]. Because homocysteine may play a role in both atherogenesis and thrombogenesis, an understanding of its metabolism and regulation is essential. With this information it should be possible to design intervention strategies for lowering total plasma homocysteine* concentrations in patients with cardiovascular disease and in subjects who are at high risk for developing cardiovascular diseases. Homocysteine is derived from the methionine in dietary protein and from methionine produced by the turnover of body proteins. Dietary protein can modulate total plasma homocysteine to some extent [3]. However, B complex vitamins, especially folic acid, $B_6$, and $B_{12}$, are major determinants of total plasma homocysteine and play important roles in maintaining homocysteine homeostasis [4]. To avoid a cytotoxic build up of intracellular homocysteine, cells have two options. They can convert homocysteine to non-cytotoxic metabolites, or they can export homocysteine to the blood where it rapidly undergoes autooxidation. There are two major metabolic pathways for homocysteine metabolism- remethylation and transsulfuration, and in cells in which both pathways are functional, newly formed homocysteine is equally distributed between the two pathways [5]. The remethylation pathway converts homocysteine back to methionine while the transsulfuration pathway converts homocysteine to the non-cytotoxic amino acid cysteine.

Defects in remethylation or transsulfuration, whether due to genetic or acquired factors, can lead to an intracellular accumulation of homocysteine followed by export to the circulation. Once in circulation homocysteine can autooxidize with itself and other low molecular weight sulfur-containing amino acids [8]. It can also interact with plasma proteins to form stable covalent

---

*Nomenclature: "Homocysteine" has a precise chemical meaning as originally described by its discoverer Vincent du Vigneaud [6,7]. Homocysteine is an amino acid in which the α-carbon side chain has the structure $-CH_2CH_2SH$. The sulfhydryl group (-SH) is a reduced form of sulfur. Because of its chemical reactivity, homocysteine can oxidize with itself (autooxidation) to form a homodimer known as "homocystine", linked by a covalent disulfide (-SS-) bond. The sulfhydryl group of homocysteine can also oxidize with the sulfhydryl group of cysteine and with the sulfhydryl groups of cysteine residues in proteins to form heterodimers known as "mixed disulfides". Thus, "total plasma homocysteine" refers to the sum of reduced (-SH) and oxidized (-S-S-) forms of homocysteine. See also note on nomenclature p.xix.

Table 1. The Methionine Content of Food Protein*

| SOURCE | | METHIONINE (g per 100 g of protein) | EXCEPTIONS |
|---|---|---|---|
| **PLANT** | Fruits | 0.9 | Peaches/grapes, 3.6 g |
| | Vegetables | 1.2 | |
| | Nuts | 1.4 | Brazil nuts, 5.6 g |
| | Cereals | 1.8 | |
| **ANIMAL** | Meat and Fish | 2.7 | |
| | Cow's milk | 2.9 | Human milk, 1.4 g |
| | Eggs | 3.2 | |

*From Reference 9.

disulfide complexes by reactions that are probably non-enzymatically driven [8]. It is commonly thought that homocysteine is the injurious agent of hyperhomocysteinemia. However, since the oxidized forms of homocysteine make up greater than 98% of total plasma homocysteine, it is possible that they too have unknown adverse effects on cardiovascular cells and tissues.

SOURCES OF HOMOCYSTEINE

Homocysteine is derived primarily from the methionine in dietary protein. Foods contain only trace amounts of homocysteine, which reflects the notion that homocysteine, albeit an essential intracellular metabolite, is maintained at low concentrations in both animal and plant cells. In contrast, the abundance of methionine, the proximal precursor of homocysteine, varies widely depending on the source of food proteins. As shown in Tab. 1, food protein derived from animal sources generally has a higher methionine content than food protein derived from plant sources [9]. Ingestion of a meal rich in protein (= 50 g) can elevate plasma homocysteine and have a significant effect on the other circulating forms of homocysteine [3]. Meals containing smaller amounts of protein (15-18 g) do not appear to significantly affect plasma homocysteine levels [3], and may actually cause a transient depression of total homocysteine [10].

The oral methionine-loading test, which is used clinically to evaluate homocysteine metabolism in subjects with cardiovascular disease [11], simulates the ingestion of a meal extremely rich in animal protein. For a 70 kg individual, 7 g of L-methionine (0.1 g/kg or 3.8 $g/m^2$) is administered which is equivalent to ingesting 200-300 g of animal-derived protein. Normally there is a 2-3-fold increase in total plasma homocysteine 6-8 hours after methionine loading, which then declines to basal levels within 24 hours [12]. Individuals with

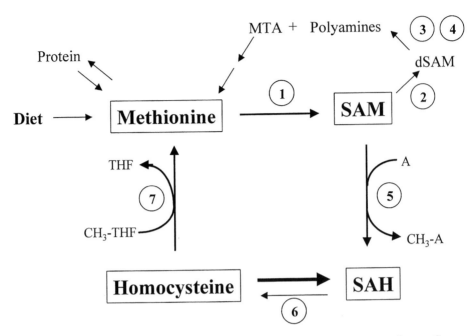

*Figure 1. The methionine cycle. Dietary methionine is converted to S-adenosylmethionine (SAM) by methionine adenosyltransferase (Reaction 1). SAM is diverted into polyamine biosynthesis by SAM decarboxylase (Reaction 2). Propylaminotransferase I (Reaction 3) and II (Reaction 4) use decarboxylated SAM as substrate for polyamine biosynthesis. Methylthioadenosine (MTA), the other product of Reactions 3 and 4, is recycled to the methionine pool. Methyltransferases (Reaction 5) use SAM as substrate for methyl-group transfers to acceptor (A) molecules and macromolecules. S-Adenosylhomocysteine (SAH) is the other product of methyltransferase activity and it undergoes hydrolysis by SAH hydrolase (Reaction 6). The methionine cycle is completed by the remethylation of homocysteine to back to methionine by $B_{12}$-dependent methionine synthase (Reaction 7) using 5-methyltetrahydrofolate ($CH_3$-THF) as substrate. In liver and kidney betaine-homocysteine methyltransferase (Reaction 10 is shown in Fig. 3) can also remethylate homocysteine back to methionine. The methionine cycle (defined by Reactions 1, 5, 6, and 7) is active in cardiovascular cells and tissues. However, Reaction 7 may be the only pathway available to the cardiovascular system for homocysteine metabolism. Reversal of Reaction 6 is undesirable in that it could lead to the accumulation of SAH and inhibition of methyltransferase activity.*

impaired homocysteine metabolism thought to be associated with the transsulfuration pathway may have significantly higher increases in the concentration of total plasma homocysteine and it may take longer for levels to normalize. Not only does the methionine-loading test illustrate the precursory relationship with homocysteine, it also serves as a useful diagnostic test to identify individuals with underlying abnormal homocysteine metabolism.


METABOLISM OF HOMOCYSTEINE

The metabolism of homocysteine is inextricably linked to methionine and one-carbon metabolism. The need for one-carbon methyl (labile methyl) groups is universal and most, if not all, cells in the body actively metabolize methionine through the methionine cycle [13]. The generation of labile methyl groups results in the generation of homocysteine, an amino acid that appears to be cytotoxic at higher concentrations. Although most cells produce homocysteine during methionine cycle activity, they differ in the expression of pathways available for the removal of homocysteine. This was clearly demonstrated by Mudd, Finkelstein and coworkers in their survey of homocysteine metabolism in rat tissues and organs [5,14-17]. Their work demonstrated that most cells and tissues expressed at least one remethylation pathway for homocysteine removal, but that transsulfuration pathway activity was limited in its distribution. Is the situation the same in human tissues? Although less data is available, human cells and tissues also have unequal potentials for metabolizing homocysteine. In particular reference to this work is the capability of cardiovascular cells and tissues to metabolize homocysteine (*vide infra*) and the implications for development of vascular disease. In this section, the methionine cycle will be briefly described, followed by a more detailed examination of the pathways used for homocysteine disposal.


**The methionine cycle**

A major portion of methionine that originates from dietary sources and from intracellular turnover of protein is funneled into the methionine cycle (Fig. 1) by the enzyme methionine adenosyltansferase (MAT) (ATP:L-methionine S-adenosyltransferase; EC 2.5.1.6) [18]. This enzyme catalyzes the transfer of the adenosyl moiety of ATP to the sulfur atom of methionine forming an energy-rich sulfonium compound S-adenosylmethionine (SAM)*. The tripolyphosphate moiety ($PPP_i$) from ATP is then hydrolyzed by the enzyme to inorganic phosphate ($P_i$) and pyrophosphate ($PP_i$) (Reaction 1) essentially assuring reaction irreversibility.

---

  * S-Adadenosylmethionine and S-adenosylhomocysteine are also abbreviated AdoMet and AdoHcy, respectively. For this chapter SAM and SAH will be used.

L-Methionine + ATP $\rightarrow$ S-Adenosylmethionine + [MAT-PPP$_i$] $\rightarrow$

MAT + P$_i$ + PP$_i$ $\hspace{10cm}$ (1)

Structural genes have been cloned and sequenced from human liver and kidney [19,20]. The isozymes MAT I, a homodimer, and MAT III, a homotetramer, are products of a gene expressed only in liver and are referred to as "intermediate K$_m$ methionine" and "high K$_m$ methionine" forms, respectively. When methionine concentrations are high, liver appears to be the only tissue in the body that continues to produce SAM, and this is carried out by MAT III, which is activated by SAM [5]. The isozyme MAT II is a product of the kidney gene, which is expressed in all tissues. MAT II is a "low K$_m$ methionine" isozyme and is inhibited by its end product SAM [5,13,18]. MAT I and MAT III activities are regulated by nitric oxide [21,22]. Thus, when specific cysteine residues in MAT I and MAT III are nitrosylated, enzyme activity is severely inhibited.

A branch point in the methionine cycle occurs with the formation of SAM (Fig. 1). In addition to serving as a methyl group donor, SAM is also an aminopropyl group donor in polyamine biosynthesis. S-Adenosylmethionine is directed towards polyamine biosynthesis by pyruvate-dependent SAM decarboxylase [23] (Reaction 2).

S-Adenosylmethionine $\rightarrow$ Decarboxylated SAM + $CO_2$ $\hspace{5cm}$ (2)

Decarboxylated SAM is used by propylamino transferase I and II as an aminopropyl-group donor for the synthesis of spermidine (Reaction 3) and spermine (Reaction 4), respectively.

Decarboxylated SAM + Putrescine $\rightarrow$ Methylthioadenosine + Spermidine $\hspace{0.5cm}$ (3)

Decarboxylated SAM + Spermidine $\rightarrow$ Methylthioadenosine + Spermine $\hspace{0.5cm}$ (4)

The other product of propylaminotransferase activity, methylthioadenosine (MTA), is conserved and metabolically recycled back to methionine (Fig. 1). The biosynthesis of polyamines is upregulated during cell proliferation. The cationic polyamines play important roles in stabilizing negatively charged nucleic acids during chromatin condensation and, for this rea-son, polyamine biosynthesis is a target for cancer chemotherapeutic agents [24].

S-Adenosylmethionine serves as the methyl-group donor substrate for the numerous methyltransferases in cells. Biological methylations are fundamental to life and involve processes such as gene expression, protein translation, chemotaxis, cellular differentiation and signal transduction [25]. The only other methyl-group donor substrate is 5-methyltetrahydrofolate, which serves as substrate for methionine synthase (*vide infra*). The SAM-dependent methyltransferases catalyze the general reaction shown in Reaction 5.

SAM + Acceptor Substrates →
S-Adenosylhomocysteine + Methylated Products                    (5)

Small molecules such as guanidioacetic acid and norepinephrine accept a methyl group from SAM to form creatine and epinephrine, respectively. Macromolecules (phospholipids, protein, DNA, RNA) are also acceptor substrates for methyl groups donated by SAM in reactions catalyzed by substrate specific methyltransferases. The other product of SAM-dependent methyltransferase activity is S-adenosylhomocysteine (SAH), the proximal precursor of homocysteine in the body.

The SAH formed because of SAM-dependent methyltransferases is hydrolyzed to homocysteine and adenosine by the enzyme SAH hydrolase (EC 3.3.1.1) (Reaction 6).

SAH + $H_2O$ ⇋ L-Homocysteine + Adenosine                    (6)

The reaction is reversible and the back reaction is actually favored thermodynamically. Therefore, to drive the reaction in the forward direction the products must be metabolized as well. Adenosine is a substrate for salvage pathway enzymes as well as for adenosine deaminase. Homocysteine serves as another branch point metabolite in the methionine cycle. It can undergo remethylation or transsulfuration. If SAH accumulates as a result of SAH hydrolase inhibition or reversal of Reaction 6, SAM-dependent methyltransferases are likely to be inhibited since SAH is a potent end-product inhibitor. In hyperhomocysteinemia intracellular accumulation of homocysteine could lead to higher SAH concentrations and impaired methyltransferase activity [26]. The methionine cycle is completed when homocysteine in remethylated back to methionine.

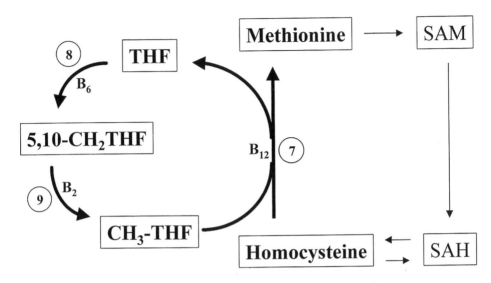

*Figure 2. The mini-folate cycle provides the substrate 5-methyltetrahydrofolate (CH₃-THF) for B₁₂-dependent remethylation of homocysteine to methionine by methionine synthase (Reaction 7). The tetrahydrofolate (THF) generated by Reaction 7 reacts with serine to form 5,10-methylenetetrahydrofolate (5,10-CH₂THF). Reaction 8 is catalyzed by B₆-dependent serine-glycine hydroxymethyltransferase. The mini-folate cycle is completed by the reduction of 5,10-CH₂THF to CH₃-THF by B₂-dependent methylenetetrahydrofolate reductase (Reaction 9).*

**Remethylation of homocysteine**

The ubiquitous methionine cycle (Fig. 2) is completed by the remethylation of homocysteine back to methionine. The enzyme that catalyzes this reaction is methionine synthase (MS) (5-methyltetrahydrofolate:homocysteine methyl-trans-ferase; EC 2.1.1.13). It converts homocysteine to methionine using 5-methyltetrahydrofolate as the methyl-group donor and methylcobalamin, a coenzyme form of cyanocobalamin (vitamin $B_{12}$), as catalyst. The enzyme also requires SAM, which serves as a "repair substrate" and is utilized approximately once every 1,000 turns of the catalytic cycle [27]. The enzyme also requires an ancillary reducing system to sustain maximal activity [28,29]. The other important product of the reaction catalyzed by MS is tetrahydrofolate, the active substrate form of folic acid that mediates one-carbon metabolism (Reaction 7).

5-Methyltetrahydrofolate + L-Homocysteine →

Tetrahydrofolate + L-Methionine                                     (7)

Thus, vitamin $B_{12}$ and folic acid play critical roles in homocysteine metabolism and a deficiency of either can lead to severe hyperhomocysteinemia. It appears that most, if not all, nucleated cells express functional $B_{12}$-dependent methionine synthase. This enzyme and its molecular biology are more comprehensively described in Chapter 17.

The 5-methyltetrahydrofolate necessary to drive homocysteine remethylation through $B_{12}$-dependent MS is provided by the "mini folate cycle" shown in Fig. 2. The tetrahydrofolate produced in Reaction 7 reacts with serine to produce glycine and 5,10-methylenetetrahydrofolate. The reaction (Reaction 8) is catalyzed by $B_6$-dependent serine:glycine hydroxymethyltransferase (SGHMT; EC 2.1.2.1).

L-Serine + Tetrahydrofolate → Glycine + 5,10-Methylenetetrahydrofolate   (8)

5,10-Methylenetetrahydrofolate is then reduced to 5-methyltetrahydro-folate by the $B_2$-dependent enzyme methylenetetra-hydrofolate reductase (MTHFR; EC 1.5.1.20) using NADPH as cosubstrate (Reaction 9).

5,10-Methylenetetrahydrofolate + NADPH → 5-Methyltetrahydrofolate     (9)

The enzyme is a homodimer with a subunit $Mr$ of  77,000 and has both a catalytic and regulatory domain [30,31]. The human gene has been cloned [32]. A common polymorphism for MTHFR is found in Caucasian populations that could contribute to elevated total plasma homocysteine, particularly in subjects with low folate status [33]. The genetics and molecular biology of MTHFR and its association with cardiovascular disease are described in Chapter 16. The mini folate cycle, consisting of MS, SGHMT and MTHFR, acts like a pump to drive the methionine cycle. The pump provides fuel in the form of 5-methyltetrahydrofolate, which then returns one-carbon units via MS to the methionine cycle for additional biological methylations or polyamine biosynthesis from the methionine carbon skeleton.

A second remethylation enzyme with very limited tissue distribution uses betaine as the methyl donor. Betaine (trimethylglycine) is a product of choline oxidation. In liver and kidney, homocysteine can be remethylated back to methionine by betaine:homocysteine methyltransferase (BHMT; EC 2.1.1.5). Dimethylglycine is the other product of the reaction (Reaction 8).

L-Homocysteine + Betaine → L-Methionine + Dimethylglycine         (10)

BHMT, which was recently cloned, is a zinc metalloprotein with a hexameric structure consisting of identical subunits ($Mr$ of 45,000) [34,35]. In a survey of human tissues by Northern analysis, BHMT mRNA was detected in liver and kidney, but not in pancreas, brain, heart, lung, and spleen [36]. The role of BHMT in homocysteine homeostasis is still under investigation. Betaine has been used for many years to lower total plasma homocysteine in homocystinurics, particularly those who are non-responsive to pyridoxine [37,38]. However, betaine therapy fails to normalize total plasma homocysteine in most individuals and its use in the treatment of inborn errors of metabolism has been questioned [39]. It seems unlikely that betaine would be used to treat hyperhomocysteinemia in subjects with cardiovascular disease since most of these individuals have mildly elevated total plasma homocysteine which can often be normalized with a combination of folic acid, vitamin $B_{12}$ and vitamin $B_6$. Nevertheless, as in homocystinuria, there may be cardiovascular patients who are non-responsive to common therapies, but who may respond to betaine.

**Transsulfuration of homocysteine**

In a limited number of human tissues and organs, homocysteine formed in the methionine cycle enters the transsulfuration pathway where it is converted to cysteine. Cysteine can undergo complete catabolism to inorganic sulfate, or it can be converted into other sulfur-containing metabolites such as taurine (Fig. 3). However, the capacity of the transsulfuration pathway to metabolize homocysteine must be limited since the pathway is apparently unable to handle the increases in intracellular homocysteine that occur when remethylation pathway activity is impaired.

Transsulfuration is initiated by the $B_6$-dependent enzyme cystathionine β-synthase (CBS; EC 4.2.1.22). With pyridoxal phosphate, the cofactor form of vitamin $B_6$, the enzyme catalyzes a β-elimination reaction between serine and homocysteine to produce the thioether cystathionine (Reaction 11).

L-Homocysteine + L-Serine → L-Cystathionine + HO⁻         (11)

The enzyme, a homotetramer with a subunit $Mr$ of 63,000, requires heme for catalytic activity in addition to pyridoxal phosphate [40]. The active site of the enzyme appears to be formed at a dimer interface since each tetramer appears to have two equivalents each of pyridoxal phosphate and heme[41]. When the heme iron is reduced to the ferrous state, CBS enzyme activity decreases approximately 2-fold [41]. The human cDNA has been cloned, and there are five MRNA isoforms, all differing at the beginning of the 5'-untranslated region [42-45]. The activity of CBS is regulated by SAM, which serves as a positive allosteric effector. When cellular and tissue extracts containing CBS are assayed in the presence SAM, enzyme activity is stimulated 3-10 fold [46]. The molecular biology and genetic variants of CBS are described in Chapter 18.

In the second step of the transsulfuration pathway, L-cystathionine is converted to L-cysteine, $\alpha$-ketobutyrate and ammonia (Reaction 12) by the $B_6$-dependent enzyme cystathionase (cystathionine $\gamma$-lyase; EC 4.4.1.1).

$$L\text{-Cystathionine} + H_2O \rightarrow L\text{-Cysteine} + \alpha\text{-Ketobutyrate} + NH_3 \qquad (12)$$

The rat liver enzyme has been cloned and shares sequence homology with other cystathionine metabolizing enzymes [47]. The full-length human cDNA has been cloned and exists in two forms, one of which contains a deletion of 132 bases compared to rat [48]. The two forms could be separate gene products or could be splice variants. After realignment the human cDNA is 84% homologous with the rat cDNA. The specific activity of the human liver enzyme, consisting of four identical subunits of $Mr = 43,000$, is approximately one-fifth of that found in rat liver and may be the rate-limiting step in glutathione biosynthesis [48,49].

The transsulfuration pathway ends with the formation of cysteine (Reaction 12). However, cysteine undergoes further metabolism and is an essential metabolite that is incorporated into protein and glutathione. Cysteine is the distal precursor of taurine and, by a separate catabolic pathway, a source of inorganic sulfate in the body (Fig. 3.).

## Organ and tissue-specific metabolism of homocysteine

Earlier work on the determination of enzyme activity in rat organ extracts demonstrated that most if not all tissues were able to remethylate homocysteine to methionine using $B_{12}$-dependent MS, but that the distribution of $B_6$-dependent CBS enzyme activity was limited to rat liver, kidney, pancreas, adipose, brain, and possibly the intestinal mucosa [5,14]. CBS enzyme activity was not detected in rat adrenal, lung, testes, or heart. These early studies also showed that human liver and brain expressed active CBS, but other organ systems were not examined. This suggests that some cells and tissues must obtain cysteine from the circulation. The concentration of total plasma cysteine ranges from 200 to 300 $\mu$M, and approximately 50% is non-protein bound.

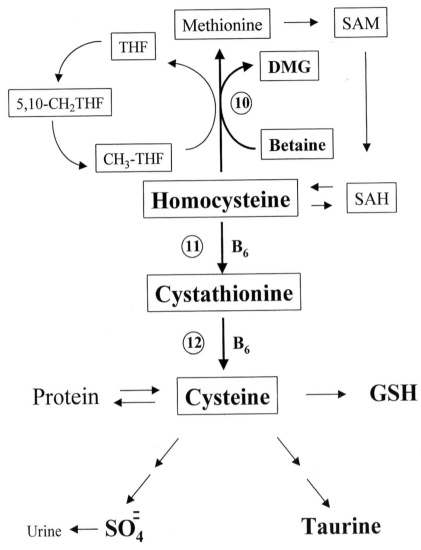

*Figure 3. The transsulfuration and alternate remethylation pathways. The former is initiated by B₆-dependent cystathionine β-synthase which catalyzes the conversion of homocysteine to cystathionine (Reaction 11). The latter is converted to cysteine by B6-dependent cystathionine γ-lyase (Reaction 12). The cysteine formed in this reaction is utilized in a variety of metabolic pathways. A second remethylation pathway using betaine as methyl-group donor is found in liver. Reaction 10 is catalyzed by BHMT as described in the text.*

Plasma cysteinyl-glycine (25-40 $\mu$M) might also serve as source of cysteine for cells lacking a transsulfuration pathway.

How does the human cardiovascular system metabolize homocysteine? Until recently there were no reports of homocysteine metabolizing enzymes in cardiovascular tissues except that extracts from cultured human umbilical vein endothelial cells had low levels of CBS activity [50,51]. Our laboratory has been unable to detect significant CBS enzyme activity in extracts of cultured human umbilical vein and aortic endothelial cells, even when assayed in the presence of the positive allosteric effector SAM [52]. Extracts prepared from human heart muscle, saphenous vein, internal mammary artery, and coronary arteries also had undetectable levels of CBS activity when assayed in the presence of SAM [46]. In addition the 63 kDa subunit of CBS was undetectable by Western blot analysis of heart muscle and aorta extracts suggesting that the CBS gene product was not expressed in these cardiovascular tissues [46]. Furthermore, the betaine-dependent remethylation pathway using BHMT is also undetectable in human cardiovascular cells and tissues [46]. None of the five isoforms of CBS mRNA are detectable in adult human heart, but fetal heart extracts contain isoforms 3 and 4 [45]. It thus appears that homocysteine metabolism in the adult human cardiovascular system, including the vascular endothelium, is limited. The only metabolic pathway available for the removal of intracellular homocysteine is $B_{12}$-dependent remethylation catalyzed by MS. Another option, yet uninvestigated, as a means to lower intracellular concentrations would be export of homocysteine to the circulation. However, in hyperhomocysteinemic individuals, export against a concentration gradient could impair this mechanism of achieving nontoxic intracellular levels.

## REGULATION OF HOMOCYSTEINE METABOLISM

### Dietary factors

The partitioning of homocysteine between the remethylation and transsulfuration pathways is dependent upon dietary intake of labile methyl donors such as methionine and choline [53]. Mudd and Poole estimated that in males and females on normal diets, the homocysteinyl moiety was remethylated 1.9 and 1.5 times, respectively, before entering the transsulfuration pathway. However, when labile methyl groups were removed from the diet, males and females recycled homocysteine back to methionine on average 3.9 and 3.0 times, respectively [53].

Dietary intake of essential micronutrients will also determine the efficiency of homocysteine metabolism in general. At least four B complex vitamins are

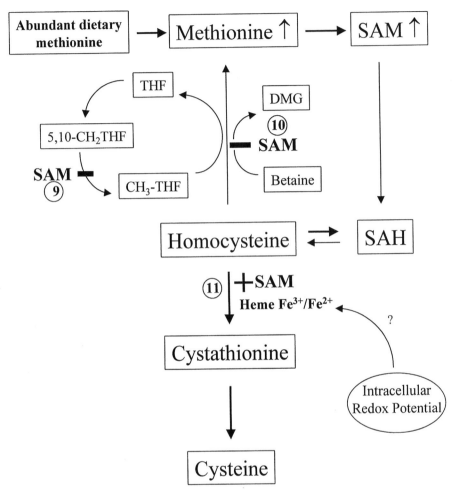

*Figure 4. Regulation of homocysteine metabolism. When dietary methionine is abundant, intracellular concentrations of SAM are likely to increase. Acting as a negative allosteric effector, SAM inhibits MTHFR (Reaction 9) thereby the supply of $CH_3$-THF for remethylation of homocysteine. SAM also inhibits BHMT, the alternate remethylation pathway using betaine as substrate (Reaction 10). In contrast SAM is a positive allosteric effector for CBS (Reaction 11) and therefore directs more homocysteine through the transsulfuration pathway. CBS, as a heme-dependent protein, may also be regulated by the oxidation state of heme iron.*

essential: folic acid, $B_{12}$, $B_6$ and $B_2$. Vitamin $B_{12}$ is converted to the cofactor methylcobalamin for MS. $B_6$ is converted to the cofactor pyridoxal phosphate for SGHMT in the remethylation pathway and for CBS and cystathionase in the transsulfuration pathway. Finally, $B_2$ is converted to the cofactor flavin adenine dinucleotide for MTHFR in the remethylation pathway. Dietary deficiencies of $B_{12}$ and $B_6$ clearly cause hyperhomocysteinemia, but there are, as of yet, no reports of $B_2$ deficiency as a cause of hyperhomocysteinemia. Folic acid is the fourth B complex micronutrient that serves not as a cofactor, but as a substrate for labile methyl group metabolism in the methionine cycle and in other folate dependent pathways requiring one-carbon groups (e.g., thymidylate and de novo purine ring biosynthesis). Of the four B complex micronutrients, low folate appears to be the strongest determinant of total plasma homocysteine [2]. In apparently healthy individuals with mid to high "normal" levels of total plasma homocysteine, it was possible to significantly lower their concentrations by daily oral supplementation with 100 to 200 µg of folic acid [54]. All residents of the United States are now receiving , on average, an additional 100 µg of folic acid daily since mandated food fortification with folic acid began in January of 1998 [55].

## S-Adenosylmethionine

The remethylation and transsulfuration pathways are regulated by SAM as shown in Fig. 4. When methionine is abundant in the diet, the intracellular concentration of SAM increases and more homocysteine is funneled through the transsulfuration pathway [5]. This occurs because SAM, a positive allosteric effector of CBS, stimulates transsulfuration pathway activity while inhibiting remethylation activity. The latter is accomplished at the level of MTHFR and BHMT where SAM is a negative allosteric effector [5,56]. Inhibition of MTHFR by SAM limits the amount of 5-methyltetrahydrofolate produced, thereby lowering the amount of substrate for $B_{12}$-dependent MS. In addition betaine-dependent remethylation of homocysteine by BHMT in the liver and kidney could be regulated by SAM acting as a negative effector on the enzyme. However, in rats the activity of BHMT is dependent upon steady-state levels of BHMT mRNA, which in turn are determined by dietary methionine, betaine and choline [57]. Thus, human homocysteine homeostasis is likely to be determined by dietary factors and their effects on gene expression as well as by pathway end products such as SAM and SAH. The latter can modulate enzyme activity by end product inhibition, or by positive or negative allosterism.

## CELLULAR TRANSPORT OF HOMOCYSTEINE

Even under apparent optimal conditions for homocysteine metabolism, that is to say when the micronutrients that drive homocysteine metabolism are not rate-limiting because of dietary abundance, the basal levels of total plasma homocysteine in most healthy adults are in the range of 4 to 12 μM [58]. It is thought that little or no homocysteine per se is of dietary origin. However, there are probably trace amounts of homocysteine in foods which could be absorbed and contribute to the "basal concentrations". Nevertheless, the bulk of circulating homocysteine must originate from the metabolism of methionine, and therefore, be of cellular origin.

## Daily turnover

In the average adult, it has been estimated that 55 μmol of homocysteine is exported to the blood every hour (equivalent to 1.32 mmol/day), but that only 0.006 mmol/day is excreted in the urine [59]. Therefore, the daily turnover of homocysteine, due largely to metabolism but not to excretion in healthy individuals, is somewhere in the range of 1 to 2 mmol. In contrast to a net arteriovenous difference (approximately 20%) of total plasma homocysteine in rat kidneys [60], there appears to be no arteriovenous difference across the human kidney [61] suggesting that homocysteine turnover must be due to liver and other organ system metabolism.

## Mechanisms of transport

Cultured human umbilical vein endothelial cells appear to transport homocysteine by the cysteine transporter systems ASC and L [62]. Conditions which impair homocysteine metabolism lead to marked increases in homocysteine export from cells. Thus, when cultured cells are treated with nitrous oxide, which irreversibly inactivates $B_{12}$-dependent methionine synthase, there is a dramatic increase in the export of homocysteine to the culture medium [63-65]. The rate of homocysteine export is dependent upon the rate of proliferation in most cell lines and is stimulated in some but not all cell types in the presence of antifols such as methotrexate [66]. The addition of 5-methyltetrahydrofolate to the culture medium drastically curtails homocysteine export in human umbilical vein endothelial cells [67]. Transformed human endothelial cells maintain very low intracellular homocysteine by exporting it to the culture medium, but are unable to reutilize exported homocysteine metabolically [68]. In comparison to HeLa and hepatoma cells, these cells are also much more sensitive to extracellular homocysteine. This could be related to their inability to metabolize homocysteine through the transsulfuration pathway [52].

BIOCHEMISTRY OF HOMOCYSTEINE IN CIRCULATION

There is still considerable uncertainty concerning the role that homocysteine plays in atherogenesis and thrombogenesis. There is also uncertainty concerning the form(s) of homocysteine that are potentially atherothrombogenic. Further studies are needed to address these issues as well as the most effective therapeutic strategies for lowering total plasma homocysteine in patients with cardiovascular disease.

## Circulating forms of homocysteine

The majority of subjects with cardiovascular disease have a mild form of hyperhomocysteinemia, with total plasma homocysteine levels rarely exceeding 25 µM. Most of the homocysteine in serum is oxidized to a disulfide form, and this occurs within a few minutes to hours after free homocysteine enters circulation [8,69,70]. The major forms of homocysteine in circulation are shown in Fig. 5. The concentration of free reduced homocysteine in healthy individuals and in vascular disease patients with mild hyperhomocysteinemia is usually less than 2% of total plasma homocysteine [71,72]. In contrast homocystinurics have much higher concentrations of free reduced homocysteine, which can account for up to 5%-20% of total plasma homocysteine [72,73]. When homocysteine oxidizes with itself the product is called *homocystine*. If homocysteine oxidizes with cysteine, the product is called *homocysteine-cysteine mixed disulfide*. Homocysteine can also oxidize with sulfhydryl groups on proteins to form *protein-bound homocysteine mixed disulfides*. The disulfide bond is a common feature of all oxidized forms of homocysteine in circulation. The low-molecular weight forms homocystine and homocysteine-cysteine mixed disulfide comprise 5%-10% of total plasma homocysteine. Protein-bound homocysteine makes up the largest fraction of total plasma homocysteine in normal and mildly hyperhomocysteinemic sera [74-77]. Thus, 80%-90% of total homocysteine in circulation is carried by disulfide linkage on serum proteins. Human serum albumin, with a single free cysteine residue at position 34, is probably the major carrier of homocysteine in circulation [74].

It has been reported that homocysteine thiolactone, the stable 5-membered ring condensation product of homocysteine, is a physiological form of homocysteine in human plasma. In 1988 it was reported that patients with cardiovascular disease had mM (millimolar) concentrations of homocysteine thiolactone in their sera [78]. However, this proved to be incorrect [79,80]. Although homocysteine thiolactone is produced physiologically due to enzyme "editing" by methionyl-tRNA aminoacyl synthetase [81], it is unlikely that homocysteine thiolactone could accumulate in the circulation. This is due to the presence of

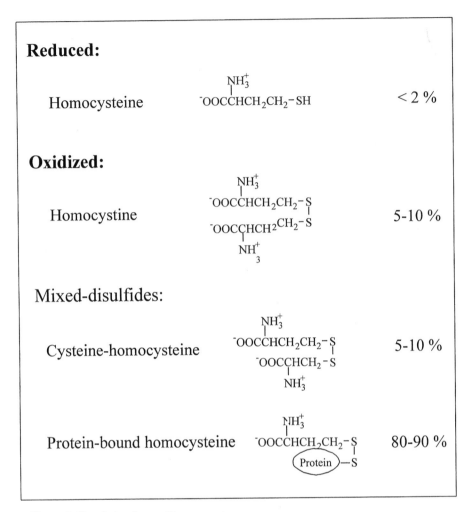

*Figure 5. Circulating forms of homocysteine.*

esterase-like activities, both soluble and vessel wall-bound, that catalyze its hydrolysis to homocysteine [82]. It has also been reported that patients with ischemic heart disease have near mM concentrations of "protein-bound homocysteine" [83], but this observation could not be substantiated by others [84].

## Mechanism of formation of circulating forms of homocysteine

Because of the reducing potential of the intracellular milieu, due largely to reduced glutathione, it is likely that homocysteine is exported from cells in a reduced state. In normal subjects a small amount of homocysteine is exported to circulation where it undergoes oxidation with itself and other sulfhydryl-containing compounds in the presence of molecular oxygen to form a disulfide (-SS-) product and hydrogen peroxide. The general reaction for sulfhydryl autooxidation is shown in Reaction 13.

$$2 \, RSH + O_2 \rightarrow RSSR + H_2O_2 \tag{13}$$

The rate of reaction is greatly accelerated by trace metals such as copper, or cobalt [85]. The copper-binding protein ceruloplasmin would be a likely candidate for catalyzing homocysteine and other thiol oxidations in vivo [86,87]. Homocysteine will oxidize with $Cys_{34}$ of serum albumin to form albumin-bound homocysteine in vitro [88]. In addition to autooxidation, albumin-bound homocysteine can also be formed by thiol-disulfide exchange reactions. At physiologic pH approximately 1% of homocysteine exists as a thiolate anion. Homocysteine thiolate anion can rapidly displace albumin-bound cysteine from $Cys_{34}$ by nucleophilic substitution according to Reaction 14 [88].

$$Homocysteine\text{-}S^- + Albumin\text{-}S\text{-}S\text{-}Cysteine \rightarrow$$
$$Cysteine\text{-}S^- + Albumin\text{-}S\text{-}S\text{-}Homocysteine \tag{14}$$

Albumin, with a free cysteine at position 34 (presumably as the $Cys_{34}$ thiolate anion), can attack homocystine to form albumin-bound homocysteine (Reaction 15) [88].

$$Albumin\text{-}Cys_{34}\text{-}S^- + Homocystine \rightarrow$$

$$Albumin\text{-}Cys_{34}\text{-}S\text{-}S\text{-}Homocysteine + Homocysteine \tag{15}$$

Thus, there appear to be multiple reactions that can lead to albumin-bound homocysteine, likely the most abundant form of homocysteine in circulation.

## IMPLICATIONS WITH RESPECT TO CARDIOVASCULAR DISEASE

We are only now beginning to understand how homocysteine is metabolized in human cardiovascular cells and tissues. Why is this important? Homocysteine is an independent risk factor for cardiovascular disease. However, the strong association between hyperhomocysteinemia and vascular disease does not necessarily mean there is a causal relationship. Nevertheless, many lines of evidence suggest that homocysteine is cytotoxic at higher concentrations and that it is capable of disrupting endothelial function both in vitro and in vivo. The underlying mechanisms of homocysteine toxicity are unexplained, and this in due in large part to a lack of understanding of homocysteine transport and metabolism in the cardiovascular system. The benefit of lowering total plasma homocysteine by therapeutic intervention, based on our understanding of homocysteine metabolism, may soon be realized in on-going and soon to be initiated clinical trials.

## ACKNOWLEDGEMENTS

I would like to knowledge the colleagues in my laboratory who participated in many aspects of this work, in particular Ranjana Poddar, Patricia M. DiBello, Rachel M. Wilson, Ping Chen and Eumelia V. Tipa. I would also like to acknowledge the financial support (RO1HL52234) of the National Institutes of Health.

## REFERENCES

1.  Mayer EL, Jacobsen DW, Robinson K. Homocysteine and coronary atherosclerosis. J Am Coll Cardiol 1996; 27:517-527.
2.  Refsum H, Ueland P, Nygård O, Vollset SE. Homocysteine and cardiovascular disease. Annu Rev Med 1998; 49:31-62.
3.  Guttormsen AB, Schneede J, Fiskerstrand T, Ueland PM, Refsum HM. Plasma concentrations of homocysteine and other aminothiol compounds are related to food intake in healthy human subjects. J Nutr 1994; 124:1934-1941.
4.  Jacobsen DW. Homocysteine and vitamins in cardiovascular disease. Clin Chem 1998; 44 Suppl.:1833-1843.
5.  Finkelstein JD. Methionine metabolism in mammals. J Nutr Biochem 1990; 1:228-237.
6.  Butz LW, du Vigneaud V. The formation of a homologue of cystine by the decomposition of methionine with sulfuric acid. J Biol Chem 1932; 99:135-142.
7.  Riegel B, du Vigneaud V. The isolation of homocysteine and its conversion to a thiolactone. J Biol Chem 1935; 112:149-154.
8.  Mansoor MA, Svardal AM, Schneede J, Ueland PM. Dynamic relation between reduced, oxidized, and protein-bound homocysteine and other thiol components in plasma during methionine loading in healthy men. Clin Chem 1992; 38:1316-1321.
9.  Anonymous . Geigy Scientific Tables, Volume 1. Units of Measurement, Body Fluids, Composition of the Body, Nutrition. 8th ed. Basal: Ciba-Geigy, 1981:241-266.

10. Ubbink JB, Vermaak WJH, van der Merwe A, Becker PJ. The effect of blood sample aging and food consumption on plasma total homocysteine levels. Clin Chim Acta 1992; 207:119-128.

11. Silberberg J, Crooks R, Fryer J, et al. Fasting and post-methionine homocysteine levels in a healthy Australian population. Aust N Z J Med 1997; 27:35-39.

12. Ueland PM, Refsum H, Brattström L. Plasma homocysteine and cardiovascular disease. In: Francis RB, ed. Atherosclerotic Cardiovascular Disease, Hemostasis, and Endothelial Function. New York: Marcel Dekker,Inc., 1992:183-236.

13. Finkelstein JD. The metabolism of homocysteine: pathways and regulation. Eur J Pediatr 1998; 157 Suppl. 2:S40-S44.

14. Mudd SH, Finkelstein JD, Irreverre F, Laster L. Transsulfuration in mammals. Microassays and tissue distribution of three enzymes of the pathway. J Biol Chem 1965; 240:4382-4392.

15. Finkelstein JD, Kyle WE, Harris BJ. Methionine metabolism in mammals. Regulation of homocysteine methyltransferases in rat tissue. Arch Biochem Biophys 1971; 146:84-92.

16. Finkelstein JD, Harris B. Methionine metabolism in mammals. Synthesis of S-adenosylhomocysteine in rat tissues. Arch Biochem Biophys 1973; 159:160-165.

17. Finkelstein JD, Martin JJ, Kyle WE, Harris BJ. Methionine metabolism in mammals: regulation of methylenetetrahyrofolate reductase content in rat tissues. Arch Biochem Biophys 1978; 191:153-160.

18. Mudd SH, Levy HL, Skovby F. Disorders of transsulfuration. In: Scriver CR, Beaudet AL, Sly WS, Valle D, eds. The Metabolic and Molecular Basis of Inherited Disease. 7th ed. New York: McGraw-Hill, Inc, 1995:1279-1327.

19. Horikawa S, Tsukada K. Molecular cloning and nucleotide sequence of cDNA encoding the human liver S-adenosylmethionine synthetase. Biochem Int 1991; 25:81-90.

20. Horikawa S, Tsukata K. Molecular cloning and developmental expression of a human kidney S-adenosylmethionine synthetase. FEBS Lett 1992;312:37-41.

21. Avila MA, Mingorance J, Martínez-Chantar ML, et al. Regulation of rat liver *S*-adenosylmethionine synthetase during septic shock: Role of nitric oxide. Hepatology 1997; 25:391-396.

22. Ruiz F, Corrales FJ, Miqueo C, Mato JM. Nitric oxide inactivates rat hepatic methionine adenosyltransferase *in vivo* by S-nitrosylation. Hepatology 1998; 28:1051-1057.

23. Stanley BA, Shantz LM, Pegg AE. Expression of mammalian *S*-adenosylmethionine decarboxylase in *Escherichia coli*. Determination of sites for putrescine activation of activity and processing. J Biol Chem 1994; 269:7901-7907.

24. Seiler N, Atanassov CL, Raul F. Polyamine metabolism as target for cancer chemoprevention. Int J Oncol 1999; 13:993-1006.

25. Chiang PK, Gordon RK, Tal J, et al. *S*-adenosylmethionine and methylation. FASEB J 1996; 10:471-480.

26. Wang H, Yoshizumi M, Lai K, et al. Inhibition of growth and p21[ras] methylation in vascular endothelial cells by homocysteine but not cysteine. J Biol Chem 1997; 272:25380-25385.

27. Banerjee RV, Matthews RG. Cobalamin-dependent methionine synthase. FASEB J 1990; 4:1450-1459.

28. Chen ZQ, Banerjee R. Purification of soluble cytochrome $b_5$ as a component of the reductive activation of porcine methionine synthase. J Biol Chem 1998; 273:26248-26255.

29. Leclerc D, Wilson A, Dumas R, et al. Cloning and mapping of a cDNA for methionine synthase reductase, a flavoprotein defective in patients with homocystinuria. Proc Natl Acad Sci USA 1998; 95:3059-3064.

30. Matthews RG, Vanoni MA, Hainfeld JF, Wall J. Methylenetetrahydrofolate reductase. Evidence for spatially distinct subunit domains obtained by scanning transmission electron microscopy and limited proteolysis. J Biol Chem 1984; 259:11647-11650.

31. Frosst P, Blom HJ, Milos R, et al. A candidate genetic risk factor for vascular disease: a common mutation in methylenetetrahydrofolate reductase. Nature Genet 1995; 10:111-113.

32. Goyette P, Sumner JS, Milos R, et al. Human methylenetetrahydrofolate reductase: Isolation of cDNA, mapping and mutation identification. Nature Genet 1994; 7:195-200.

33. Rozen R. Genetic predisposition to hyperhomocysteinemia: Deficiency of methylenetetrahydrofolate reductase (MTHFR). Thromb Haemost 1997; 78:523-526.

34. Garrow TA. Purification, kinetic properties, and cDNA cloning of mammalian betaine-homocysteine methyltransferase. J Biol Chem 1996; 271:22831-22838.

35. Millian NS, Garrow TA. Human betaine-homocysteine methyltransferase is a zinc metalloenzyme. Arch Biochem Biophys 1998; 356:93-98.

36. Sunden SLF, Renduchintala MS, Park EI, Miklasz SD, Garrow TA. Betaine-homocysteine methyltransferase expression in porcine and human tissues and chromosomal localization of the human gene. Arch Biochem Biophys 1997; 345:171-174.

37. Smolin LA, Benevenga NJ, Berlow S. The use of betaine for the treatment of homocystinuria. J Pediatr 1981; 99:467-472.

38. Wilcken DEL, Wilchen B, Dudman NPB, Tyrrell PA. Homocystinuria - the effects of betaine on the treatment of patients not responsive to pyrodoxine. N Engl J Med 1983; 309:448-453.

39. Allen RH, Stabler SP, Lindenbaum J. Serum betaine, $N,N$-dimethylglycine and $N$-methylglycine levels in patients with cobalamin and folate deficiency and related inborn errors of metabolism. Metabolism 1993; 42:1448-1460.

40. Kery V, Bukovska G, Kraus JP. Transsulfuration depends on heme in addition to pyridoxal 5'-phosphate. Cystathionine β-synthase is a heme protein. J Biol Chem 1994; 269:25283-25288.

41. Taoka S, Ohja S, Shan XY, Kruger WD, Banerjee R. Evidence for heme-mediated redox regulation of human cystathionine β-synthase activity. J Biol Chem 1998; 273:25179-25184.

42. Kraus JP, Le K, Swaroop M, et al. Human cystathionine β-synthase cDNA: Sequence, alternative splicing and expression in cultured cells. Hum Mol Genet 1993; 2:1633-1638.

43. Kruger WD, Cox DR. A yeast system for expression of human cystathionine β-synthase: Structural and functional conservation of the human and yeast genes. Proc Natl Acad Sci USA 1994; 91:6614-6618.

44. Chasse JF, Paly E, Paris D, et al. Genomic organization of the human cystathionine β-synthase gene: evidence for various cDNAs. Biochem Biophys Res Commun 1995; 211:826-832.

45. Bao LM, Vlcek C, Paces V, Kraus JP. Identification and tissue distribution of human cystathionine β-synthase mRNA isoforms. Arch Biochem Biophys 1998; 350:95-103.

46. Chen P, Poddar R, Tipa EV, et al. Homocysteine metabolism in cardiovascular cells and tissues: implcations for hyperhomocysteinemia and cardiovascular disease. Adv Enz Regul 1999; 39:(in press)

47. Erickson PF, Maxwell IH, Su L-J, Bauman M, Golde LM. Sequence of cDNA for rat cystathionine γ-lyase and comparison of deduced amino acid sequence with related *Escheriche coli* enzymes. Biochem J 1990; 269:335-340.

48. Lu Y, O'Dowd BF, Orrego H, Israel Y. Cloning and nucleotide sequence of human liver cDNA encoding for cystathionine γ-lyase. Biochem Biophys Res Commun 1992; 189:749-758.

49. Braunstein AE, Goryachenkova EV. The β-replacement-specific pyridoxal-P-dependent lyases. Adv Enzymol Relat Areas Mol Biol 1984; 56:1-89.

50. Wang J, Dudman NPB, Wilcken DEL, Lynch JF. Homocysteine catabolism: levels of 3 enzymes in cultured human vascular endothelium and their relevance to vascular disease. Atherosclerosis 1992; 97:97-106.

51. Van der Molen EF, Hiipakka MJ, Van Lith-Zanders H, et al. Homocysteine metabolism in endothelial cells of a patient homozygous for cystathionine β-synthase (CS) deficiency. Thromb Haemost 1997; 78:827-833.

52. Jacobsen DW, Savon SR, Stewart RW, et al. Limited capacity for homocysteine catabolism in vascular cells and tissues: a pathophysiologic mechanism for arterial damage in hyperhomocysteinemia? Circulation 1995; 91:29.(abstract)

53. Mudd SH, Poole JR. Labile methyl balances for normal humans on various dietary regimens. Metabolism 1975; 24:721-735.

54. Ward M, McNulty H, McPartlin J, Strain JJ, Weir DG, Scott JM. Plasma homocysteine, a risk factor for cardiovascular disease, is lowered by physiological doses of folic acid. Q J Med 1997; 90:519-524.

55. Food and Drug Administration. Food standards: amendment of standards of identity for enriched grain products to require addition of folic acid. Final rule. Federal Register 1996; 61:8781-8807.

56. Selhub J, Miller JW. The pathogenesis of homocysteinemia: interruption of the coordinate regulation by S-adenosylmethionine of the remethylation and transsulfuration of homocysteine. Am J Clin Nutr 1992; 55:131-138.

57. Park EI, Renduchintala MS, Garrow TA. Diet-induced changes in hepatic betaine-homocysteine methyltransferase activity are mediated by changes in the steady-state level of its mRNA. J Nutr Biochem 1997; 8:541-545.

58. Rasmussen K, Moller J, Lyngbak M, Pedersen AMH, Dybkjær L. Age and gender specific reference intervals for total homocysteine and methylmalonic acid in plasma before and after vitamin supplementation. Clin Chem 1996; 42:630-636.

59. Guttormsen AB, Ueland PM, Svarstad E, Refsum H. Kinetic basis of hyperhomocysteinemia in patients with chronic renal failure. Kidney Int 1997; 52:495-502.

60. Bostom A, Brosnan JT, Hall B, Nadeau MR, Selhub J. Net uptake of plasma homocysteine by the rat kidney in vivo. Atherosclerosis 1995; 116:59-62.

61. Van Guldener C, Donker AJM, Jakobs C, Teerlink T, De Meer K, Stehouwer CDA. No net renal extraction of homocysteine in fasting humans. Kidney Int 1998; 54:166-169.

62. Ewadh MJA, Tudball N, Rose FA. Homocysteine uptake by human umbilical vein endothelial cells in culture. Biochim Biophys Acta 1990; 1054:263-266.

63. Christensen B, Refsum H, Garras A, Ueland PM. Homocysteine remethylation during nitrous oxide exposure of cells cultured in media containing various concentrations of folates. J Pharmacol Exp Ther 1992; 261:1096-1105.

64. Christensen B, Ueland PM. Methionine synthase inactivation by nitrous oxide during methionine loading of normal human fibroblasts. Homocysteine remethylation as determinant of enzyme inactivation and homocysteine export. J Pharmacol Exp Ther 1993; 267:1298-1303.

65. Christensen B, Rosenblatt DS, Chu RC, Ueland PM. Effect of methionine and nitrous oxide on homocysteine export and remethylation in fibroblasts from cystathionine synthase-deficient, cb1G, and cb1E patients. Pediatr Res 1994; 35:3-9.

66. Refsum H, Christensen B, Djurhuus R, Ueland PM. Interaction between methotrexate, "rescue" agents and cell proliferation as modulators of homocysteine export from cells in culture. J Pharmacol Exp Ther 1991; 258:559-566.

67. Van der Molen EF, Van den Heuvel LPWJ, Te Poele Pothoff MTWB, Monnens LAH, Eskes TKAB, Blom HJ. The effect of folic acid on the homocysteine metabolism in human umbilical vein endothelial cells (HUVECs). Eur J Clin Invest 1996; 26:304-309.

68. Hultberg B, Andersson A, Isaksson A. Higher export rate of homocysteine in a human endothelial cell line than in other human cell lines. Biochim Biophys Acta Mol Cell Res 1998; 1448:61-69.

69. Mansoor MA, Guttormsen AB, Fiskerstrand T, Refsum H, Ueland PM, Svardal AM. Redox status and protein binding of plasma aminothiols during the transient hyperhomocysteinemia that follows homocysteine administration. Clin Chem 1993; 39:980-985.

70. Guttormsen AB, Mansoor AM, Fiskerstrand T, Ueland PM, Refsum H. Kinetics of plasma homocysteine in healthy subjects after peroral homocysteine loading. Clin Chem 1993; 39:1390-1397.

71. Mansoor MA, Bergmark C, Svardal AM, Lonning PE, Ueland PM. Redox status and protein binding of plasma homocysteine and other aminothiols in patients with early-onset peripheral vascular disease. Homocysteine and peripheral vascular disease. Arterioscler Thromb Vasc Biol 1995; 15:232-240.

72. Andersson A, Lindgren A, Hultberg B. Effect of thiol oxidation and thiol export from erythrocytes on determination of redox status of homocysteine and other thiols in plasma from healthy subjects and patients with cerebral infarction. Clin Chem 1995; 41:361-366.

73. Mansoor MA, Ueland PM, Aarsland A, Svardal AM. Redox status and protein binding of plasma homocysteine and other aminothiols in patients with homocystinuria. Metabolism 1993; 42:1481-1485.

74. Refsum H, Helland S, Ueland PM. Radioenzymic determination of homocysteine in plasma and urine. Clin Chem 1985; 31:624-628.

75. Kang S-S, Wong PWK, Cook HY, Norusis M, Messer JV. Protein-bound homocysteine: A possible risk factor for coronary artery disease. J Clin Invest 1986; 77:1482-1486.

76. Sartorio R, Carrozzo R, Corbo L, Andria G. Protein-bound plasma homocyteine and identification of heterozygotes for cystathionine-synthase deficiency. J Inherit Metab Dis 1986; 9:25-29.

77. Wiley VC, Dudman NPB, Wilcken DEL. Interrelations between plasma free and protein-bound homocysteine and cysteine in homocystinuria. Metabolism 1988; 37:191-195.

78. McCully KS, Vezeridis MP. Homocysteine thiolactone in arteriosclerosis and cancer. Res Commun Chem Pathol Pharmacol 1988; 59:107-119.

79. Mudd SH, Matorin AI, Levy HL. Homocysteine thiolactone: failure to detect in human serum or plasma. Res Commun Chem Pathol Pharmacol 1989; 63:297-300.

80. McCully KS. Homocysteinemia and arteriosclerosis: failure to isolate homocysteine thiolactone from plasma and lipoproteins. Res Commun Chem Pathol Pharmacol 1989; 63:301-304.

81. Jakubowski H, Goldman E. Synthesis of homocysteine thiolactone by methionyl-tRNA synthetase in cultured mammalian cells. FEBS Lett 1993; 317:237-240.

82. Dudman NPB, Hicks C, Lynch JF, Wilcken DEL, Wang J. Homocysteine thiolactone disposal by human arterial endothelial cells and serum in vitro. Arterioscler Thromb 1991; 11:663-670.

83. Olszewski AJ, Szostak WB. Homocysteine content of plasma proteins in ischemic heart disease. Atherosclerosis 1988; 69:109-113.

84. Dudman NPB, Lynch J, Wang J, Wilcken DEL. Failure to detect homocysteine in the acid-hydrolyzed plasmas of recent myocardial infarct patients. Atherosclerosis 1991; 86:201-209.

85. Jacobsen DW, Troxell LS, Brown KL. Catalysis of thiol oxidation by cobalamins and cobinamides: reaction products and kinetics. Biochemistry 1984; 23:2017-2025.

86. Starkebaum G, Harlan JM. Endothelial cell injury due to copper-catalyzed hydrogen peroxide generation from homocysteine. J Clin Invest 1986; 77:1370-1376.

87. Chidambaram MV, Zgirski A, Frieden E. The reaction of cysteine with ceruloplasmin copper. J Inorg Biochem 1984; 21:227-239.

88. Chen H, Robinson K, Jacobsen DW. Model studies on the formation of protein-bound homocysteine in hyperhomocysteinemia. FASEB J 1997; 11:A1264.(abstract)

# 4. REFERENCE RANGES FOR HOMOCYSTEINE CONCENTRATIONS

JOHAN B. UBBINK AND RHENA DELPORT

## SUMMARY

Reference ranges are used to interpret results, to confirm a diagnosis and to define levels at which a certain blood component may increase risk of a disease. Therefore care should be taken in defining the range in which the results of 95% of a healthy population would be expected to fall. Subjects should constitute a random sample of the healthy population and the procedure should be standardized to exclude pre-analytical factors that may impact on the assay result. When the distribution of the data is parametric, the central 95% interval may be calculated as mean ± 2 standard deviations of the mean, and if the data distribution is non-parametric, as is the case with plasma total homocysteine, the central 95% interval is obtained by computing the 2.5$^{th}$ and the 97.5$^{th}$ percentiles. It may however be inappropriate to generate reference data from populations who have a high incidence of CHD and who may have sub-clinical disease. Furthermore, the validity of the plasma homocysteine reference range may be affected by certain confounding variables, e.g. use of different analytical methods and standards, gender, age, vitamin nutritional status, and race. In this chapter the plasma homocysteine reference range is redefined by taking vitamin nutritional status into consideration. Different models indicate that the upper limit of normal for the plasma homocysteine concentration is 12 µmol/L. The clinical relevance of this cutoff value is tested by evaluating the outcome of studies that applied similar cutoff values in assessing CHD risk. Standardization of the ana-

K. Robinson (ed.), Homocysteine and Vascular Disease, 41-57.

lytical method is required before a reference range for plasma tHcy can be applied universally.

## INTRODUCTION: THE PHILOSOPHY BEHIND REFERENCE VALUES

When only one of two results are possible in laboratory analysis, it is easy to interpret the result and to diagnose the patient's condition. For example, a qualitative test for human antibodies against the human immunodeficiency virus (HIV) can only be positive or negative and the interpretation of the result is straight forward. The results obtained from quantitative analysis of serum or blood components are often more difficult to interpret. How does one know whether the obtained result is indicative of disease? To assist in the interpretation of these results, comparisons are usually made with reference data obtained from an appropriate reference group. Some blood components are not measured for diagnostic purposes, but are monitored because they are causally related to a specific disease (e.g. serum cholesterol levels and CHD) and may either increase risk of the disease or may accelerate the disease process. Reference values may aid in defining levels at which interventional measures are instigated.

Blood samples from young, apparently healthy volunteers (at least 120) are often utilized to generate reference data. The sampling scheme should be as random as possible, pre-analytical factors that may impact on the assay results should be standardized for and the sampling process should be described and made available to the end user [1].

A list of reference values obtained by analysis of blood samples from a selected reference population is of little use in the interpretation of patient derived results. Therefore, the reference values are usually summarized as a central 95% interval. When the data distribution is parametric, the central 95% interval may be calculated as mean ± 2 standard deviations of the mean. This approach is however not valid for non-parametric data distributions. In the latter case logarithmic or square root transformation of the data may be performed to normalise the distribution, or preferably, the central 95% interval is obtained by computing the 2.5th and the 97.5th percentiles [1].

The basic, simple approach as outlined above has been used to define reference ranges for a large number of analytes. However, it should be realized that this approach is not suitable for all the biological variables that may be measured in serum. For example, some serum components (eg testosterone) may require sex and age specific reference ranges and criteria have been published to identify analytes for which population specific reference ranges may be useful [2]. Furthermore, when determining reference ranges for variables that may be causally related to the expression of chronic diseases of lifestyle, random sample selection may be inappropriate to define normal (disease free) levels of the variable. For example, even a young, apparently healthy population sample from an industrialized western country will include an undisclosed number of individuals with subclinical coronary heart disease (CHD). It would therefore be inappropriate to use the above mentioned group together with a pure statistical approach to define e.g. serum cholesterol reference ranges. It has in fact been shown that serum cholesterol concentrations that confer a higher-than-basal risk for premature CHD start well below the upper limit of the statistical reference range calculated in a "healthy" population with a high CHD prevalence [3,4]. Therefore, optimal values for serum cholesterol associated with good health have been derived from cholesterol concentrations in populations with a low CHD incidence and from serum cholesterol concentrations in the lowest-risk segment of populations with a high CHD incidence [3].

In this chapter the utility of reference data published for serum or plasma total homocysteine concentrations will be discussed. Is it appropriate to use statistical reference ranges for homocysteine concentrations, or should the reference range be adjusted according to the models used for serum cholesterol? Do we require age and sex specific homocysteine reference ranges? Provided that appropriate reference ranges are defined, how should a result outside the reference range be interpreted?

## STATISTICAL REFERENCE RANGES FOR SERUM OR PLASMA HOMOCYSTEINE CONCENTRATIONS

Reference values for serum or plasma homocysteine concentrations published before 1993 have been summarized by Ueland et al [5]. In general, these earlier studies were performed on small groups that did not meet the criterion of the International Federation of Clinical Chemistry (IFCC) that data from at least 120 individuals are required to define a reference interval. Nevertheless, these earlier studies indicated that the normal reference range for plasma homocysteine would probably be between 5--15 µmol/L.

Table 1 summarizes a number of studies that included at least 100 subjects in the generation of reference data. It is clear from Table 1 that a considerable variability exists between plasma homocysteine levels published from different laboratories. This may reflect methodological differences that are aggravated by the absence of international reference material and the lack of standardization for the homocysteine assay. However, some of the variation may be due to real population differences. For example, the plasma homocysteine concentrations in free-living elderly Britons are notably higher compared to their peers in Norway [6,7]. This is unlikely to be ascribed to methodological differences inasmuch as

*Table 1: Adult reference ranges for plasma homocysteine concentrations.*

| Population description | Sex | n | Sample | Analytical Method | Mean (SD) (µmol/L) | Non parametric 95% reference range | Reference |
|---|---|---|---|---|---|---|---|
| Elderly British subjects (> 65 y) [a] | — | 375 | Heparinized plasma | Monobromobimane derivatisation + HPLC | 15.7 (7.4) | 7.6-30.0 | 6 |
| | — | 373 | | | 14.7 (6.3) | 6.9-31.9 | |
| Elderly Norwegians from Hordaland (40-67y) | — | 941 | EDTA plasma | Monobromobimane derivatisation + HPLC | 12.9 (6.7) | 8.0-21.5 | 7 |
| | — | 1410 | | | 11.6 (4.7) | 6.7-21.0 | |
| Middle aged Norwegians from Hordaland (40-42 yr) | — | 4260 | EDTA plasma | Monobromobimane derivatisation + HPLC | 11.3 (4.3) | 6.9 - 20.9 | 7 |
| | — | 4905 | | | 9.6 (4.1) | 5.6 - 17.4 | |
| South African urban whites | — | 1437 | EDTA plasma | SBDF derivatisation + HPLC | 12.0 (6.7) | 5.4 - 30.1 | 8 |
| South African rural blacks from the Venda/Shangaan tribes | — | 117 | EDTA plasma | SBDF derivatisation + HPLC | 9.7 (3.4) | | 9 |
| | — | 107 | | | 7.5 (1.9) | | |
| Danish subjects (20 - 85 y) | — | 109 | Fluoride plasma | Stable isotope dilution | 9.9 (2.5) | 6.3 - 15.7 | 10 |
| | — | 126 | | | 8.7 (2.5) | 4.9 - 14.9 | |
| White-collar workers, Montreal, Canada [b] | — | 380 | EDTA plasma | SBDF derivatisation + HPLC | 9.7 (4.9) | 3.6 - 22.7 | 11 |
| | — | 204 | | | 7.6 (4.1) | 3.3 - 18.4 | |

Additional calculations of data not reported [a] in reference 6 was kindly provided by Dr. CJ Bates, Medical Research Council Dunn Nutrition Unit, Cambridge, UK, and [b] in reference 11 by Dr S Lussier-Cacan, Clinical Research Institute of Montreal, Quebec, Canada.

both sets of samples were analysed with monobromobimane derivatisation and HPLC. Similarly, South African Whites and Blacks differ significantly with respect to plasma homocysteine concentrations [8,9]. Age and gender are further causes of variation in plasma homocysteine concentrations [10-12]. It is interesting to note that the gender difference exists in all the population groups studied, even those characterized by low circulating homocysteine levels.

Certain population groups differ distinctly with respect to the shape of the plasma homocysteine concentration frequency distribution curve. In most populations the distribution of data points is positively skewed [11,13] (Fig. 1 and 2), but in others, namely the Finns [14] and South African Blacks [9], the data distribution is essentially parametric. In the latter two populations the reference range may be calculated as the population mean $\pm$ 2 SD. However, for nonparametric data distribution the central 95% interval is obtained by computing the 2.5[th] and the 97.5[th] percentiles [1]. The value of the 97.5[th] percentile will depend heavily on the number of individuals with plasma homocysteine concentrations in the long drawn-out tail of the markedly skewed plasma homocysteine frequency distribution. A comparison of figures 1 and 2 illustrates the point. Although the bulk of the distribution points in both the Canadian and South African white populations are < 20 μmol/L, the tail of the frequency distribution is more pronounced in the South African group. This implies that the 97.5[th] percentile is notably higher in South Africans than in Canadians, thus explaining the considerable difference in the central 95% intervals as determined for the two populations (Tab. 1). Furthermore, the exclusion of statistical outliers in some studies contributes to the impression that there is a considerable variation of the 97.5[th] percentile amongst different population groups. For example, Rasmussen et al. [10] excluded 6 individuals identified as outliers in their study; with the outliers removed, the 97.5[th] percentile was 15.7 μmol/L in men, which is nearly 50% lower than the 97.5[th] percentile of 30.1 in white South Africans, where no outliers wereexcluded.

It is clear that small differences in the marked positive skewness of the plasma homocysteine concentration frequency distribution can result in substantially different reference ranges for distinct population groups. This complicates the comparison of reference intervals from different laboratories. A degree of inter-laboratory standardization could be achieved if statistical outliers are excluded before computing the reference interval. It should be noted, however, that statistical outliers (data points > mean + 3SD) are usually retained in establishing reference levels. Both the IFCC and the National Committee for Clinical Laboratory Standards (NCCLS) have very conservative recommendations with respect to the exclusion of outliers. Both recommend Dixon's "one-third" rule to identify outliers [15]. This rule states that if the difference between the extreme value and the next observation is greater than one third of the entire range of all observations, the extreme observation may be omitted [15]. In computing the

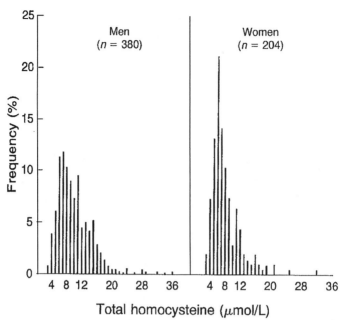

*Figure 1. Frequency distribution of plasma total homocysteine concentrations in healthy Canadian subjects. (Reprinted with permission from reference 11).*

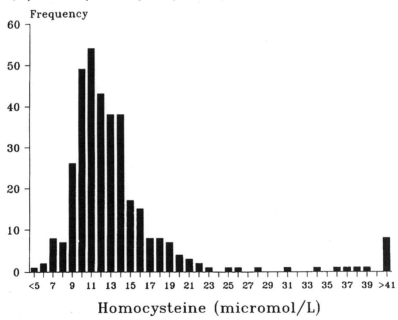

*Figure 2. Frequency distribution of plasma total homocysteine concentrations in adult South African men (n = 349). (Reprinted with permission from reference 13).*

statistical reference range in white South Africans, no data point qualified as an outlier according to Dixon's rule.

Another interesting point that emerges from Tab. 1 is the consistent gender differences with respect to plasma homocysteine concentrations. Some authors therefore recommend the use of gender specific reference ranges [10,11]. However, the clinical utility of separate reference ranges for plasma homocysteine determination remains to be investigated. The main objective for partitioning reference data into more homogenous subgroups is to reduce the between-person variability and to reduce the variance or spread of the data. Partitioning of reference data will only be useful if it allows a more meaningful interpretation of a single laboratory result from the patient. The mere existence of significant differences between subgroups (gender or age) in mean plasma homocysteine concentrations does not per se justify separate reference ranges, because the very nature of statistics dictates that any difference, no matter how small or clinically irrelevant, can become statistically significant provided that the sample sizes are large enough [16].

Tab. 2 summarizes reference values for children. Only a few studies have been performed in children [9,17], but available data indicate that plasma homocysteine levels at birth (cord blood) are low [18], and that plasma homocysteine levels rise steadily during childhood to reach adult levels in late adolescence (Fig. 3). No statistically significant gender differences were observed with respect to paediatric plasma homocysteine concentrations [17]. For both white and black South African children, parametric frequency distributions were observed [9].

## ADJUSTING THE STATISTICAL REFERENCE RANGE FOR PLASMA HOMOCYSTEINE CONCENTRATIONS

The skew (tailed) frequency distributions of plasma homocysteine concentrations summarized in Tab. 1 may be typical of coronary heart disease - prone western populations. According to the Physicians Health Study [19], the risk for myocardial infarction increased 3.4 fold in cases with plasma homocysteine concentrations in the tailed part of the homocysteine frequency distribution curve. It may therefore be inappropriate to include the tail of the plasma homocysteine distribution curve in a definition of plasma homocysteine concentrations associated with good health. Furthermore, individuals with plasma homocysteine concentrations in the tailed part of the distribution curve generally have a sub-optimal vitamin (folate, vitamin $B_{12}$, vitamin $B_6$) nutritional status [13], thus supporting the suggestion that the marked positive skewness of the homocysteine frequency distribution curve is abnormal. It may therefore be more appropriate to account for vitamin nutritional status in the definition of the ho-

*Table 2: Paediatric reference ranges for the plasma homocysteine assay*

| Population description | Sex | n | Mean (SD) Age | Mean (SD) homocysteine (µmol/L) | Median homocysteine (µmol/L) | Non-parametric reference range | Reference |
|---|---|---|---|---|---|---|---|
| Children from Mediterranean countries, aged 2mo-18y[a] | — | 112 | 8.6 (1.6) | 6.4 (1.6) | 6.0 | 3.5 - 9.8 | 17 |
| | — | 83 | 10.2 (1.7) | 6.7 (1.7) | 6.3 | 3.8 - 10.8 | |
| Black South African children from Venda/Shangaan tribes, aged 7-15 y | — | 127 | 10.2 (2.6) | 5.9 (1.6) | 5.7 | 3.3 - 9.5 | 9 |
| | — | 139 | 10.3 (2.6) | 5.5 (1.5) | 5.4 | 3.2 - 9.6 | |
| White urban South African children, aged 7 - 15 y | — | 49 | 10.7 (2.4) | 5.2 (0.9) | 5.1 | 3.4 - 7.5 | 9 |
| | — | 74 | 10.4 (1.6) | 5.0 (0.9) | 4.9 | 3.3 - 7.1 | |

[a] Additional calculations of data not reported in ref.17 were kindly provided by Dr. A Vilaseca, Hospital Sant Joan de Déu, Barcelona, Spain.

mocysteine reference range. Several approaches have been used to redefine the plasma homocysteine reference rangewith respect to vitamin nutritional status.

Ubbink et al [20] utilized data from 75 subjects who had been treated with various vitamin supplements to determine the relationship between plasma homocysteine concentrations before and after vitamin supplementation. A scatter plot was constructed of pretreatment plasma homocysteine concentrations versus the ratio of post and pretreatment plasma homocysteine concentrations. Using the method of least squares, a piecewise linear regression [21] line with one node at a pretreatment homocysteine concentration of 26 µmol/L was fitted to the data (Fig. 4).

The node at 26 µmol/L corresponds to the piecewise linear regression line with the smallest mean square error. The regression line is described by the equation

$$Y = 1.0089 - 0.022\ X_1 + 0.0144\ X_2$$

where     $Y$ = ratio of post-treatment to pretreatment homocysteine concentrations

$X_1$ = pretreatment homocysteine concentration.

$X_2 = 0$ if pretreatment homocysteine$\leq$ 26.0 µmol/L, or

$X_2$ = pretreatment homocysteine concentration - 26, if pretreatment homocysteine > 26.0 µmol/L.

The regression equation was used to calculate the estimated plasma homocysteine concentration for each individual in a population sample (South African white men, n = 1437), as if he had been treated with a suitable vitamin formulation for 6 weeks. In effect, the population plasma homocysteine concentrations were therefore adjusted for an optimal vitamin nutritional status.

The calculations showed that vitamin therapy could be expected to reduce the mean(SD) plasma homocysteine concentration from 12.0 (6.7) to 8.3 (1.7) µmol/L. Furthermore, the distribution of adjusted plasma homocysteine concentrations is Gaussian (Fig. 5), implying that the plasma homocysteine reference range will then be 4.9 - 11.7 µmol/L (mean $\pm$ 2 SD). This calculated upper normal limit is considerably lower when compared to the non-parametric definition of the upper normal limit on the unadjusted data.

Support for an approach in which nutritional considerations are accounted for in the definition of the plasma homocysteine reference range has been forthcoming from other researchers in this field. Lussier-Cacan et al [11] excluded subjects with plasma folate and/or vitamin $B_{12}$ levels in the lowest quartile of the plasma vitamin frequency distribution. In the remainder of the population sample, mean plasma homocysteine concentrations were 8% and 11% lower in

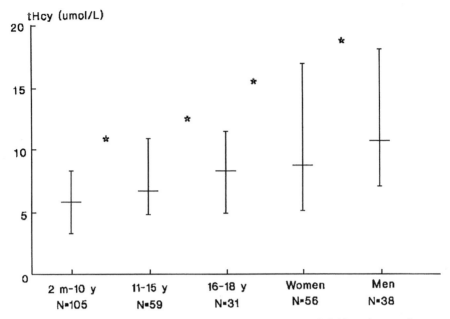

*Figure 3. Total homocysteine concentrations in three age groups of children (m, month; y, years) and male and female control adults (20-65 years old). (Reprinted with permission from reference 17).*

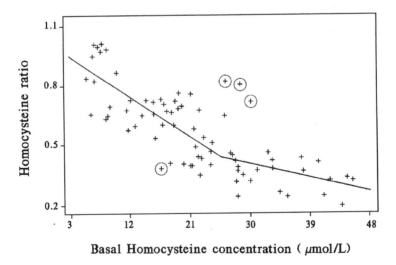

*Figure 4. Scatter plot of pretreatment plasma total homocysteine concentrations vs the ratio of post- and pretreatment plasma homocysteine concentrations. (Reprinted with permission from reference 20).*

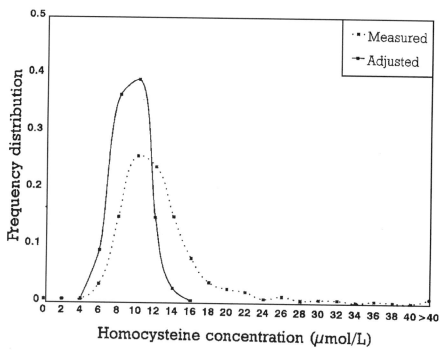

*Figure 5. Smoothed frequency distribution of measured and adjusted plasma homocysteine concentrations in South African white men. (Reprinted with permission from reference 20).*

men and women, respectively, than in the entire groups. The exclusion of subjects with subnormal vitamin nutritional status may be used in a population-based approach to define the plasma homocysteine reference range.

Rasmussen et al. computed the plasma homocysteine reference interval in 235 volunteers before and after vitamin (1 mg of cyanocobalamin/day for one week followed by 10 mg of folate/day for one week) supplementation [10]. Vitamin supplementation resulted in a more symmetrical plasma homocysteine concentration frequency distribution, but, in contrast to the mathematical projections by Ubbink et al [20], some positive skewness remained (Fig. 6). The central 0.95 reference interval of 5.0 - 12.1 µmol/L for the vitamin-supplemented men in the study of Rasmussen et al [10], corresponds closely to the extrapolated reference interval (4.9 - 11.7 µmol/L) after data adjustment as suggested by Ubbink et al [20]. This close agreement is particularly noteworthy, considering the remarkable difference in the upper normal limit for plasma homocysteine concentration as reported by the two groups before vitamin status was accounted for (Tab. 1).

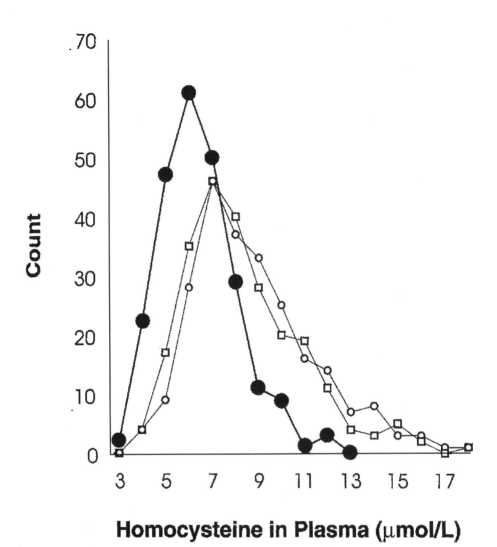

*Figure 6. Distribution of plasma homocysteine concentrations in adults before (O) and after supplementation with cyanocobalamin (□), and after supplementation with folic acid (●) (n = 235). (Reprinted with permission from reference 10).*

## HOW RELEVANT IS A VITAMIN STATUS ADJUSTED PLASMA HOMOCYSTEINE REFERENCE RANGE?

Both the work of Rasmussen et al [10] and Ubbink, et al. [20] on vitamin status-adjusted plasma homocysteine concentration reference ranges indicate that a fasting plasma homocysteine concentration > 12.0 µmol/L should be considered as elevated. But what evidence would support the clinical validity of the above defined cutoff value?

In the European Concerted Action Project involving 750 patients with vascular disease and 800 controls, Graham and co-workers [22] found that CHD risk started to rise from the middle of the plasma homocysteine distribution. The most apparent increase in CHD risk was beyond the eighth decile of the plasma homocysteine frequency distribution; the eighth decile corresponded with a plasma homocysteine concentration of 12.0 µmol/L [22]. Malinow et al recently found that the risk of having a thickened carotid artery wall was significantly increased when the plasma homocysteine concentrations were > 10.5 µmol/L [23]. Selhub et al also studied the association between carotid artery stenosis and plasma homocysteine concentrations and found that the risk of stenosis was elevated in subjects with homocysteine concentrations above 11.4 µmol/L [24]. Pancharuniti et al studied patients with angiographically demonstrated CHD and found that CHD-risk started to increase from plasma homocysteine concentrations ≥ 11.7 µmol/L [25]. Nygård prospectively investigated the relation between plasma homocysteine concentrations and mortality among 587 patients with angiographically confirmed CHD [26]. Using individuals with a plasma homocysteine concentration < 9.0 µmol/L as reference group, they found that the CHD mortality ratio already doubled for the next category which included individuals with plasma homocysteine concentrations between 9.0 - 14.9 µmol/L.

From the examples cited above it becomes clear that the association between increased CHD risk and plasma homocysteine concentrations is noted at much lower levels than suggested by the upper reference limits computed from unadjusted plasma homocysteine concentrations as summarized in Tab. 1. In fact, the plasma homocysteine concentrations associated with increased CHD risk closely resemble the upper normal limit as derived from vitamin adjusted data by two independent procedures as discussed above [10,20]. This suggests that an adult upper normal limit for plasma homocysteine concentration of 12 µmol/L is appropriate, but it does not suggest that lowering an individual's plasma homocysteine concentration to <12.0 µmol/L will be protective against CHD. Only the long awaited intervention trials will supply us with the real benefit that may be achieved by maintaining homocysteine concentrations < 12µmol/L.

## VALUES OUTSIDE THE REFERENCE RANGE.

A scientifically validated plasma homocysteine reference ranges will be of little use if it is not appropriately utilized. How, for example, should an elevated

*Table 3. Variability components for plasma homocysteine measurement*

| Parameter | Data according to Garg et al [27] | Data according to Cob baert et al [28] |
|---|---|---|
| $CV_A$ | 4.3 % | 3.70 % |
| $CV_I$ | 7.03 % | 9.40 % |
| $CV_G$ | 33.5 % | 23.9 % |
| Possible % difference from homeostatic set point if: | | |
| n = 1 | 16.1 % | 18.4 % |
| n = 3 | 9.3 % | 10.6 % |
| n = 5 | 7.2 % | 8.2 % |

plasma homocysteine concentration be interpreted? The significance of a single observation of plasma homocysteine concentration above the upper limit of normal should be interpreted in terms of the biological and analytical variation of this assay. Tab. 3 summarizes data on the variability of the plasma homocysteine measurement as determined by Garg and coworkers [27] and by Cobbaert, et al. [28].

Knowledge of the analytical and within-subject variance relates the observed value(s) to the individual's homeostatic set point [29].

This is given by the formula:

$$n = \frac{z^2 (CV_A^2 + CV_I^2)}{D^2}$$

where     n = the number of specimens analyzed
          z = number of standard deviations required for a stated probability (for p = 0.05; z = 1.96)
          D = percentage closeness to the homeostatic set point
          $CV_A^2$ = analytical coefficient of variation
          $CV_I^2$ = within-subject coefficient of variation.

Using the data published by Garg et al., simple substitution in the equation above indicates that a single plasma homocysteine determination (n = 1) produces a result with a 95% probability to be within ± 16.1% of the individual's homeostatic set point. It should therefore be realized that an individual presenting with a mildly elevated plasma homocysteine concentration may still have a set point below the upper limit of normality. Repeat measurements are required to obtain a more accurate assessment of an individual's homocysteine status. Tab. 3 indicates that the mean of 3 plasma homocysteine determinations will be within 10% of an individual's homeostatic set point.

It is generally important to be aware of biological variation and that it is often undesirable to commence treatment upon a single observation of an abnormal analyte blood concentration. This of less relevance for an elevated homocysteine level, inasmuch as the therapy (folic acid) is both innocuous and cheap. However the concept of biological variation is very relevant with respect to prospective epidemiological studies relating homocysteine concentrations to premature coronary heart disease. These studies normally rely on a single homocysteine determination per individual, which is related to the homeostatic set point by a large error margin.

CONCLUSION

It is clear from the discussion above that a universally accepted reference range for total plasma homocysteine does not yet exist. Indeed, this cannot come into existence without proper standardization of the homocysteine analytical method. Standardization requires consistent, stable, human plasma-based reference material, the definition of a reference method and comparisons of the alternative methods with the reference method. With the accumulating evidence that homocysteine is involved in the pathogenesis of vascular disease, it is trusted that national and international regulatory bodies will proceed on the standardization of plasma homocysteine determinations.

REFERENCES

1. Solberg HE, Grüsbeck R. Reference values. Adv Clin Chem 1989;27:1-79
2. Harris EK, Boyd JC. On dividing reference data into subgroups to produce separate reference ranges. Clin Chem 1990;36:265-70.
3. The Expert Panel. Report on the National Cholesterol Education Program Expert Panel on detection, evaluation and treatment of high blood cholesterol in adults. Arch Intern Med 1988;148:36-69.
4. Rossouw JE, Steyn K, Berger GMB, Vermaak WJH, Kock J, Seftel HC, Gevers W. Action limits for serum total cholesterol. S Afr Med J 1988;73:693-700.
5. Ueland PM, Refsum H, Stabler SP, Malinow MR, Andersson A, Allen RH. Total homocysteine in plasma or serum: Methods and clinical applications. Clin Chem 1993;39:1764-79.

6.  Bates CJ, Mansoor MA, Van der Pols J, Prentice A, Cole TJ, Finch S. Plasma total homocysteine in a representative sample of 972 British men and women aged 65 and over. Eur J Clin Nutr 1997;51:691-7.

7.  Nygård O, Refsum H, Ueland PM, Vollset SE. Major lifestyle determinants of plasma total homocysteine distribution: the Hordaland Homocysteine Study. Am J Clin Nutr 1988;67:263-70.

8.  Ubbink JB, Vermaak WJH, Delport R, Van der Merwe A, Becker PJ, Potgieter H. Effective homocysteine metabolism may protect South African Blacks against coronary heart disease. Am J Clin Nutr 1995;62:802-8.

9.  Ubbink JB, Delport R, Vermaak WJH. Plasma homocysteine concentrations in a population with a low coronary heart disease prevalence. J Nutr 1996;126:1254S-1257S.

10. Rasmussen K, Møller J, Lyngbak M, Holm Pedersen A-M, Dybkjaer L. Age and gender-specific reference intervals for total homocysteine and methylmalonic acid in plasma before and after vitamin supplementation. Clin Chem 1996;42:360-6.

11. Lussier-Cacan S, Xhignesse M, Piolot A, Selhub J, Davignon J, Genest J. Plasma total homocysteine in healthy subjects - sex-specific relation with biological traits. Am J Clin Nutr 1996;64:587-93.

12. Joosten E, Lesaffre R, Riezler R. Are different reference intervals for methylmalonic acid and total homocysteine necessary in elderly people ? Eur J Haematol 1996;57:222-6.

13. Ubbink JB, Vermaak WJH, Van der Merwe A, Becker PJ. Vitamin B-12, vitamin B-6 and folate nutritional status in men with hyperhomocysteinemia. Am J Clin Nutr 1993;57:47-53.

14. Alfthan G, Pekkanen J, Jauhiainen J, Pitkäniemi J, Karvonen M, Toumilehto J, Salonen, JT, Ehnholm C. Relation of serum homocysteine and lipoprotein (a) concentrations to atherosclerotic disease in a prospective Finnish population based study. Atherosclerosis 1994;106:9-19.

15. Dixon WJ. Processing data for outliers. Biometrics 1953;9:74-89.

16. Harris EK, Boyd JC. On dividing reference data into subgroups to produce separate reference ranges. Clin Chem 1990;36:265-70.

17. Vilaseca MA, Moyano D, Ferrer I, Artuch R. Total homocysteine in pediatric patients. Clin Chem 1997;43:690-2.

18. Malinow MR, Rajkovic A, Duell PB, Hess DL, Upson BM. The relationship between maternal and neonatal umbilical cord plasma homocysteine suggests a potential role for maternal homocysteine in fetal metabolism. Am J Obst Gynecol 1998;178:228-33.

19. Stampfer MJ, Malinow R, Willet WC, Newcomer LM, Upson B, Ullmann D, Tischler PV, Hennekens CH. A prospective study of plasma homocysteine and risk of myocardial infarction in US physicians. JAMA 1992;268:877-81.

20. Ubbink JB, Becker PJ, Vermaak WJH, Delport R. Results of B-vitamin supplementation study used in a prediction model to define a reference range for plasma homocysteine. Clin Chem 1995;41:1033-7.

21. Montgomery DC, Peck EA. Introduction to linear regression analysis. New York: John Wiley & Sons,1982;19:15-8.

22. Graham IM, Daly LE, Refsum HM, et al. The European Concerted Action Project. Plasma homocysteine as a risk factor for vascular disease. JAMA 1997;277:1775-81.

23. Malinow MR, Nieto J, Szklo M, Chambless LE, Bond G. Carotid artery intimal-medial wall thickening and plasma homocysteine in asymptomatic adults. Circulation 1993;87:1107-13.
24. Selhub JS, Jacques PF, Bostom AG, et al. Association between plasma homocysteine concentrations and extra-cranial carotid-artery stenosis. N Engl J Med 1995;332:286-91.
25. Pancharuniti N, Lewis CA, Sauberlich HE, Perkins LL, Go RCP, Alvarez JO, Maculuso M, Acton RT, Copeland RB, Cousins AL, Gore TB, Cornwell PE, Roseman JM. Plasma homocysteine, folate and vitamins B-12 concentrations and risk of early coronary artery disease. Am J Clin Nutr 1994;59:940-8.
26. Nygård O, Vollset SE, Refsum H, Stesvold I, Tverdal A, Nordrehaug JE, Ueland PM, Kvåle G. Total plasma homocysteine and cardiovascular risk profile. The Hordaland Homocysteine Study. JAMA 1995;274:1526-33.
27. Garg UC, Zheng Z-J, Folsom AR, Moyer YS, Tsai MY, McGovern P, Eckfeldt JH. Short-term and long-term variability of plasma homocysteine measurement. Clin Chem 1997;43:141-5.
28. Cobbaert C, Arentsen JC, Mulder P, Hoogerbruggen, Lindemans J. Significance of various parameters derived from biological variability of lipoproteina, homocysteine, cysteine, and total antioxidant status. Clin Chem 1997;43:1958-64.
29. Frazer CG, Harris EK. Generation and application of data on biological variation in clinical chemistry. CRC Lab Sci 1989;27:409-37.

# 5. DETERMINANTS OF PLASMA HOMOCYSTEINE

PER MAGNE UELAND, HELGA REFSUM AND JØRN SCHNEEDE

## SUMMARY

The concentration of total homocysteine in plasma is influenced by a diversity of genetic and acquired factors, and by interactions between such factors. The most prevalent genetic cause of hyperhomocysteinemia is the C677T polymorphism of the methylenetetrahydrofolate reductase gene, which predisposes to hyperhomocysteinemia under conditions of impaired folate status. Among the physiological and life-style determinants, increasing age, male sex, poor nutrition with low vitamin intake, smoking, heavy coffee consumption cause high homocysteine, whereas young age, premenopausal state, pregnancy, vitamins like folate and cobalamin, and exercise are associated with low homocysteine. Several drugs may influence the homocysteine level by acting as vitamin antagonists, and among these, methotrexate and nitrous oxide cause a rapid increase in homocysteine by interfering with folate and cobalamin functions, respectively. Some sulfhydryl-containing drugs reduce homocysteine, probably via disulphide exchange reactions, whereas the effect of steroid hormones on homocysteine is complex and their mechanisms are conjectural. Cyclosporin A increases homocysteine, possibly by a mechanism independent of interference with renal function. The diseases which most often and profoundly increase homocysteine are folate and cobalamin deficiencies and renal failure. Some proliferative (psoriasis) and malignant (leukemia) diseases may increase homocysteine, probably by directing folates towards DNA synthesis. Hyperhomocysteinemia has been

*K. Robinson (ed.), Homocysteine and Vascular Disease, 59-84.*
© 2000 *Kluwer Academic Publishers. Printed in the Netherlands.*

associated with diabetes, but this is most likely secondary to impaired renal function, since factors like insulin itself and glomerular hyperfiltration seem to reduce homocysteine.

*Table 5-1.* Categorization of plasma homocysteine determinants

| **Categories** |
| --- |
| Genetic factors |
| Physiological determinants |
| Life-style factors |
| Diseases |
| Drugs |

Other states that affect homocysteine are thyroid dysfunction, heart transplantation and the acute phase after a cardiovascular event. The implications of variations of homocysteine according to various determinants are threefold. First, elevated homocysteine may be useful for diagnosis or follow up of some diseases or drug therapies, as for example folate or cobalamin deficiencies or nitrous oxide anaesthesia. Secondly, high homocysteine may itself be hazardous by predisposing to occlusive vascular disease, and may contribute to the increased prevalence of cardiovascular disease in conditions like renal failure or hypothyroidism. Finally, strategies to modify factors predisposing to hyperhomocysteinemia may have a health promoting effect, and are actually in line with established guidelines promoting good health.


INTRODUCTION

Plasma total homocysteine levels are determined by a variety of factors. These factors are categorized in table 1. This chapter will focus on physiological and life-style determinants, effect of drugs and various diseases, with emphasis on the Hordaland Homocysteine study, a population based screening of 18043 healthy subjects aged 40-67 years. The relation of plasma homocysteine to genetic factors, vitamin status and renal function will be addressed in detail in Chapters 6 and 15-18 are only briefly summarized here.

GENETICS

Heterozygosity for cystathionine ß-synthase (CBS) deficiency was established as a cause of elevated post-methionine loading plasma homocysteine more than 30 years ago (1). The fasting levels in these individuals seem to be normal or slightly elevated (2). It has been suggested that heterozygosity for CBS deficiency explains hyperhomocysteinemia in most vascular patients (3, 4), but this conclusion has later been refuted (5). Although post loading homocysteine seems to be partly a genetic trait (6), the frequency of carriers of CBS deficiency is not sufficiently high to account for hyperhomocysteinemia in either a normal (7) or vascular population (8).

Inheritance as a factor influencing fasting plasma homocysteine was suggested by the finding of a correlation between the homocysteine levels in monozygotic and dizygotic healthy twins (9, 10), and between family members with heart disease (6, 11, 12). Healthy children (13) and children with familiar hypercholesterolemia (14) who have relatives with cardiovascular disease, have higher fasting homocysteine than children with healthy relatives, suggesting that the fasting level is a genetic transmittable risk factor.

The common C677T polymorphism of the methylenetetrahydrofolate reductase (MTHFR) gene has been established as an important genetic determinant of elevated fasting homocysteine. Homozygosity for this polymorphism (TT genotype) predisposes to hyperhomocysteinemia under conditions of impaired folate status (Chapter 16). Also in children, homocysteine is determined by the MTHFR status, and the highest levels are observed in TT subjects with low serum folate (15). Mutations in the methionine synthase gene causing moderate hyperhomocysteinemia have hitherto not been identified (16).

PHYSIOLOGICAL DETERMINANTS (FIG. 5-1).

Plasma homocysteine increases throughout life in both sexes. Before puberty, homocysteine in children is similar in boys and girls (about 5 µmol/L). The levels show a marked increase, particularly in boys, between pubertal stages 1 and 2-5. By puberty, the plasma homocysteine level has increased to about 6-7 µmol/L (13-15, 17-19), and the characteristic skew distribution (13) and the sex difference observed in adults have been established.

In adults, the plasma homocysteine levels are usually about 1-2 µmol/L higher in men than in women. In the Norwegian Hordaland cohort, the geometric means were 10.8 µmol/L in 5918 healthy men and 9.1 µmol/L in 6348 women aged 40-42 years (7). From puberty to old age, mean homocysteine increases (about 3-5 µmol/L) in both sexes (7, 20), but homocysteine seems to

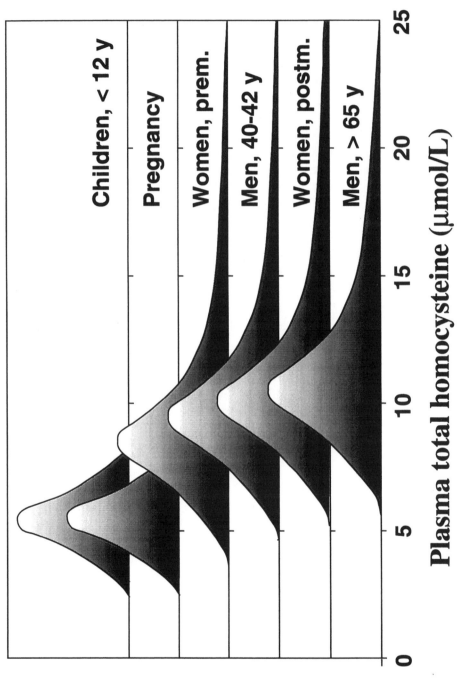

*Figure 5-1. Plasma homocysteine level and distribution according to physiological factors.*

decline in the very old (21). The age-related increase in homocysteine is steeper in women than in men. This is at least partly seems to be related to menopause. Both fasting and post methionine load homocysteine are higher in postmenopausal than in premenopausal women (20, 22). The age-dependent increase may be attributed to deterioration of renal function (23, 24)_and impaired folate status (25, 26), whereas the sex-related differences are explained by the effects of sex steroids on homocysteine or possibly higher homocysteine production (linked to creatine-creatinine synthesis (2)) in men due to higher muscle mass (see later).

There are consistent reports of a substantial reduction (by about 50%) of homocysteine during pregnancy (27, 28). The reduction seems independent of folate status (29). homocysteine decreases between the first and second trimester, and thereafter remains essentially stable throughout the rest of the pregnancy (28). After delivery, the maternal homocysteine level is inversely related to neonatal weight and gestational age (30). Normal homocysteine concentrations are attained 2-4 days post-partum (28). An umbilical vein to artery homocysteine decrement and a relation between homocysteine and neonatal weight and gestational age have been interpreted as fetal uptake of maternal homocysteine (30). Alternatively, low homocysteine may represent physiological adaption to pregnancy (31), which may support adequate placental circulation.

## LIFE-STYLE AND DIET (FIG. 5-2)

The metabolic relations between homocysteine and methionine (Chapter 3) and the metabolic adaption to methionine excess in the rats (32), raise the possibility that methionine intake may influence fasting or post methionine load homocysteine. Plasma homocysteine increases by about 14% 8 hours after a protein rich meal (33). However, neither the homocysteine response after loading (34, 35) nor fasting homocysteine (36) seems to be related to the daily dietary methionine or protein content. On the contrary, there are two reports suggesting that high dietary protein intake (37) or methionine intake (38) may actually decrease fasting homocysteine. This observation is in accordance with infrequent elevation of homocysteine and positive cobalamin status in high meat-eaters (39).

Folate and cobalamin deficiencies are common causes of moderate to severe fasting hyperhomocysteinemia (40, 41), whereas vitamin $B_6$ deficiency normally results in increased post methionine load homocysteine only (42). Fasting plasma homocysteine correlated negatively with both intake and serum levels of folate, cobalamin and vitamin $B_6$ (36, 43). These relations between vitamin status and homocysteine are corroborated by supplementation studies

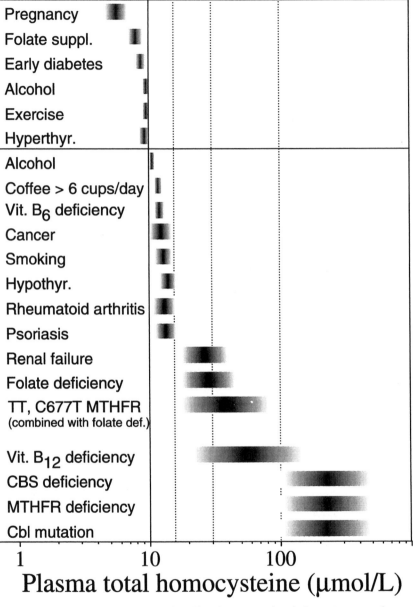

*Figure 5-2. Schematic representation of the effect from an isolated determinant on the expected mean homocysteine level. Normal value for homocysteine is defined as 10 μmol/L, and factors that reduce and increase homocysteine are sorted and separated by the horizontal line. The width of the bars does not indicate the range of homocysteine values but rather the uncertainty of the estimate, related to the extent or severity of disease or variable response. The estimates are not based on published data, but rather reflect an overall impression of the authors. Relevant literature is quoted in the text.*

showing that folate is the most efficient means to reduce fasting homocysteine (41, 44), whereas vitamin $B_6$ does not affect fasting homocysteine (45) but selectively influences post load homocysteine (41).

Folic acid supplementation seems to be more efficient in lowering homocysteine than folate derived from food (46, 47), and a meta-analysis of intervention studies demonstrated that increasing the folic acid dose above 0.5 mg/d does not further reduce the homocysteine concentration (44). The effectiveness of folate supplementation seems to reach a plateau at about 0.4 mg/day (47), and 0.2-0.4 mg/day have been reported to maintain a positive folate homeostasis and thereby optimal homocysteine remethylation in healthy subjects (48, 49). A similar dose-response relationship has recently been observed for folic acid fortified cereals demonstrating maximal homocysteine lowering effect between 0.5 and 0.665 mg folic per 30 gram cereal (50).

The homocysteine distribution in the general population is skew with a marked tail towards higher homocysteine values (7). There are consistent reports that homocysteine is reduced and approaches normal distribution both after folic acid supplementation and in subgroups with adequate vitamin status (51-53). In the Hordaland Homocysteine cohort, we could distinguish between the reduction of high homocysteine to normal levels, which is usually conferred by folate derived from food, and the reduction from normal to subnormal levels which is attributable to intake of folic acid containing supplements (54).

In addition to the expected effect of dietary folate, recent studies have also provided data which demonstrate that life-style significantly affects the plasma homocysteine level (54).

Higher levels of homocysteine in smokers than in non-smokers have been demonstrated in some (12, 55, 56) but not all (8) smaller studies. The Hordaland Homocysteine study demonstrated a strong dose-response relationship between the number of cigarettes and homocysteine levels, independent of age and sex (7), also in subjects with high folate intake (54). Notably, smoking increases mean homocysteine and causes a shift of the whole homocysteine distribution curve to higher levels, similar to that observed in populations with low folate intake (54). This may suggest an influence of smoking on folate function. However, smokers generally consume a less healthy diet containing less vegetables and more fat than non-smokers (57-59), and smokers have reduced intake and blood levels of several vitamins involved in homocysteine metabolism, including vitamins $B_{12}$ (60) and $B_6$ (61, 62). In addition, tobacco smoke contains abundant free radicals that confer oxidative stress and thereby may affect redox status of thiols (63), including homocysteine (64).

Heavy coffee consumption was among the strongest life-style determinants of homocysteine in the Hordaland Homocysteine cohort (65). A dose-response relation was observed, and in individuals drinking more than 6 cups each day, the mean homocysteine level was 2-3 $\mu$mol/L higher than in coffee abstainers.

In contrast, in US participants in the ARIC study, there was no relation between homocysteine and moderate coffee consumption. A recent study demonstrated homocysteine elevation in the elderly consuming 4 or more cups daily (37).

Coffee consumption is known to be associated with unhealthy life-style and poor nutrition (57, 66, 67), but the homocysteine-coffee relation reported in the Hordaland Study was also found in non-smokers and at both high and low folate intake. Heavy coffee consumption increases mean homocysteine by decreasing the proportion with low and intermediate homocysteine, and in this respect can be distinguished from folate deficiency and cigarette smoking (54). Notably, the effect was observed with filtered coffee and thus is not mediated by the cholesterol-raising diterpenes. As the consumption of decaffeinated coffee did not have an effect on homocysteine, caffeine may play a mechanistic role (65). The caffeine effect may be related to its influence on the cardiovascular system or kidney function (68). Another possibility is interference with vitamin $B_6$ function, as reported for another xanthine, theophylline (69), but such a mechanism implies a predominant effect on post methionine load homocysteine.

In the Hordaland study, a life-style profile, which reflects the combined effect of the three major modifiable homocysteine determinants, folate intake, smoking and coffee consumption, is strongly correlated with homocysteine (54). Subjects with a contrasting life-style have a difference of 3-5 μmol/L in homocysteine which is larger than the effect attributable to each factor alone. This supports the notion of different mechanisms underlying the homocysteine elevating effects of smoking, low folate intake and heavy coffee consumption. Furthermore, homocysteine is essentially normally distributed in a population characterized by a healthy life-style profile (54).

Among the 18043 subjects investigated in the Hordaland Homocysteine study, only 67 (0.4%) had homocysteine equal or higher than 40 μmol/L (70). Compared to controls, these subjects had lower plasma folate and cobalamin levels, lower intake of vitamin supplements, consumed much coffee and were frequently (60%) smokers. When 7 subjects with cobalamin deficiency were excluded, 92% of these hyperhomocysteinemic subjects (compared to 10.4% controls) were homozygous for the C677T MTHFR polymorphism. These findings demonstrate a strong positive interaction between MTHFR genotype and life-style determinants of homocysteine (70).

Both exercise and moderate alcohol consumption are weak but significant determinants of homocysteine in the Hordaland cohort (7, 71). The difference in homocysteine between subjects with sedentary life-style compared with those doing exercise on a daily basis is most pronounced in the elderly, and approaches 1 μmol/L. Exercise reduces the skewness of the homocysteine distribution curve, and therefore seems to lower homocysteine in subjects with

*Table 5-2. Drug effects on plasma total homocysteine*

| Class Drug | homocysteine response | Possible mechanism |
|---|---|---|
| Folate antagonists | | |
| Methotrexate | Increase | Inhibition of DHFR[a], depletion of reduced folates |
| Anticonvulsants | Increase | Inhibition of polyglutamation, folate depletion |
| Colestipol | Increase | Inhibition of folate absorption |
| Cholestyramine | Increase | Inhibition of folate absorption |
| Cobalamin antagonists | | |
| Nitrous oxide | Increase | Inactivation of methionine synthase |
| Nitric oxide | ND[a] | Inactivation of methionine synthase |
| Metformin | Increase | Inhibition of cobalamin absorption |
| H2-receptor antag. | ND | Inhibition of cobalamin absorption |
| Omeprazole | ND | Inhibition of cobalamin absorption |
| Cholestyramine | ND | Inhibition of cobalamin absorption |
| Vitamin $B_6$ antagonists | | |
| Niacin | Increase | Inhibition of pyridoxal kinase |
| Azauridine | Increase | Inhibition of pyridoxal kinase |
| Isoniazid | ND | Inhibition of pyridoxal kinase |
| Theophylline | Increase | Inhibition of pyridoxal kinase |
| Homocysteine production | | |
| Adenosine analogues | Decrease | Inhibition AdoHcy[a] hydrolase |
| L-Dopa | Increase | Substrate for AdoMet[a]-dependent transmethylation |
| Sulfhydryl compounds | | |
| D-Penicillamine | Decrease | Disulphide exchange, displacement |
| N-Acetylcysteine | Decrease | Disulphide exchange, displacement |
| Mesna | Decrease | Disulphide exchange, displacement |
| Sex steroids | | |
| Contraceptives | Increase, variable | Not known, interference with vitamin |
| Estrogens (postm.) | Decrease | Not known, interference with vitamin function |
| Androgens | Increase | Increased muscle mass and creatinine synthesis |
| Antiestrogens | | |
| Tamoxifen | Decrease | Not known |
| Aminoglutethimide | Increase | Induction of liver metabolism |
| Others | | |
| Cyclosporin A | Increase | Impaired renal function |
| Betaine | Decrease | Enhancement of remethylation |

[a] Abbreviations: ND, not determined; DHFR, dihydrofolate reductase; AdoHcy, S-adenosylhomocysteine; AdoMet, S-adenosylmethionine

hyperhomocysteinemia (7). In subjects aged 40-42 years, and in particular among smokers, the relation between homocysteine levels and long-term alcohol consumption forms a weak U-shaped curve with reduction in homocysteine up to 14 alcohol units per week. Higher alcohol intake increases homocysteine (71).

Plasma homocysteine shows a transient increase during acute alcohol intoxication in alcoholics (72), and direct inhibition of methionine synthase by acetaldehyde (73) should be considered as a possible mechanism. Chronic alcoholism seems to be associated with hyperhomocysteinemia (74), but only in subjects with poor nutrition (72). This may be explained by impaired folate, vitamin $B_{12}$ or vitamin $B_6$ status (74).


DRUGS (TABLE 5-2)


A variety of drugs affect  homocysteine levels. They act via different mechanisms, including inhibition of vitamin (folate, cobalamin or vitamin $B_6$) function, by affecting homocysteine production, undergoing thiol-disulphide exchange reactions, interfering with renal function and influencing hormonal status. Most literature on homocysteine and drugs has been reviewed previously (75-77). The effects of various drugs on homocysteine are summarized in Table 5-2.

The antifolate drug methotrexate (MTX) induces elevated homocysteine within hours after high-dose infusions (up to 33.6 grams $/m^2$) used for cancer chemotherapy, and this effect is subsequently reversed by rescue therapy with high doses of folinic acid (78, 79). In leukemia patients, the marked increase in plasma homocysteine was associated a 4-fold increase in cerebrospinal fluid homocysteine and a massive build-up (from undetectable levels to about 30-100 µmol/L) of homocysteic and cysteic acid in the cerebrospinal fluid. Accumulation of these neuroexcitatory amino acids is related to and may be responsible for neurological toxicity (80).

In psoriasis patients treated with low doses of methotrexate (10-25 mg), homocysteine increases slowly over a period of several days (81). In rheumatoid arthritis patients treated with 1 mg/day methotrexate, elevated homocysteine seems to develop slowly between 3-6 months (82) and one year (83). Folic acid (5-27.6 mg/week) improves folate status and prevents the methotrexate-induced hyperhomocysteinemia (83) and toxicity, but preserves the therapeutic efficacy in rheumatoid arthritis patients (84).

Several other drugs may cause hyperhomocysteinemia through interference with folate metabolism. This has been demonstrated for phenytoin and other anticonvulsants (75, 85, 86), which probably act by depleting liver folate stores by inhibiting polyglutamation (87). Plasma homocysteine is also elevated following therapy with niacin in combination with the bile sequestrant colestipol.

The latter agent may interfere with folate absorption (88). Notably, elevation of homocysteine following treatment with another bile resin, cholestyramine, was largely confined to subjects with the C677T transition in the MTHFR gene (89). This genotype predisposes to hyperhomocysteinemia under conditions of impaired folate status.

Plasma homocysteine increases within hours in patients exposed to the anaesthetic gas, nitrous oxide (90-94). The increase reflects irreversible oxidation of cob(I)alamin formed as a transient intermediate of the methionine synthase reaction. This, in addition to the irreversible inactivation of the enzyme methionine synthase itself, is assumed to be responsible for the side effects from bone marrow and central nervous system observed after prolonged nitrous oxide exposure (95). The deleterious effect of nitrous oxide on methionine synthase may be alleviated by methionine loading prior to anaesthesia (91).

The endothelial-derived relaxing factor, nitric oxide, has a similar effect on isolated methionine synthase (96, 97) and on the enzyme in isolated hepatocytes (98), but the significance of this interaction in vivo remains to be established.

In contrast to the rapid increase in homocysteine observed during nitrous oxide exposure, a slow increase over months to years is expected during prolonged intake of drugs interfering with cobalamin absorption. Such interference with cobalamin absorption has been reported for cholestyramine (99), histamine H2-receptor antagonists (100), omeprazole (101) and the antidiabetic metformin, but elevation of homocysteine has hitherto only been reported for cholestyramine (89) and metformin (102, 103). The latter two drugs may also affect folate absorption.

Several drugs interfere with the function of vitamin $B_6$. A common mechanism involves inhibition of pyridoxal kinase (104). High plasma or urinary homocysteine or homocystine has been reported following treatment with azauridine (105), isoniazid (106), niacin (107) and theophylline (69).

Some drugs may influence homocysteine production. Several adenosine analogues with antiviral properties inhibit S-adenosylhomocysteine hydrolase (108) and may thereby decrease homocysteine production. Such drugs are not widely used, and low plasma homocysteine has only been demonstrated for the antimetabolite, 2-deoxycoformycin (109). Enhanced homocysteine production may occur following intake of drugs that serve as a substrate for S-adenosylmethionine-dependent transmethylation reaction, as demonstrated for the antiparkinson drug, L-dopa, in rats (110) and humans (Miller and Brattström, unpublished). One may speculate whether a similar mechanism contributes to the hyperhomocysteinemia induced by niacin (107).

Three sulfhydryl-containing drugs, D-penicillamine (111, 112), N-acetylcysteine (113) and 2-mercaptoethane sulfonate (mesna) (114, 115), have been found to reduce plasma homocysteine. These drugs probably act by a thiol-disulphide exchange reaction, which may enhance excretion, lower plasma protein-binding or alter distribution of homocysteine (77).

The effect of sex steroid hormones on homocysteine is indicated by sex differences in homocysteine level and by the observation of low homocysteine levels in premenopausal women (20, 116) and during pregnancy (27, 28). Inconsistent data (117-119) have been published on change in plasma homocysteine of women taking oral contraceptives (117), the effect of which seems to depend on the hormonal phase (118). Replacement therapy containing estrogen in postmenopausal women results in a decrease in plasma homocysteine within 3-6 months of treatment (120), after which the homocysteine returns to baseline in some (121) but not all patients (122). The mean decrease in homocysteine was 13.5%, but the largest reduction was obtained in women with highest base-line values (123).

Estrogen treatment reduces homocysteine of healthy men (124) and men with prostatic carcinoma (117), whereas short-term treatment of normal men with supraphysiological doses of testosterone is without effect (125). A recent cross-sex hormone study in transsexual males and females demonstrates that plasma homocysteine decreases after estrogen plus antiandrogen administration to male subjects, and increases after androgen administration to female subjects (126). This study suggests that physiological levels of sex hormones affect plasma homocysteine concentration. A positive correlation between homocysteine and plasma creatinine levels during androgen administration (126) suggests that androgens act by enhancing synthesis of creatinine and thereby homocysteine secondary to increase in muscle mass (126). In addition, sex hormones and contraceptives may impair folate (127), cobalamin (128) and vitamin $B_6$ status (129), which may predispose to hyperhomocysteinemia.

In postmenopausal breast cancer patients, the antiestrogens tamoxifen and aminoglutethimide have opposite effects on the homocysteine levels. Tamoxifen lowers plasma homocysteine after 6-12 months of treatment, particularly in subjects with high pre-treatment levels (130, 131). The drug also possesses estrogen agonist effect, and the mechanism behind the homocysteine reduction is uncertain (130). Among three aromatase inhibitors which block the androgen to estradiol conversion, only aminoglutethimide causes a substantial increase in homocysteine. Thus, this effect is probably not related to low estrogen levels, but may be due to the ability of aminoglutethimide to induce hepatic mixed function oxidase (132), which has been associated with enhanced folate turnover (133).

The immunosuppressive drug cyclosporine A (CyA) increases plasma homocysteine. Renal transplant patients receiving CyA have significantly higher homocysteine than both non-treated renal transplant recipient, and patients without a renal graft but matched for glomerular filtration rate (134). In renal patients, it may be difficult to distinguish high homocysteine caused by CyA interference with renal function from high homocysteine related to impaired renal function from other causes (135). Hyperhomocysteinemia also develops in cardiac transplant patients, and high homocysteine is predicted by both serum creatinine and serum CyA concentration (136), suggesting that the CyA effect is independent of renal function. The usual correlation between homocysteine and serum folate was absent in the CyA-treated renal transplant recipients, which may suggest a mechanism involving interference with folate-dependent remethylation (134). This conclusion has been refuted by a recent study (135), and is not supported by the observation of a reduction of homocysteine in CyA-treated renal transplant recipients by high-dose folic acid (137).

Betaine is the co-substrate in the betaine-homocysteine methyltransferase reaction (32), and has been extensively used as a safe and effective homocysteine lowering agent in homocystinuria. In contrast to vitamin $B_6$, folate or cobalamin, betaine is effective in all forms of homocystinuria (2). Data on betaine treatment of moderate hyperhomocysteinemia are sparse. Betaine in doses up to 6 g/day has been shown to reduce (138) or normalize (139, 140) post load homocysteine in vascular patients, but has essentially no effect on fasting homocysteine level in renal patients receiving folic acid (141). Betaine as possible means to reduce homocysteine should be further investigated.


DISEASES (FIG. 5-2)

Folate and cobalamin deficiencies and renal failure (142, 143) are the clinical states most often responsible for markedly elevated homocysteine. These conditions are discussed in detail in chapters 6 and 14.

High homocysteine has been demonstrated in children with acute lymphoblastic leukemia (79) and in patients with psoriasis (81). These are conditions with a large burden of proliferating cells which export more Hcy than resting cells (144), possibly due to drainage of the folate pool in the direction of DNA synthesis at the expense of homocysteine remethylation.

Data on homocysteine levels in rheumatoid patients are somewhat controversial, probably because of frequent systemic manifestations combined with variable and extensive drug treatment. In patients not receiving methotrexate, one small study has reported an elevated post load homocysteine level, attributable to impaired vitamin $B_6$ status often seen in rheumatoid arthritis (145). Normal fasting homocysteine has been found in patients not receiving long-term methotrexate (82, 145), whereas elevated fasting levels have been reporting in patients with severe and long-standing rheumatoid arthritis associated with impaired cobalamin absorption and function (146).

In type I diabetes, hyperhomocysteinemia occurs at an advanced stage and is characterized by elevated creatinine or macroalbuminuria. Elevated homocysteine is attributable to impaired renal function (147-149), but marginal folate deficiency may also contribute (150). In both type 1 and 2 diabetes, elevated fasting (151-153) or post methionine load homocysteine (152, 154) are associated with macroangiopathy, whereas a relation between homocysteine and microangiopathy (152, 155, 156) or microalbuminuria (157, 158) has been demonstrated in some but not all (148) studies. In type I diabetes patients with normal creatinine (159) and in non-diabetic hyperinsulinemic subjects (160), subnormal homocysteine has been reported. Low homocysteine may be due to the glomerular hyperfiltration observed in early diabetes (173) or is possibly a metabolic effect of high insulin level. The latter possibility is in agreement with elevated homocysteine in insulin-resistant subjects (161) and with reduction of homocysteine by insulin, as demonstrated during hyperinsulinemic-euglycemic clamp. The homocysteine reduction was not observed in type 2 diabetes, suggesting impaired insulin effects on homocysteine in these patients (162).

Homocysteine has recently been reported to be moderately elevated in hypothyroidism and low in hyperthyroidism (163). This may be related to the influence of thyroid status on riboflavin (164) or folate function, GFR or creatinine synthesis.

There are consistent reports on higher homocysteine in heart transplant recipients than in controls (165, 166), and close to 70% of these patients have values higher than the 90th percentile of controls. The increase in homocysteine takes place in the early postoperative phase and persists thereafter, and may be partly related to impaired functions of folate, $B_6$ status (167) or possibly vitamin $B_{12}$ (166). Elevated homocysteine was related to vascular complications in one (168) but not all (167, 169) studies, and underlying low $B_6$ may be an independent predictor of cardiovascular morbidity and mortality (169).

Plasma homocysteine is low in the acute phase (first days) after myocardial infarction (38, 170, 171) or stroke (172) compared to the convalescent stage. In patients with infarction, homocysteine increases by about 40% within 7 days, and thereafter is essentially stable for at least 6 months or decreases slightly (171). The low homocysteine level in the acute phase is probably a response to the acute stress causing both hemodynamic and hormonal changes, but the possibility that the low homocysteine reflects the pre-infarction level cannot be ruled out.

*Table 5-3. Common causes of various degrees of hyperhomocysteinemia.*

| homocysteine level | Prevalence[a] | Common cause[a] |
|---|---|---|
| Moderate elevation (15-30 μmol/L) | ≤10% | Unhealthy life-style, including poor nutrition |
| | | MTHFR[b] polymorphism combined with low folate status (S-folate in lower normal range) |
| | | Folate deficiency |
| | | Mild cobalamin deficiency |
| | | Renal failure |
| | | Hyperproliferative disorders |
| | | Drug effects |
| Intermediate elevation (30-100 μmol/L) | ≤1% | MTHFR polymorphism combined with folate deficiency |
| | | Moderate cobalamin deficiency |
| | | Severe folate deficiency |
| | | Severe renal failure |
| Severe elevation (>100 μmol/L) | ≤0.02% | Severe cobalamin deficiency |
| | | CBS[b]-deficiency (homozygous) |

[a] Prevelance data (for a normal population) taken from ref. 7. The prevalence and causes of high homocysteine may vary according to population investigated.

[b] Abbreviations: MTHFR, 5,10-methylenetetrahydrofolate reductase; CBS, cystathionine-ß-synthase.


SUMMARY AND CONCLUSION

Plasma homocysteine levels are related to physiological parameters like age, gender, and altered hormonal status during pregnancy and after menopause (Fig. 5-1). Knowledge of such variations forms the basis for the assessment of homocysteine status and for establishing reference intervals. Moderate changes of homocysteine concentrations of 1-4 μmol/L are secondary to several modifiable life-style factors, such as smoking, nutrition, vitamin intake, coffee consumption and exercise, and reduction of homocysteine should be an incentive to improve life-style. Such recommendations should be given irrespective of homocysteine being a cause or indicator of cardiovascular or other diseases, since they conform with established guidelines promoting good health. Some diseases, like renal failure and hypothyroidism, are associated with hyperhomocysteinemia, which may contribute to the increased cardiovascular morbidity in these patients. Several drugs elevate homocysteine. For methotrexate and nitrous oxide, homocysteine may be a valuable indicator of pharmacodynamics, and high homocysteine induced by some drugs may confer increased cardiovascular risk (77). Folate and cobalamin deficiencies and some inborn errors of homocysteine metabolism cause a sub- stantial elevation of homocysteine, which serves as a disease indicator useful for diagnosis and follow-up. Finally, knowledge of the expected mean homocysteine level in the presence of various determinants (Fig. 5-2) and the prevalence of the determinants forms the basis of the diagnostic value of elevated homocysteine (Table 5-3).

## REFERENCES

1.    Brenton DP, Cusworth DC, Dent CE, Jones EE. Homocystinuria: Clinical and dietary studies. Q. J. Med. 1966;35:325-346.
2.    Mudd SH, Levy HL, Skovby F. Disorder of transsulfuration. In: Scriver CR, Beaudet AL, Sly WS, Valle D, eds. The metabolic and molecular bases of inherited disease. New York: McGraw-Hill, 1995:1279-1327.
3.    Clarke R, Daly L, Robinson K, et al. Hyperhomocysteinemia: An independent risk factor for vascular disease. N. Engl. J. Med. 1991;324:1149-1155.
4.    Boers GHJ, Smals AGH, Trijbels FJM, et al. Heterozygosity for homocystinuria in premature peripheral and cerebral occlusive arterial disease. N. Engl. J. Med. 1985;313:709-715.
5.    Engbersen AMT, Franken DG, Boers GHJ, Stevens EMB, Trijbels FJM, Blom HJ. Thermolabile 5,10-methylenetetrahydrofolate reductase as a cause of mild hyperhomocysteinemia. Am. J. Hum. Genet. 1995;56:142-150.
6.    Franken DG, Boers GHJ, Blom HJ, Cruysberg JRM, Trijbels FJM, Hamel BCJ. Prevalence of familial mild hyperhomocysteinemia. Atherosclerosis 1996;125:71-80.
7.    Nygård O, Vollset SE, Refsum H, et al. Total plasma homocysteine and cardiovascular risk profile. The Hordaland homocysteine study. JAMA 1995;274:1526-1533.
8.    Ueland PM, Refsum H, Brattström L. Plasma homocysteine and cardiovascular disease. In: Francis RBJr, ed. Atherosclerotic Cardiovascular Disease, Hemostasis, and Endothelial Function. New York: Marcel Dekker, inc, 1992:183-236.
9.    Reed T, Malinow MR, Christian JC, Upson B. Estimates of heritability for plasma homocyst(e)ine levels in aging adult male twins. Clin. Genet. 1991;39:425-428.
10.   Berg K, Malinow MR, Kierulf P, Upson B. Population variation and genetics of plasma homocyst(e)ine (H(e)) level. Clin. Genet. 1992;41:315-321.
11.   Genest JJJr, McNamara JR, Upson B, et al. Prevalence of familial hyperhomocyst(e)inemia in men with premature coronary artery disease. Arterioscler. Thromb. 1991;11:1129-1136.
12.   Wu LL, Wu J, Hunt SC, et al. Plasma homocyst(e)ine as a risk factor for early familial coronary artery disease. Clin. Chem. 1994;40:552-561.
13.   Tonstad S, Refsum H, Sivertsen M, Christophersen B, Ose L, Ueland PM. Relation of total homocysteine and lipid levels in children to premature cardiovascular death in male relatives. Pediatr. Res. 1996;40:47-52.

14. Tonstad S, Refsum H, Ueland PM. Association between plasma total homocysteine and parental history of cardiovascular disease in children with familial hypercholesterolemia. Circulation 1997;96:1803-1808.

15. Bjørke-Monsen AL, Vollset SE, Ueland PM, Refsum H. Plasma total homocysteine, vitamin status and the 5,10-methylenetetrahydrofolate reductase polymorphism in children. Netherl. J. Med. 1998;51:S50.

16. van der Put NMJ, van der Molen EF, Kluijtmans LAJ, et al. Sequence analysis of the coding region of human methionine synthase: relevance to hyperhomocysteinemia in neural-tube defects and vascular disease. Qjm-Mon J Assoc Physician 1997;90:511-517.

17. Vilaseca MA, Moyano D, Ferrer I, Artuch R. Total homocysteine in pediatric patients. Clin. Chem. 1997;43:690-692.

18. Reddy MN. Reference ranges for total homocysteine in children. Clin. Chim. Acta 1997;262:153-155.

19. Graf WD, Oleinik OE, Jack RM, Eder DN, Shurtleff DB. Plasma homocysteine and methionine concentrations in children with neural tube defects. Eur. J. Pediatr. Surg. 1996;6,Suppl:7-9.

20. Andersson A, Brattström L, Israelsson B, Isaksson A, Hamfelt A, Hultberg B. Plasma homocysteine before and after methionine loading with regard to age, gender, and menopausal status. Eur. J. Clin. Invest. 1992;22:79-87.

21. Rea IM, McMaster D, Doherty G, et al. Plasma homocysteine, folate, vitamin $B_{12}$ and $B_6$ status in the oldest old. Netherl. J. Med. 1998;52:S12.

22. van der Mooren MJ. Homocysteine: influences of menopausal hormone replacement therapy. Netherl. J. Med. 1998;52:S44.

23. Arnadottir M, Hultberg B, Nilsson Ehle P, Thysell H. The effect of reduced glomerular filtration rate on plasma total homocysteine concentration. Scand. J. Clin. Lab. Invest. 1996;56:41-46.

24. Norlund L, Grubb A, Fex G, et al. The increase of plasma homocysteine concentrations with age is partly due to the deterioration of renal function as determined by plasma cystatin C. Clin. Chem. Lab. Med. 1998;36:175-178.

25. Tucker KL, Selhub J, Wilson PW, Rosenberg IH. Dietary intake pattern relates to plasma folate and homocysteine concentrations in the Framingham Heart Study. J. Nutr. 1996;126:3025-3031.

26. Koehler KM, Pareo-Tubbeh SL, Romero LJ, Baumgartner RN, Garry PJ. Folate nutrition and older adults: challenges and opportunities. J. Am. Diet. Assoc. 1997;97:167-173.

27. Kang S-S, Wong PWK, Zhou J, Cook HY. Preliminary report: Total homocyst(e)ine in plasma and amniotic fluid of pregnant women. Metabolism 1986;35:889-891.

28. Andersson A, Hultberg B, Brattström L, Isaksson A. Decreased serum homocysteine in pregnancy. Eur. J. Clin. Chem. Clin. Biochem. 1992;30:377-379.

29. Bonnette RE, Caudill MA, Boddie AM, Hutson AD, Kauwell GP, Bailey LB. Plasma homocyst(e)ine concentrations in pregnant and nonpregnant women with controlled folate intake. Obstet. Gynecol. 1998;92:167-170.

30. Malinow MR, Rajkovic A, Duell PB, Hess DL, Upson BM. The relationship between maternal and neonatal umbilical cord plasma homocyst(e)ine suggests a potential role for maternal homocyst(e)ine in fetal metabolism. Am. J. Obstet. Gynecol. 1998;178:228-233.

31.  Bailey LB, Kauwell GPA. Homocysteine concentration in pregnant and nonpregnant women on folate controlled diet. Netherl. J. Med. 1998;52:S18.

32.  Finkelstein JD. Methionine metabolism in mammals. J. Nutr. Biochem. 1990;1:228-237.

33.  Guttormsen AB, Schneede J, Fiskerstrand T, Ueland PM, Refsum H. Plasma concentrations of homocysteine and other aminothiol compounds are related to food intake in healthy subjects. J. Nutr. 1994;124:1934-1941.

34.  Andersson A, Brattström L, Israelsson B, Isaksson A, Hultberg B. The effect of excess daily methionine intake on plasma homocysteine after a methionine loading test in humans. Clin. Chim. Acta 1990;192:69-76.

35.  den Heijer M, Bos GMJ, Brouwer IA, Gerrits WBJ, Blom HJ. Variability of the methionine loading test: no effect of a low protein diet. Ann. Clin. Biochem. 1996;33:551-554.

36.  Shimakawa T, Nieto FJ, Malinow MR, Chambless LE, Schreine PJ, Szklo M. Vitamin intake: a possible determinant of plasma homocyst(e)ine among middle-aged adults. Ann. Epidemiol. 1997;7:285-293.

37.  Stolzenberg-Solomon RZ, Miller ER 3rd, Maguire MG, Selhub J, Apple LJ. Association of dietary protein intake and coffee consumption with serum homocysteine concentrations in an older population. Am. J. Clin. Nutr. 1999;69:467-475.

38.  Verhoef P, Stampfer MJ, Buring JE, et al. Homocysteine metabolism and risk of myocardial infarction: relation with vitamins B-6, B-12, and folate. Am. J. Epidemiol. 1996;143:845-859.

39.  Mann NJ, Dudman N, Guo XW, Li D, Sinclair AJ. The effect of diet on homocysteine levels in healthy male subjects. Netherl. J. Med. 1998;52:S10.

40.  Allen RH, Stabler SP, Savage DG, Lindenbaum J. Metabolic abnormalities in cobalamin (vitamin-$B_{12}$) and folate deficiency. FASEB J. 1994;7:1344-1353.

41.  Ubbink JB. The role of vitamins in the pathogenesis and treatment of hyperhomocyst(e)inemia. J. Inherit. Metab. Dis. 1997;20:316-325.

42.  Miller JW, Nadeau MR, Smith D, Selhub J. Vitamin B-6 deficiency vs folate deficiency - comparison of responses to methionine loading in rats. Am. J. Clin. Nutr. 1994;59:1033-1039.

43.  Selhub J, Jacques PF, Wilson PWF, Rush D, Rosenberg IH. Vitamin status and intake as primary determinants of homocysteinemia in an elderly population. JAMA 1993;270:2693-2698.

44.  Brattström L, Landgren F, Israelsson B, et al. Lowering blood homocysteine with folic acid based supplements: meta-analysis of randomized trials. Br. Med. J. 1998;316(7135):894-898.

45.  Dierkes J, Kroesen M, Pietrzik K. Folic acid and Vitamin $B_6$ supplementation and plasma homocysteine concentrations in healthy young women. Int. J. Vitam. Nutr. Res. 1998;68:98-103.

46.  Wei MM, Gregory JF. Organic acids in selected foods inhibit intestinal brush border pteroylpolyglutamate hydrolase in vitro: potential mechanism affecting the bioavailability of dietary polyglutamyl folate. J. Agr. Food Chem. 1998;46:211-219.

47.  Omenn GS, Beresford SAA, Motulsky AG. Preventing coronary heart disease: B vitamins and homocysteine. Circulation 1998;97:421-424.

48. Jacob RA, Wu MM, Henning SM, Swendseid ME. Homocysteine increases as folate decreases in plasma of healthy men during short-term dietary folate and methyl group restriction. J. Nutr. 1994;124:1072-1080.
49. O'Keefe CA, Bailey LB, Thomas EA, et al. Controlled dietary folate affects folate status in nonpregnant women. J. Nutr. 1995;125:2717-2725.
50. Malinow MR, Duell PB, Hess DL, et al. Reduction of plasma homocyst(e)ine levels by breakfast cereal fortified with folic acid in patients with coronary heart disease. N. Engl. J. Med. 1998;338:1009-1015.
51. Ubbink JB, Becker PJ, Vermaak WJH, Delport R. Results of B-vitamin supplementation study used in a prediction model to define a reference range for plasma homocysteine. Clin. Chem. 1995;41:1033-1037.
52. Rasmussen K, Møller J, Lyngbak M, Holm Pedersen A-M, Dybkjær L. Age and gender specific reference intervals for total homocysteine and methylmalonic acid in plasma before and after vitamin supplementation. Clin. Chem. 1996;42:630-636.
53. Joosten E, Lesaffre E, Riezler R. Are different reference intervals for methylmalonic acid and total homocysteine necessary in elderly people? Eur. J. Haematol. 1996;57:222-226.
54. Nygård O, Refsum H, Ueland PM, Vollset SE. Major life-style determinants of plasma total homocysteine distribution: the Hordaland Homocysteine Study. Am. J. Clin. Nutr. 1998;67:263-270.
55. Bergmark C, Mansoor MA, Swedenborg J, de Faire U, Svardal AM, Ueland PM. Hyperhomocysteinemia in patients operated for lower extremity ischemia below the age of 50. Effect of smoking and extent of disease. Eur. J. Vasc. Surgery 1993;7:391-396.
56. Mansoor AM, Bergmark C, Svardal AM, Lønning PE, Ueland PM. Redox status and protein-binding of plasma homocysteine and other aminothiols in patients with early-onset peripheral vascular disease. Arterioscler. Thromb. Vasc. Biol. 1995;15:232-240.
57. Berger J, Wynder EL. The correlation of epidemiological variables. J. Clin. Epidemiol. 1994;47:941-952.
58. Preston AM. Cigarette smoking-nutritional implications. Prog. Food. Nutr. Sci. 1991;15:183-217.
59. Oshaug A, Bugge KH, Refsum H. Diet, an independent determinant for plasma total homocysteine. A cross sectional study of Norwegian workers on platforms in the North Sea. Eur. J. Clin. Nutr. 1998;52:7-11.
60. Piyathilake CJ, Macaluso M, Hine RJ, Richards EW, Krumdieck CL. Local and systemic effects of cigarette smoking on folate and vitamin B-12. Am. J. Clin. Nutr. 1994;60:559-566.
61. Vermaak WJH, Ubbink JB, Barnard HC, Potgieter GM, van Jaarsveld H, Groenewald AJ. Vitamin B-6 nutrition status and cigarette smoking. Am. J. Clin. Nutr. 1990;51:1058-1061.
62. Giraud DW, Martin HD, Driskell JA. Erythrocyte and plasma B-6 vitamer concentrations of long-term tobacco smokers, chewers, and nonusers. Am. J. Clin. Nutr. 1995;62:104-109.
63. Eiserich JP, Vandervliet A, Handelman GJ, Halliwell B, Cross CE. Dietary antioxidants and cigarette smoke-induced biomolecular damage: a complex interaction. Am. J. Clin. Nutr. 1995;62:S1490-S1500.

64.  Ueland PM. Homocysteine species as components of plasma redox thiol status. Clin. Chem. 1995;41:340-342.
65.  Nygård O, Refsum H, Ueland PM, et al. Coffee consumption and total plasma homocysteine. The Hordaland homocysteine study. Am. J. Clin. Nutr. 1997;65:136-143.
66.  Jacobsen BK, Thelle DS. The Tromso Heart Study: is coffee drinking an indicator of a life-style with high risk for ischemic heart disease? Acta Med. Scand. 1987;222:215-221.
67.  Schwarz B, Bischof HP, Kunze M. Coffee, tea, and life-style. Prev. Med. 1994;23:377-384.
68.  Holycross BJ, Jackson EK. Effects of chronic treatment with caffeine on kidney responses to angiotensin II. Eur. J. Pharmacol. 1992;219:361-367.
69.  Ubbink JB, van der Merwe, A., Delport, R., Allen, R.H., Stabler, S.P., Riezler, R., and Vermaak, W.J.H. The effect of a subnormal vitamin B-6 status on homocysteine metabolism. J. Clin. Invest. 1996;98:177-184.
70.  Guttormsen AB, Ueland PM, Nesthus I, et al. Determinants and vitamin responsiveness of intermediate hyperhomocysteinemia ($\geq$40 µmol/liter). The Hordaland homocysteine study. J. Clin. Invest. 1996;98:2174-2183.
71.  Vollset SE, Nygård O, Kvåle G, Ueland PM, Refsum H. The Hordaland homocysteine study: Life-style and total plasma homocysteine in Western Norway. In: Graham I, Refsum H, Rosenberg IH, Ueland PM, eds. Homocysteine Metabolism. From Basic Science to Clinical Medicine. Boston, Dordrecht, London: Kluwer Academic Publisher, 1997:177-182.
72.  Hultberg B, Berglund M, Andersson A, Frank A. Elevated plasma homocysteine in alcoholics. Alcohol Clin. Exp. Res. 1993;17:687-689.
73.  Kenyon SH, Nicolaou A, Gibbons WA. The effect of ethanol and its metabolites upon methionine synthase activity in vitro. Alcohol 1998;15:305-309.
74.  Cravo ML, Gloria LM, Selhub J, et al. Hyperhomocysteinemia in chronic alcoholism: correlation with folate, vitamin B-12, and vitamin B-6 status. Am. J. Clin. Nutr. 1996;63:220-224.
75.  Ueland PM, Refsum H. Plasma homocysteine, a risk factor for vascular disease: Plasma levels in health, disease, and drug therapy. J. Lab. Clin. Med. 1989;114:473-501.
76.  Refsum H, Ueland PM. Clinical significance of pharmacological modulation of homocysteine metabolism. Trends Pharmacol. Sci. 1990;11:411-416.
77.  Ueland PM, Fiskerstrand T, Lien EA, Refsum H. Homocysteine and drug therapy. In: Graham I, Refsum H, Rosenberg IH, Ueland PM, eds. Homocysteine Metabolism. From Basic Science to Clinical Medicine. Boston, Dordrecht, London: Kluwer Academic Publisher, 1997:145-152.
78.  Refsum H, Ueland PM, Kvinnsland S. Acute and long-term effects of high-dose methotrexate treatment on homocysteine in plasma and urine. Cancer Res. 1986;46:5385-5391.
79.  Refsum H, Wesenberg, F, and Ueland, PM Plasma homocysteine in children with acute lymphoblastic leukemia. Changes during a chemotherapeutic regimen including methotrexate. Cancer Res. 1991;51:828-835.
80.  Quinn CT, Griener JC, Bottiglieri T, Hyland K, Farrow A, Kamen BA. Elevation of homocysteine and excitatory amino acid neurotransmitters in the CSF of children who receive methotrexate for the treatment of cancer. J. Clin. Oncol. 1997;15:2800-2806.

81. Refsum H, Helland S, Ueland PM. Fasting plasma homocysteine as a sensitive parameter to antifolate effect. A study on psoriasis patients receiving low-dose methotrexate treatment. Clin. Pharmacol. Ther. 1989;46:510-520.

82. Morgan SL, Baggott JE, Refsum H, Ueland PM. Homocysteine levels in rheumatoid arthritis patients treated with low-dose methotrexate. Clin. Pharmacol. Ther. 1991;50:547-556.

83. Morgan SL, Baggott JE, Lee JY, Alarcon GS. Folic acid supplementation prevents deficient blood folate levels and hyperhomocysteinemia during longterm, low dose methotrexate therapy for rheumatoid arthritis: implications for cardiovascular disease prevention. J. Rheumatol. 1998;25:441-446.

84. Morgan SL, Baggott JE, Vaughn WH, et al. Supplementation with folic acid during methotrexate therapy for rheumatoid arthritis. A double-blind, placebo-controlled trial. Ann. Intern. Med. 1994;121:833-841.

85. James GK, Jones MW, Pudek MR. Homocyst(e)ine levels in patients on phenytoin therapy. Clin. Biochem. 1997;30:647-649.

86. Ono H, Sakamoto A, Eguchi T, et al. Plasma total homocysteine concentrations in epileptic patients taking anticonvulsants. Metabolism 1997;46:959-962.

87. Carl GF, Hudson FZ, Mcguire BS. Phenytoin-induced depletion of folate in rats originates in liver and involves a mechanism that does not discriminate folate form. J. Nutr. 1997;127:2231-2238.

88. Blankenhorn DH, Malinow MR, Mack WJ. Colestipol plus niacin therapy elevates plasma homocyst(e)ine levels. Coron. Art. Dis. 1991;2:357-360.

89. Tonstad S, Refsum H, Ose L, Ueland PM. The C677T mutation in the methylenetetrahydrofolate reductase gene predisposes to hyperhomocysteinemia in children with familial hypercholesterolemia treated with cholestyramine. J. Pediatr. 1998;132:365-368.

90. Ermens AAM, Schoester M, Spijkers LJM, Lindemans J, Abels J. Toxicity of methotrexate in rats preexposed to nitrous oxide. Cancer Res. 1989;49:6337-6341.

91. Christensen B, Guttormsen AB, Schneede J, et al. Preoperative methionine-loading enhances restoration of the cobalamin-dependent enzyme methionine synthase after nitrous oxide anesthesia. Anesthesiology 1994;80:1046-1056.

92. Guttormsen AB, Refsum H, Ueland PM. The interaction between nitrous oxide and cobalamin. Biochemical effects and clinical consequences. Acta Anaesthesiol. Scand. 1994;38:753-756.

93. Landon MJ, Toothill VJ. Effect of nitrous oxide on placental methionine synthase activity. Br. J. Anaesth. 1986;58:524-527.

94. Frontiera MS, Stabler SP, Kolhouse JF, Allen RH. Regulation of methionine metabolism - effects of nitrous oxide and excess dietary methionine. J. Nutr. Biochem. 1994;5:28-38.

95. Koblin DD. Toxicity of nitrous oxide. In: Rice SA, Fish KJ, eds. Anesthetic Toxicity. New York: Raven Press, 1994:135-155.

96. Nicolaou A, Kenyon SH, Gibbons JM, Ast T, Gibbons WA. In vitro inactivation of mammalian methionine synthase by nitric oxide. Eur. J. Clin. Invest. 1996;26:167-170.

97. Brouwer M, Chamulitrat W, Ferruzzi G, Sauls DL, Weinberg JB. Nitric oxide interactions with cobalamins: biochemical and functional consequences. Blood 1996;88:1857-1864.

98. Nicolaou A, Waterfield CJ, Kenyon SH, Gibbons WA. The inactivation of methionine synthase in isolated rat hepatocytes by sodium nitroprusside. Eur. J. Biochem. 1997;15:876-882.

99. Coronato A, Glass GB. Depression of the intestinal uptake of radio-vitamin B 12 by cholestyramine. Proc Soc Exp Biol Med 1973;142:1341-4.

100. Force RW, Nahata MC. Effect of histamine H2-receptor antagonists on vitamin $B_{12}$ absorption. Ann Pharmacother 1992;26:1283-6.

101. Bellou A, Aimone-Gastin I, De Korwin JD, et al. Cobalamin deficiency with megaloblastic anemia in one patient under long-term omeprazole therapy. J Intern Med 1996;240:161-4.

102. Carlsen SM, Følling I, Grill V, Bjerve KS, Schneede J, Refsum H. Metformin increases total serum homocysteine levels in non-diabetic male patients with coronary heart disease. Scand J Clin Lab Invest 1997;57:521-7.

103. Hoogeveen EK, Kostense PJ, Jakobs C, Bouter LM, Heine RJ, Stehouwer CD. Does metformin increase the serum total homocysteine level in non- insulin-dependent diabetes mellitus? J Intern Med 1997;242:389-94.

104. Laine-Cessac P, Cailleux A, Allain P. Mechanisms of the inhibition of human erythrocyte pyridoxal kinase by drugs. Biochem. Pharmacol. 1997;54:863-870.

105. Drell W, Welch AD. Azaribine-homocystinemia-thrombosis in historical perspectives. Pharmac. Ther. 1989;41:195-206.

106. Krishnaswamy K. Isonicotinic acid hydrazide and pyridoxine deficiency. Int. J. Vitam. Nutr. Res. 1974;44:457-465.

107. Basu TK, Mann S. Vitamin B-6 normalizes the altered sulfur amino acid status of rats fed diets containing pharmacological levels of niacin without reducing niacin's hypolipidemic effects. J. Nutr. 1997;127:117-121.

108. Ueland PM. Pharmacological and biochemical aspects of S-adenosylhomocysteine and S-adenosylhomocysteine hydrolase. Pharmacol. Rev. 1982;34:223-253.

109. Kredich NM, Hershfield MS, Falletta JM, Kinney TR, Mitchell B, Koller C. Effects of 2'-deoxycoformycin on homocysteine metabolism in acute lymphoblastic leukemia. Clin. Res. 1981;29:541A.

110. Miller JW, Shukitt-Hale B, Villalobos-Molina R, Nadeau MR, Selhub J, Joseph JA. Effect of L-Dopa and the catechol-O-methyltransferase inhibitor Ro 41-0960 on sulfur amino acid metabolites in rats. Clin. Neuropharmacol. 1997:55-66.

111. Kang S-S, Wong PWK, Curley K. The effect of D-penicillamine on protein-bound homocyst(e)ine in homocystinurics. Pediatr. Res. 1982;16:370-372.

112. Kang S-S, Wong PWK, Glickman PB, MacLeod CM, Jaffe IA. Protein-bound homocyst(e)ine in patients with rheumatoid arthritis undergoing D-penicillamine treatment. J. Clin. Pharmacol. 1986;26:712-715.

113. Hultberg B, Andersson A, Masson P, Larson M, Tunek A. Plasma homocysteine and thiol compound fractions after oral administration of n-acetylcysteine. Scand. J. Clin. Lab. Invest. 1994;54:417-422.

114. Stofer-Vogel B, Cerny T, Küpfer A, Junker E, Lauterburg BH. Depletion of circulating cyst(e)ine by oral and intravenous mesna. Br. J. Cancer 1993;68:590-593.

115. Lauterburg BH, Nguyen T, Hartmann B, Junker E, Kupfer A, Cerny T. Depletion of total cysteine, glutathione, and homocysteine in plasma by ifosfamide/mesna therapy. Cancer Chemother. Pharmacol. 1994;35:132-136.

116. Wouters MGAJ, Moorrees MTEC, van der Mooren MJ, et al. Plasma homocysteine and menopausal status. Eur. J. Clin. Invest. 1995;25:801-805.

117. Brattström L, Israelsson B, Olsson A, Andersson A, Hultberg B. Plasma homocysteine in women on oral oestrogen-containing contraceptives and in men with oestrogen-treated prostatic carcinoma. Scand. J. Clin. Lab. Invest. 1992;52:283-287.

118. Steegers-Theunissen RPM, Boers GHJ, Steegers EAP, Trijbels FJM, Thomas CMG, Eskes TKAB. Effects of sub-50 oral contraceptives on homocysteine metabolism - A preliminary study. Contraception 1992;45:129-139.

119. Green TJ, Houghton LA, Donovan U, Gibson RS, O'Connor DL. Oral contraceptives did not affect biochemical folate indexes and homocysteine concentrations in adolescent females. J. Am. Diet. Assoc. 1998;98:49-55.

120. 120.van der Mooren MJ, Wouters MGAJ, Blom HJ, Schellekens LA, Eskes TKAB, Rolland R. Hormone replacement therapy may reduce high serum homocysteine in postmenopausal women. Eur. J. Clin. Invest. 1994;24:733-736.

121. van der Mooren MJ, Demacker PN, Blom HJ, de Rijke YB, Rolland R. The effect of sequential three-monthly hormone replacement therapy on several cardiovascular risk estimators in postmenopausal women. Fertil. Steril. 1997;67:67-73.

122. Mijatovic V, Kenemans P, Jakobs C, van Baal WM, Peters-Muller ER, van der Mooren MJ. A randomized controlled study of the effects of 17beta-estradiol-dydrogesterone on plasma homocysteine in postmenopausal women. Obstet. Gynecol. 1998;91:432-436.

123. Mijatovic V, Kenemans P, Netelenbos C, et al. Postmenopausal oral 17beta-estradiol continuously combined with dydrogesterone reduces fasting serum homocysteine levels. Fertil. Steril. 1998;69:876-882.

124. Giri S, Thompson PD, Taxel P, et al. Oral estrogen improves serum lipids, homocysteine and fibrinolysis in elderly men. Atherosclerosis 1998;137:359-366.

125. Zmuda JM, Bausserman LL, Maceroni D, Thompson PD. The effect of supraphysiologic doses of testosterone on fasting total homocysteine levels in normal men. Atherosclerosis 1997;130:199-202.

126. Giltay EJ, Hoogeveen EK, Elbers JMH, Gooren LJG, Asscheman H, Stehouwer CDA. Effects of sex steroids on plasma total homocysteine levels: a study in transsexual males and females. J. Clin. Endocrinol. Metab. 1998;83:550-553.

127. Steegers-Theunissen RPM, van Rossum JM, Steegers EAP, Thomas CMG, Eskes TKAB. Sub-50 oral contraceptives affect folate kinetics. Gynecol. Obstet. Invest. 1993;36:230-233.

128. Shojania AM. Oral contraceptives: Effects on folate and vitamin $B_{12}$ metabolism. Can. Med. Assoc. J. 1982;126:244-247.

129. Miller LT. Do oral contraceptive agents affect nutrient requirements--vitamin B-6. J Nutr. 1986;116:1344-1345.

130. Anker G, Lønning PE, Ueland PM, Refsum H, Lien EA. Plasma levels of the atherogenic amino acid homocysteine in post-menopausal women with breast cancer treated with tamoxifen. Int. J. Cancer 1995;60:365-368.

131. Cattaneo M, Baglietto L, Zighetti ML, et al. Tamoxifen reduces plasma homocysteine levels in healthy women. Br. J. Cancer 1998;77:2264-2266.
132. Anker GB, Refsum H, Ueland PM, Johannessen DC, Lien EA, Lønning PE. Influence of aromatase inhibitors on plasma total homocysteine levels in postmenopausal breast cancer patients. Clin. Chem. 1999;45:252-256.
133. Kishi T, Fujita N, Eguchi T, Ueda K. Mechanism for reduction of serum folate by antiepileptic drugs during prolonged therapy. J. Neurol. Sci. 1997;145:109-112.
134. Arnadottir M, Hultberg B, Vladov V, Nilsson-Ehle P, Thysell H. Hyperhomocysteinemia in cyclosporine-treated renal transplant recipients. Transplantation 1996;61:509-512.
135. Ducloux D, Fournier V, Rebibou JM, Bresson-Vautrin C, Gibey R, Chalopin JM. Hyperhomocyst(e)inemia in renal transplant recipients with and without cyclosporine. Clin. Nephrol. 1998;49:232-235.
136. Cole DEC, Ross HJ, Evrovski J, et al. Correlation between total homocysteine and cyclosporine concentrations in cardiac transplant recipients. Clin. Chem. 1998;44:2307-2312.
137. Arnadottir M, Hultberg B. Treatment with high-dose folic acid effectively lowers plasma homocysteine concentration in cyclosporine-treated renal transplant recipients. Transplantation 1997;64:1087.
138. Dudman NP, Wilcken DE, Wang J, Lynch JF, Macey D, Lundberg P. Disordered methionine/homocysteine metabolism in premature vascular disease. Its occurrence, cofactor therapy, and enzymology. Arterioscler. Thromb. 1993;13:1253-1260.
139. Franken DG, Boers GH, Blom HJ, Trijbels FJ, Kloppenborg PW. Treatment of mild hyperhomocysteinemia in vascular disease patients. Arterioscler. Thromb. 1994;14:465-470.
140. van den Berg M, Franken DG, Boers GH, et al. Combined vitamin B$_6$ plus folic acid therapy in young patients with arteriosclerosis and hyperhomocysteinemia. J. Vasc. Surg. 1994;20:933-940.
141. Bostom AG, Shemin D, Nadeau MR, et al. Short term betaine therapy fails to lower elevated fasting total plasma homocysteine concentrations in hemodialysis patients maintained on chronic folic acid supplementation. Atherosclerosis 1995;113:129-132.
142. Dennis VW, Robinson K. Homocysteinemia and vascular disease in end-stage renal disease. Kidney Int. 1996;50:S11-S17.
143. Bostom AG, Lathrop L. Hyperhomocysteinemia in end-stage renal disease (ESRD): Prevalence, etiology, and potential relationship to arteriosclerotic outcomes. Kidney Int. 1997;52:10-20.
144. Christensen B, Refsum H, Vintermyr O, Ueland PM. Homocysteine export from cells cultured in the presence of physiological or superfluous levels of methionine: Methionine loading of non-transformed, transformed, proliferating and quiescent cells in culture. J. Cell. Physiol. 1991;146:52-62.
145. Roubenoff R, Dellaripa P, Nadeau MR, et al. Abnormal homocysteine metabolism in rheumatoid arthritis. Arthritis. Rheum. 1997;40:718-722.
146. Pettersson T, Friman C, Abrahamsson L, Nilsson B, Norberg B. Serum homocysteine and methylmalonic acid in patients with rheumatoid arthritis and cobalaminopenia. J. Rheumatol. 1998;25:859-863.

147. Hultberg B, Agardh E, Andersson A, et al. Increased levels of plasma homocysteine are associated with nephropathy but not severe retinopathy in type 1 diabetes mellitus. Scand. J. Lab. Clin. Invest. 1991;51:277-282.

148. Agardh CD, Agardh E, Andersson A, Hultberg B. Lack of association between plasma homocysteine levels and microangiopathy in type 1 diabetes mellitus. Scand. J. Clin. Lab. Invest. 1994;54:637-641.

149. Chico A, Perez A, Cordoba A, et al. Plasma homocysteine is related to albumin excretion rate in patients with diabetes mellitus: a new link between diabetic nephropathy and cardiovascular disease? Diabetologia 1998;41:684-693.

150. Hultberg B, Agardh CD, Agardh E, Lovestamadrian M. Poor metabolic control, early age at onset, and marginal folate deficiency are associated with increasing levels of plasma homocysteine in insulin-dependent diabetes mellitus. a five-year follow-up study. Scand. J. Clin. Lab. Inves.t 1997;57:595-600.

151. Araki A, Sako Y, Ito H. Plasma homocysteine concentrations in Japanese patients with non-insulin-dependent diabetes mellitus: effect of parenteral methylcobalamin treatment. Atherosclerosis 1993;103:149-157.

152. Hofmann MA, Kohl B, Zumbach MS, et al. Hyperhomocyst(e)inemia and endothelial dysfunction in IDDM. Diabetes Care 1998;21:841-848.

153. Hoogeveen EK, Kostense PJ, Beks PJ, et al. Hyperhomocysteinemia is associated with an increased risk of cardiovascular disease, especially in non-insulin-dependent diabetes mellitus - a population-based study. Arterioscler. Thromb. Vasc. Biol. 1998;18:133-138.

154. Munshi MN, Stone A, Fink L, Fonseca V. Hyperhomocysteinemia following a methionine load in patients with non-insulin-dependent diabetes mellitus and macrovascular disease. Metabolism 1996;45:133-135.

155. Vaccaro O, Ingrosso D, Rivellese A, Greco G, Riccardi G. Moderate hyperhomocysteinemia and retinopathy in insulin-dependent diabetes. Lancet 1997;349:1102-1103.

156. Neugebauer S, Baba T, Kurokawa K, Wantanabe T. Defective homocysteine metabolism as a risk factor for diabetic retinopathy. Lancet 1997;349:473-474.

157. Lanfredini M, Fiorina P, Peca MG, et al. Fasting and post-methionine load homocyst(e)ine values are correlated with microalbuminuria and could contribute to worsening vascular damage in non-insulin-dependent diabetes mellitus patients. Metabolism 1998;47:915-921.

158. Hoogeveen EK, Kostense PJ, Jager A, et al. Serum homocysteine level and protein intake are related to risk of microalbuminuria: the Hoorn Study. Kidney Int. 1998;54:203-209.

159. Robillon JF, Canivet B, Candito M, et al. Type 1 diabetes mellitus and homocyst(e)ine. Diabete Metab. 1994;20:494-496.

160. Bar-On H, Kidron M, Friedlander Y, et al. Plasma total homocysteine in subjects with hyperinsulinemia. J. Intern. Med. 1998:in press.

161. Giltay EJ, Hoogeveen EK, Elbers JM, Gooren LJ, Asscheman H, Stehouwer CD. Insulin resistance is associated with elevated plasma total homocysteine levels in healthy, non-obese subjects. Atherosclerosis 1998;139:197-8.

162. Fonseca VA, Mudaliar S, Schmidt B, Fink LM, Kern PA, Henry RR. Plasma homocysteine concentrations are regulated by acute hyperinsulinemia in nondiabetic but not type 2 diabetic subjects. Metabolism 1998;47:686-689.

163. Nedrebø B, Ericsson UB, Nygård O, et al. Plasma total homocysteine in hyperthyroid and hypothyroid patients. Metabolism 1998;47:89-93.

164. Cimino JA, Jhangiani S, Schwartz E, Cooperman JM. Riboflavin metabolism in the hypothyroid human adult. Proc Soc Exp Biol Med 1987;184:151-3.

165. Ambrosi P, Barlatier A, Habib G, et al. Hyperhomocysteinemia in heart transplant recipients. Eur. Heart. J. 1994;15:1191-1195.

166. Berger PB, Jones JD, Olson LJ, et al. Increase in total plasma homocysteine concentration after cardiac transplantation. Mayo Clin. Proc. 1995;70:125-131.

167. Gupta A, Moustapha A, Jacobsen DW, et al. High homocysteine, low folate, and low vitamin B-6 concentrations - prevalent risk factors for vascular disease in heart transplant recipients. Transplantation 1998;65:544-550.

168. Ambrosi P, Garcon D, Riberi A, et al. Association of mild hyperhomocysteinemia with cardiac graft vascular disease. Atherosclerosis 1998;138:347-50.

169. Nahlawi M, Naso A, Boparai N, et al. Low vitamin $B_6$: An independent predictor of cardiovascular morbidity and mortality in heart transplant patients. Circulation 1998;abstract:in press.

170. Landgren F, Israelsson B, Lindgren A, Hultberg B, Andersson A, Brattström L. Plasma homocysteine in acute myocardial infarction: homocysteine-lowering effect of folic acid. J. Intern. Med. 1995;237:381-388.

171. Egerton W, Silberberg J, Crooks R, Ray C, Xie LJ, Dudman N. Serial measures of plasma homocyst(e)ine after acute myocardial infarction. Am. J. Cardiol. 1996;77:759-761.

172. Lindgren A, Brattström L, Norrving B, Hultberg B, Andersson A, Johansson BB. Plasma homocysteine in the acute and convalescent phases after stroke. Stroke 1995;26:795-800.

173. Wollesen F, Brattström L, Refsum H, Ueland PM, Berglund L, Berne C. Plasma total homocysteine and cysteine in relation to glomerular filtration rate in diabetes mellitus.Kidney Int. 1999;55:1028-1035.

# 6. EPIDEMIOLOGY OF HOMOCYSTEINE LEVELS AND RELATION TO VITAMINS

PETER W. F. WILSON AND PAUL F. JACQUES

## SUMMARY

The epidemiology of homocysteine levels is explored from the experience of large scale population-based samples. Higher levels in adults have been associated consistently with lower levels of the B group vitamins–folate, vitamin B6 and vitamin $B_{12}$. The most consistent associations have been described for lower folate intake and lower folate levels in the blood, and approximately 20-30 percent of the adult U.S. population may be affected. Fortification of the U.S. food supply, originally announced in 1996, promises to lead to greater intakes of folate and a reduced prevalence of elevated homocysteine levels in the adult population. Fortified cold cereals, multivitamins and orange juice are important sources of folate intake in men and women and appear to account for approximately 40 percent of folate consumed.

## INTRODUCTION

Since the late 1960s a marked increase of homocysteine in the blood and urine have been known to be associated with a dramatic increase in risk of arterial and venous disease (1), but more recent research has demonstrated that moderate elevations in homocysteine concentrations are associated with a moderately increased risk of atherosclerotic disease (2). This chapter will focus on the nutritional determinants of homocysteine concentrations in free-living

85

*K. Robinson (ed.), Homocysteine and Vascular Disease, 85-95.*
© 2000 *Kluwer Academic Publishers. Printed in the Netherlands.*

*Table 1. Mean Homocysteine Levels in Framingham Cohort Participants*

| | Age | n | Mean Homocysteine (μmol/L) | Homocysteine >14 μmol/L (percent) |
|---|---|---|---|---|
| Men | | | | |
| | 65-74 | 239 | 11.8 | 25.3 |
| | 75-79 | 110 | 11.9 | 26.7 |
| | 80+ | 108 | 14.1 | 48.3 |
| P (for trend by age) | | | <0.001 | <0.001 |
| Women | | | | |
| | 65-74 | 310 | 10.7 | 19.5 |
| | 75-79 | 204 | 11.9 | 28.9 |
| | 80+ | 189 | 13.2 | 41.4 |
| P(for trend by age) | | | <0.001 | <0.001 |
| P (sex) | | | 0.003 | 0.09 |

populations, emphasizing the experience of cross-sectional community and national surveys that have been conducted recently.

The role of folate and vitamin $B_{12}$ in homocysteine metabolism is well-established, and numerous trials have shown that intervention with folate and vitamin $B_{12}$ can lower homocysteine concentrations in patients with elevated homocysteine concentrations. However, less is known regarding the prevalence of inadequate folate and vitamin $B_{12}$ levels, and the importance of these nutrients in elevated homocysteine concentrations, at the population level.

Population-based information concerning homocysteine concentrations, as well as various B vitamins that are associated with homocysteine metabolism are especially helpful in the assessment of public health strategies. The clinician is primarily interested in the sick patient, an individual with an extremely elevated concentration of a risk factor such as blood cholesterol, arterial blood pressure, or homocysteine concentration. On the other hand, the epidemiological perspective considers the overall distribution of a risk factor in the population. Such an approach may suggest public health strategies that might shift the entire distribution of a factor.

This chapter will consider the population assessment of blood homocysteine concentrations and demonstrate the importance of vitamin intake and levels as risk factors for elevated homocysteine concentrations in populations. Data derived from a variety of recently conducted surveys will focus on specimens obtained casually or in the fasting state, without consideration of methionine load, to characterize homocysteine and vitamin status.

## DETERMINANTS OF HOMOCYSTEINE CONCENTRATIONS

Age and sex are two of the stronger determinants of fasting homocysteine concentrations, which are higher in the elderly and greater in men than in women (3,4). Homocysteine concentrations, as well as levels of vitamin $B_{12}$, folate, and pyridoxal-5'-phosphate (the active circulating form of vitamin $B_6$), were measured from casually obtained blood samples collected as part of the regular Framingham Heart Study visit for the study's original cohort in the late 1980's. Samples were available for approximately one thousand adult men and women age 67 and older (mean age 75 y). In these Framingham participants, the levels of homocysteine were positively correlated with age in both sexes (table 1). The mean homocysteine levels in men 67-74, 75-79, and 80+ years were 11.8, 11.9, and 14.1 μmol/L respectively. Mean homocysteine levels at each of these age groups were about 1 μmol/L lower in the female participants. The prevalence of elevated homocysteine (>14 μmol/L) a level typically observed in persons who had experienced a coronary attack in other studies, increased with age in both sexes (3).

The first data on homocysteine concentrations in a nationally representative sample of 8,585 Americans from the third National Health and Nutrition Examination Survey confirm the age and sex differences previously reported in non-representative population samples. The age-adjusted geometric mean total serum homocysteine concentrations were 9.6 and 7.9 μmol/L in non-Hispanic white males and females, 9.8 and 8.2 μmol/L in non-Hispanic black males and females, and 9.4 and 7.4 μmol/L in Mexican American males and females, respectively. The age-adjusted geometric mean total homocysteine concentrations were significantly lower in females than in males in each race-ethnicity group. There was also a significant age-sex interaction reflecting the fact that homocysteine concentrations in females tended to diverge from those in males at younger ages and converge with those in males at older ages (5).

Investigators have shown consistently that plasma homocysteine levels are inversely correlated with vitamin intake (6,7). Vitamins $B_1$, $B_2$, $B_6$, $B_{12}$, folate,

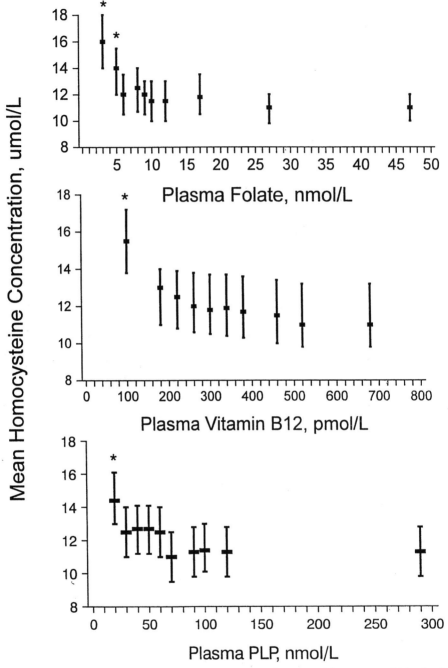

*Figure 1: Mean plasma homocysteine concentrations (and 95% confidence intervals) by deciles of plasma folate (top), vitamin B$_{12}$ (center), and pyridoxal-5'-phosphate (PLP) (bottom) concentrations. Means are adjusted for age, sex, and other plasma vitamins. Asterisk indicates significantly different from mean in highest decile (P<0.01). From Selhub(3)*

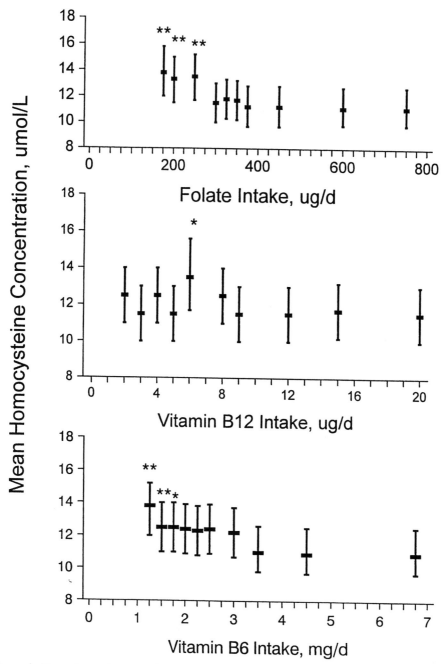

Figure 2: Mean plasma homocysteine concentrations (and 95% confidence intervals) by deciles of intake of folate (top), vitamin $B_{12}$ (center), and pyridoxal-5'-phosphate (PLP) (bottom) concentrations. Means are adjusted for age, sex, and other plasma vitamins. Asterisk indicates significantly different from mean in highest decile (P<0.05); and double asterisk, significantly different from mean in the highest decile (P<.01). From Selhub(3)

Table 2. Elevated Homocysteine Concentrations by B Vitamin Status and Intake

| B Vitamin Index* | n | Mean Homocysteine μmol/L | Prevalence (percent) | Prevalence Rate Ratio | Pop. Attributable Percent |
|---|---|---|---|---|---|
| Plasma levels | | | | | |
| Highest 1 | 89 | 9.4 | 10.1 | 1 | 0 |
| 2 | 128 | 9.8 | 12.5 | 1.2 | 1.0 |
| 3 | 534 | 11.9‡ | 28.7‡ | 2.8 | 33.7 |
| 4 | 144 | 14.9‡ | 52.1‡ | 5.2 | 20.6 |
| Lowest 5 | 70 | 16.5‡ | 58.6‡ | 5.8 | 11.6 |
| | | | | | **66.9** (total) |
| Dietary Intake | | | | | |
| Highest 1 | 138 | 9.5 | 9.4 | 1 | 0 |
| 2 | 128 | 10.4 | 15.6 | 1.7 | 3.4 |
| 3 | 369 | 11.7‡ | 25.5‡ | 2.7 | 25.6 |
| 4 | 155 | 13.0‡ | 35.5‡ | 3.8 | 17.4 |
| Lowest 5 | 94 | 14.8‡ | 53.2‡ | 5.7 | 17.7 |
| | | | | | **64.1** (total) |

*1 (highest) indicates three B vitamins >70th percentile; 2, all vitamins >50th, at least 1 <70th percentile; 3, vitamins both >50th and <50 percentile; 4, all vitamins <50th percentile, at least 1 >30th percentile; and 5 (lowest), al three vitamins < 30th percentile
‡ Significantly different from category 1 (P<0.01)

niacin, retinol, vitamin C, and vitamin E have all been studied, but the greatest interest has been shown for the vitamins that have been closely linked to homocysteine metabolic pathways. Such studies were undertaken in Framingham, where the mean levels of plasma homocysteine in the Framingham cohort survey were analyzed according to deciles of plasma folate, vitamin $B_{12}$, and pyridoxal phosphate concentrations (figure 1), as well as the corresponding nutrient intakes of folate, vitamin $B_{12}$ and vitamin $B_6$ estimated using the Willett food frequency questionnaire (figure 2). The plots show the mean concentrations and their 95% confidence intervals by deciles of the plasma levels, with adjustment for age, sex, and other plasma vitamins. For the plasma measures, the two lowest deciles of folate, the lowest decile of vitamin $B_{12}$ and the lowest decile of pyridoxal phosphate were associated with a different mean level of homocysteine relative to the highest decile of the vitamin intake. Similarly, the nutrient analyses showed the lowest three deciles of folate intake, the fifth decile of vitamin $B_{12}$ intake and the lowest two deciles of vitamin $B_6$ intake were associated with differences in mean homocysteine concentrations. It is interesting to point out that the estimated mean folate intake for approximately 50,000 members of the Boston Area Health Professionals study cohort was 451 µg/d (total) and 334 µg/d among persons not taking any folate supplements (6). These folate intakes were estimated by methods similar to what was used in Framingham and suggest that some segments of the population, such as health professionals consume greater amounts of folate than general population samples, such as Framingham participants. Homocysteine concentrations were elevated among participants who consumed up to 280 µg/day of folate, a level lower than the recently updated United States recommended dietary allowance (RDA) of 400 µg/day for adult men and women, and vitamin $B_6$ intakes as high as 1.92 mg/day, a level higher than the RDA of 1.7 and 1.5 mg/day for older men and women, respectively.

The Framingham analyses demonstrated on a population basis that lower levels of vitamin B intake or plasma vitamin B levels could contribute to elevated homocysteine concentrations and a plasma vitamin index was used as a composite measure of folate, $B_{12}$ and $B_6$ status to test for associations with elevated homocysteine concentrations (table 2). In comparisons with persons who had relatively high intake for all three vitamins, the relative odds for an increased homocysteine level was associated with lesser amounts of vitamin intake. The analyses yielded similar results and conclusions when composite measures of blood vitamin levels were considered, and it was concluded that not only was suboptimal vitamin status, assessed by dietary intake or blood levels, relatively common, but also suboptimal vitamin status was independently associated with elevated homocysteine in approximately two-thirds of the persons with homocysteine >14 µmol/L (table 2).

*Table 3. Major contributors to folate intake in the Framingham Heart Study cohort men and women aged 67-95 years*

| Both sexes (rank) | Source | Percent contribution (%) | Men (rank) | Women (rank) |
|---|---|---|---|---|
| 1 | Cold cereal | 13.3 | 1 | 2 |
| 2 | Multivitamins | 12.8 | 3 | 1 |
| 3 | Orange juice | 12.4 | 2 | 3 |
| 4 | Pizza | 3.3 | 4 | 5 |
| 5 | Iceberg lettuce | 3.2 | 7 | 4 |
| 6 | Spinach, cooked | 2.8 | 6 | 6 |
| 7 | White bread | 2.6 | 5 | 10 |
| 8 | Bananas | 2.6 | 8 | 7 |
| 9 | Romaine/leaf lettuce | 2.4 | 9 | 9 |
| 10 | Oranges | 2.3 | 13 | 8 |
| Cumulative | | 88 | | |

Lower folate levels and lower estimated folate intake were felt to be most consistently associated with higher homocysteine levels in the Framingham cohort population survey and follow-up analyses investigated the specific food groups that contributed to folate intake, as shown in table 3 (8). Individuals who regularly took vitamin supplements, ate breakfast cereals or consumed green, leafy vegetables had higher plasma folate and lower homocysteine levels than non-users in this elderly population sample. The strong positive association between cereal consumption and plasma folate levels was thought to be due to folic acid fortification of cereal products, and the relation plateaued near 5 to 6 servings per week of cereal. Interestingly, orange juice consumption was strongly associated with overall folate consumption but not significantly related to homocysteine concentrations. Overall intake of fruit and vegetable intake was highly associated with higher plasma folate levels and lower homocysteine concentrations, and this summary measure was significantly associated with more favorable vitamin and homocysteine levels. Approximately a quarter of this population sample consumed vitamin supplements and these participants had the lowest homocysteine levels.

Complementary population sample data from the Hordaland Homocysteine Study showed that higher homocysteine levels were associated with male sex, age, folate intake, smoking, and coffee intake in a multivariate analysis that included information from more than 11,000 middle aged Norwegians (9). As in the Framingham Study data the folate intake was estimated from the use of vitamin supplements as well as dietary sources, and fruit, vegetables, oranges, juices, eggs and meat were important food elements that contributed to overall folate intake. The Hordaland investigators also reported a significant association between cobalamin intake, but this nutrient was not associated with homocysteine levels in the multivariate analyses (9).

Dietary intake of folate and its plasma levels are highly correlated (10). Inadequate consumption of folate-rich foods is primarily responsible for low folate status at the population level, and an important cause of higher homocysteine concentrations (3). In contrast, low vitamin $B_{12}$ status is commonly associated with gastrointestinal conditions. Inadequate production of intrinsic factor in the stomach can result in a severe vitamin $B_{12}$ deficiency with substantially elevated homocysteine concentrations. However, this is an infrequent cause of low vitamin $B_{12}$ status and inadequate intrinsic factor was present in only 1 of 67 vitamin $B_{12}$-deficient Framingham participants (11). Hypochlorhydria and achlorhydria are much more common than inadequate intrinsic factor, especially in older individuals, and can lead to impaired absorption of found-found vitamin $B_{12}$ because low pH is needed to dissociate vitamin $B_{12}$ from food. The prevalence of hyposecretion of acid associated with atrophic gastritis ranges from approximately 10% (12) up to 30% (13) for individuals 60 years of age and older. Approximately 15% of the elderly Framingham population had low blood levels of vitamin $B_{12}$ and high methylmalonic acid or homocysteine concentrations, indicating vitamin $B_{12}$ deficiency (11).

These studies of nutrient intake and surveys of the association of homocysteine levels with vascular disease led to the conclusion that increasing folate intake in the population at large would benefit homocysteine levels and reduce vascular disease incidence. Nutritional education, supplements, and food fortification of cereal and flour products were all thought to be possible and the experience of observational studies of coronary heart disease, homocysteine, and nutrient status were used to predict the potential impact (14). Inadequate folate intake in the early stages of pregnancy was shown to be associated with fetal abnormalities such as spina bifida and anencephaly, and in 1996 the Food and Drug Administration mandated fortification of American flour and cereal products on or before January 1, 1998. Framingham intake data were used to model the population impact of various fortification levels, as seen in figure 3. It was estimated from these extrapolations that the fraction of persons with a dietary folate intake less than 200 µg/day would decline from 18 percent to 8 percent and that the prevalence of homocysteine levels > 14 µmol/L would decrease from 26 percent to 22 percent of the population (10). Investigations currently underway will test for the actual changes associated with folate fortification in recent years, drawing on survey information obtained from the second generation Framingham Offspring concerning dietary folate, plasma folate, and plasma homocysteine.

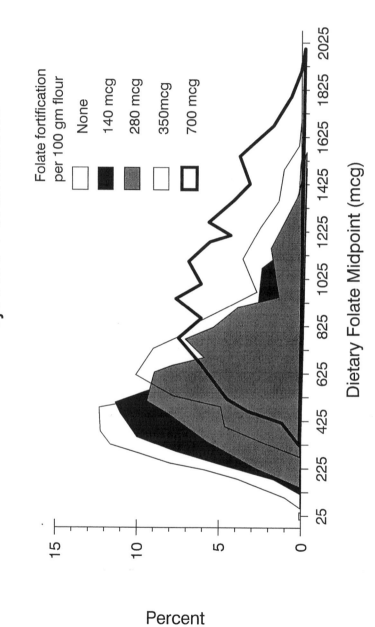

*Figure 3: Distribution of Folate intake in Framingham cohort and estimates of the distributions after projected fortification of flour with varying amounts of folate. After Tucker 1996.(10)*

## REFERENCE LIST

1.  McCully KS. Vascular pathology of homocysteinemia: implications for the pathogenesis of arteriosclerosis. Am.J.Pathol. 1969;56(1):111-28.
2.  Genest JJ, Jr., Malinow MR. Homocyst(e)ine and coronary artery disease. Curr Opinion Lipid 1992;3:295-9.
3.  Selhub J, Jacques PF, Wilson PWF, Rush D, Rosenberg IH. Vitamin status and intake as primary determinants of homocysteinemia in the elderly. JAMA 1993;270:2693-8.
4.  Selhub J, Jacques PF, Bostom AG, D'Agostino RB, Wilson PWF, Belanger AJ, O'Leary DH, Wolf PA, Schaefer EJ, Rosenberg IH. Association between plasma homocysteine and extracranial carotid stenosis. N Engl J Med 1995;332:286-91.
5.  Jacques, P. F., Rosenberg, I. H., Rogers, G., Selhub, J., Bowman, B. A., Gunter, E. W., Wright, J. D., and Johnson, C. L. Serum total homocysteine concentrations in adolescent and adult Americans: results from the third National Health and Nutrition Examination Survey (NHANES III). Am J Clin Nutr. 1999;69:482-89.
6.  Rimm EB, Giovannucci EL, Stampfer MJ, Colditz GA, Litin LB, Willett WC. Reproducibility and validity of an expanded self-administered semiquantitative food frequency questionnaire among male health professionals. Am.J.Epidemiol. 1992;135:1114-26
7.  Stampfer MJ, Malinow MR, Willett WC, Newcomer LM, Upson B, Ullmann D, Tishler PV, Hennekens CH. A prospective study of plasma homocyst(e)ine and risk of myocardial infarction in US Physicians. JAMA 1992;268:877-81.
8.  Tucker KL, Selhub J, Wilson PW, Rosenberg IH. Dietary intake pattern relates to plasma folate and homocysteine concentrations in the Framingham Heart Study. J.Nutr. 1996;126:3025-31.
9.  Nygard O, Refsum H, Ueland PM, Vollset SE. Major lifestyle determinants of plasma total homocysteine distribution: the Hordaland Homocysteine Study [see comments]. Am.J.Clin.Nutr. 1998;67:263-70.
10. Tucker KL, Mahnken B, Wilson PW, Jacques P, Selhub J. Folic acid fortification of the food supply. Potential benefits and risks for the elderly population. JAMA 1996;276:1879-85.
11. Lindenbaum J, Rosenberg IH, Wilson PWF, Saha JR, Stabler SP, Allen RH. Prevalence of cobalamin deficiency in the Framingham elderly population. Amer.J.Clin.Nutr. 1994;20:2-11.
12. Hurwitz A, Brady DA, Schaal SE, Samloff IM, Dedon J, Ruhl CE. Gastric acidity in older adults. JAMA 1997;278:659-62.
13. Krasinski SD, Russell RM, Samloff IM, Jacob RA, Dallal GE, McGandy RB, Hartz SC. Fundic atrophic gastritis in an elderly population. Effect on hemoglobin and several serum nutritional indicators. J Am Geriatr.Soc. 1986;34:800-6.
14. Boushey CJ, Beresford SAS, Omenn GS, Motulsky AG. A quantitative assessment of plasma homocysteine as a risk factor for vascular disease: Probable benefits of increasing folic acid intakes. JAMA 1995;274:1049-57.

# 7. VASCULAR PATHOLOGY OF HYPERHOMOCYSTEINEMIA

KILMER S. M$^C$CULLY

## SUMMARY

The first descriptions of vascular pathology in patients with hyper-homocysteinemia caused by cystathionine synthase deficiency emphasized the prominent thrombosis occurring in arteries and veins to major organs. Rediscovery of the index case of this disease, as first published in 1933, called attention to the similarities of the arterial pathology associated with hyperhomocysteinemia and arteriosclerosis of the elderly as it occurs in the general population. Discovery of rapidly progressive arteriosclerosis in the index case of cobalamin C disease, caused by methionine synthase deficiency, led to the conclusion that hyperhomocysteinemia causes arteriosclerosis by a direct effect of homocysteine derivatives on the cells and tissues of the arteries. The finding of essentially identical arteriosclerotic plaques in a patient with a third type of hyperhomocysteinemia, caused by methylenetetrahydrofolate reductase deficiency, confirmed the association between arteriosclerosis and hyperhomocysteinemia, regardless of which particular inherited enzyme abnormality causes the elevation of blood homocysteine levels. The vascular pathology associated with moderate hyperhomocysteinemia in subjects with dietary deficiencies of vitamin $B_6$, folic acid, or vitamin $B_{12}$ is essentially identical with arteriosclerosis as it occurs in the general population. The development of atherosclerotic plaques is related to the effects of homocysteine on aggregation of lipoprotein particles, intimal damage, hyperplasia of smooth muscle cells, formation of sulfate extracellular matrix,

K. Robinson (ed.), Homocysteine and Vascular Disease, 97-116.

calcification, degeneration of elastic fibers, effects on platelets and blood coagulation factors, and deposition of cholesterol and lipids in developing atheromas.

## VASCULAR PATHOLOGY IN CYSTATHIONINE SYNTHASE DEFICIENCY

Following the discovery of homocystinuria in mentally retarded children in 1962, the first detailed description of the vascular pathology of this disease emphasizes the possible relation to Marfan's syndrome (1). In this first published autopsy of a case of homocystinuria in a 7-year-old boy, the aorta is focally dilated with areas of intimal fibrosis and occlusion by adherent mural thrombus in the distal aorta extending into the iliac arteries. The walls of the major branches of aorta are thickened by fibrous tissue, and a fusiform aneurysm involves the superior mesenteric artery. One renal artery is occluded by a mixed thrombus. The histology reveals fibrous intimal pads associated with metachromatic extracellular matrix, splitting and fragmentation of elastica interna, and deposition of collagen fibers. In the common iliac arteries, concentric intimal fibrosis is associated with "fatty atheromatous plaques." In the aorta deposits of metachromatic matrix lie between elastic lamellae, and ridges of concentric intimal fibrous tissue contain cellular fibrous tissue thickly interspersed with elastic fibers. Pulmonary artery contains deposits of metachromatic matrix between elastic fibers of media. In a nephrectomy specimen from another case of homocystinuria in a 15-year-old boy, fibrous intimal pads with splitting of elastic fibers and deposition of metachromatic matrix are demonstrated. In a second autopsied case of homocystinuria in a 9-year-old girl, similar pathological findings are demonstrated in the arteries, and a recent organizing thrombus is found in the dural sinuses (2).

Another major series of 38 patients with homocystinuria reports fatal coronary occlusion in a 20-year-old woman with angina and previous myocardial infarction, non-fatal myocardial infarction in a 31-year-old woman, death from presumed coronary occlusion in an 18-year-old boy, and death from bilateral thrombosis of carotid arteries in a 12-year-old girl (3). Other patients exhibit thrombosis in the terminal aorta, iliac and subclavian arteries with loss of pulses and ischemic symptoms. Renal artery narrowing with renal atrophy is demonstrated in an 18-year-old with hypertension. An 8-year-old boy with a history of stroke is pulseless because of recurrent arterial thromboses. Recurrent thrombophlebitis of the extremities with pulmonary embolism occurred in several cases, and a 28-year-old man died of portal vein thrombosis. Intracranial thromboses, both venous and arterial, led to death in a 3-year-old child. The vascular pathology in many of these cases demonstrates concentric fibroelastic intimal rings severely narrowing the lumen, associated with thinning of the media. Sections of carotid artery demonstrate recent thrombosis, eccentric fibrous plaques, and reduplicated elastic lamellae, suggesting recurrent episodes of thrombosis. Autopsy findings in an additional case of homocystinuria in an 11-year-old girl reveal similar vascular pathology (4). The discussion of these cases attributes the frequent thromboses to changes in the walls of the blood vessels.

In these initial descriptive reports of the clinical and pathological findings in homocystinuria (1-4), there was no attempt to relate the vascular pathology to arteriosclerosis as found in the general population. Although the prominent episodes of both arterial and venous thrombosis implies a relation to arteriosclerotic vascular disease, the description of fibrous intimal thickening is compared to the vascular changes in Marfan's syndrome. In that condition, the vascular pathology of the aorta consists of cystic medial necrosis, dilation and dissecting aneurysm, changes which are not found in homocystinuria. Moreover, venous and arterial thromboses are not characteristic of Marfan's syndrome. In the discussion of the pathogenesis of the vascular pathology, a lathyrogenic effect of homocysteine is considered as a possible explanation of the origin of the pathological changes in arteries and connective tissues (1). However, it was not clear from these early studies whether excess homocysteine or methionine or deficiencies of cystathionine or other sulfur amino acid metabolites might be of pathogenic significance (2,3). In some patients abnormal adhesiveness of platelets is related to increased tendency to thrombosis (1).

The possible relation of homocystinuria to arteriosclerosis was clarified in 1965, when a case published in 1933 (5) was identified retrospectively by discovery of homocystinuria in a living relative (6). The index case from 1933 was an 8-year-old boy who died of thrombotic occlusion of a carotid artery and a cerebral infarct. In the discussion of the pathological findings, the pathologist suggested that the sclerotic changes in carotid arteries are similar to the changes of arteriosclerosis typically found in the elderly. Re-examination of this case of homocystinuria from 1933 revealed fibrous arteriosclerotic plaques in arteries in multiple organs, as well as carotid arteriosclerosis and thrombosis (7). These observations suggest that the vascular pathology in hyperhomocysteinemia caused by cystathionine synthase deficiency bears a relationship to the pathogenesis of arteriosclerosis as it occurs in the general population.

The typical vascular pathology in homocystinuria caused by deficiency of cystathionine synthase consists of fibrous arteriosclerotic plaques causing narrowing of the lumen (Fig 1,2). These plaques are formed by hyperplasia of smooth muscle cells, deposition of collagen fibers and extracellular matrix, associated with fragmentation, splitting, and degeneration of elastica interna

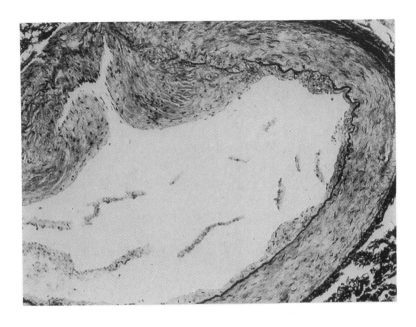

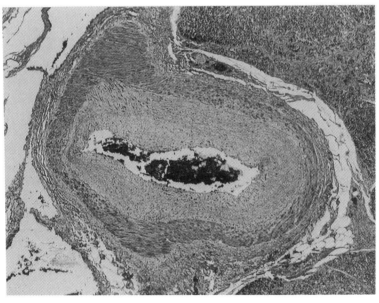

*Figure 1. Artery of pancreas is narrowed by concentric fibrous intimal plaques in cystathionine synthase deficiency. H&E x36.*

*Figure 2. Artery of heart is narrowed by eccentric fibrous intimal plaques in cystathionine synthase deficiency. Elastin x200.*

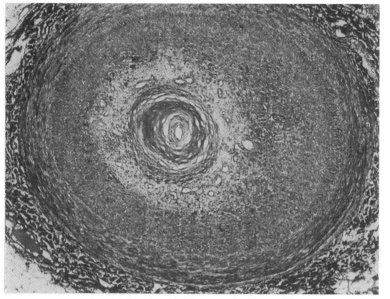

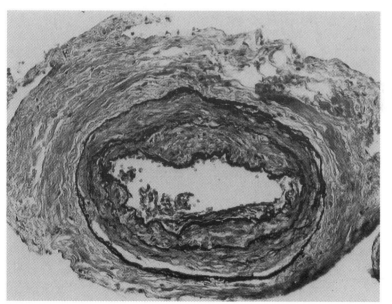

*Figure 3. Branch of carotid artery is narrowed by fibrous intimal plaque containing degenerative elastica interna in cystathionine synthase deficiency. Elastin X150.*

*Figure 4. Coronary artery is occluded by concentric fibrous intimal plaques in cystathionine synthase deficiency. Trichrome x36.*

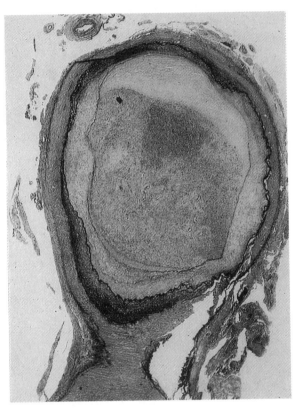

*Figure 5. Carotid artery is occluded by fibrous intimal plaques, degenerative elastica interna and organizing thrombus in cystathionine synthase deficiency. Elastin x15.*

(Fig. 3). Some arteries are severely narrowed by concentric layers of fibrous connective tissue (Fig. 4). In many cases the arteriosclerotic plaques are asso ciated with intravascular thrombosis, causing complete occlusion of the lumen by acute or organizing thrombi (Fig. 5). Deposition of cholesterol and lipids in these plaques is only occasionally observed, particularly in children. However, typical aortic aneurysm with pathological features of atherosclerosis is observed in adults with homocystinuria (8). Venous thrombosis, thrombophlebitis, and pulmonary embolism are observed in many cases of homocystinuria. Thrombosis of cerebral dural sinuses, renal vein, portal vein or other major veins are observed in some cases. In summary, the vascular pathology of hyperhomocysteinemia caused by deficiency of cystathionine synthase consists of fibrous arteriosclerotic plaques with little lipid deposition, associated with severe narrowing and thrombotic occlusions of aorta, major muscular arteries and arterioles in organs throughout the body.

## DISCOVERY OF ACCELERATED ARTERIOSCLEROSIS IN METHIONINE SYNTHASE DEFICIENCY

The index case of cobalamin C disease, caused by deficiency of methyltetrahydrofolate-homocysteine methyltransferase (methionine synthase), was described in a 2-month-old boy with growth failure and aspiration pneumonia (9). This infant was found to excrete homocystine, cystathionine and methylmalonic acid in his urine, attributed to deficiency of methionine synthase. In contrast to cases of hyperhomocysteinemia caused by deficiency of cystathionine synthase, the plasma concentration of cystathionine was elevated in this child, and the concentration of methionine was decreased rather than elevated. In addition, methylmalonic acid was highly elevated in plasma, a finding not encountered in cystathionine synthase deficiency.

The autopsy findings in the index case of methionine synthase deficiency revealed rapidly progressive arteriosclerotic plaques involving arteries and arterioles in multiple organs (7). This observation is critical because arteriosclerosis could be related directly to hyperhomocysteinemia, regardless of the enzyme deficiency which caused it, leading to the conclusion that homocysteine causes arteriosclerotic plaques by a direct effect of the amino acid on the cells and tissues of the arteries. The observation of differing concentrations of methionine and cystathionine in cystathionine synthase deficiency and methionine synthase deficiency supports the conclusion that the vascular pathology is attributable to hyperhomocysteinemia, regardless of the etiologically responsible inherited enzyme deficiency. Review of the literature also supports the atherogenic role of homocysteine, since elevation of methionine, cystathionine, or methylmalonic acid in plasma without hyperhomocysteinemia is not associated with arteriosclerotic plaques in published cases (7). The vascular pathology of methionine synthase deficiency is interpreted as rapidly progressive arteriosclerosis in a reexamination of the index case of this disease (10).

The vascular pathology of hyperhomocysteinemia caused by methionine synthase deficiency consists of widespread fibrous intimal plaques affecting arteries and arterioles in major organs throughout the body (7). Typical fibrous plaques are composed of focal proliferation of smooth muscle cells, associated with deposition of metachromatic extracellular matrix, deposition of collagen fibers, and splitting and degeneration of elastica interna (Fig 6). In some plaques the elastica interna is encrusted with calcium salts, presenting an

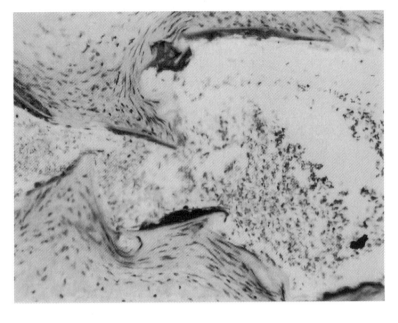

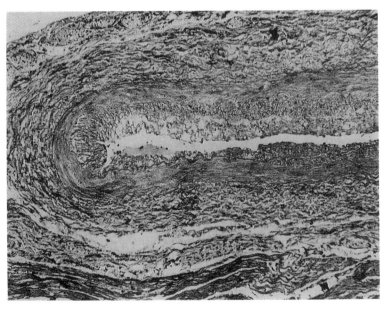

*Figure 6. Artery of heart of narrowed by proliferative smooth muscle cells, deposition of extracellular matrix and collagen, and degeneration of elastica interna in methionine synthase deficiency. H&E x200.*

*Figure 7. Artery of basal ganglia is narrowed by fibrous intimal plaques and irregular calcified elastica interna in methionine synthase deficiency. H&Ex200.*

irregular, angulated and distorted fibrocalcific intimal plaque (Fig 7). These fibrous and fibrocalcific plaques narrow the lumens of coronary, cerebral, renal, and pulmonary arteries. In some arterioles hyperplastic smooth muscle cells narrow the lumen, and vacuolated endothelial cells further compromise the lumen. In addition to these fibrous and fibrocalcific plaques, focal degenerative lesions of arterioles and small arteries are demonstrated in brain, testis and other organs. In small arterioles of brain the lumens are narrowed by fibrinous thickening associated with vacuolization of endothelial cells and hyperplasia of smooth muscle cells. In larger arterioles of brain the degenerative changes include microthrombi and focal disruption of arteriolar wall with surrounding focal hemorrhage (Fig.8). Irregular small foci of cerebral infarction are interpreted as small infarcts secondary to these vascular changes (10). Additional extensive areas of degeneration of white and gray matter are considered to be of metabolic origin. In a medium sized artery of testis, focal necrosis of arterial wall is associated with hyperplasia of smooth muscle cells, degeneration of endothelial cells, and deposition of fibrin. These vascular changes are interpreted as vascular injury caused by rapidly progressive arteriosclerosis (11).

Important confirmation of vascular lesions in methionine synthase deficiency is demonstrated in two additional cases of the rare form of hyperhomocysteinemia caused by methionine synthase deficiency (12,13). In one case vascular changes are confined to brain, where extensive fibrinoid necrosis of arteriolar walls is associated with foci of demyelination and fibrillary gliosis (12). In addition other arterioles are narrowed by prominent proliferation of smooth muscle cells or occluded by fibrin thrombi. Similar vascular lesions are not demonstrated in organs other than brain. In the other case, vascular lesions are demonstrated in organs throughout the body, but no vascular changes are found in brain (13). In this case the aorta contains foci of splitting and degeneration of elastic lamellae associated with intimal fibrous plaques. Coronary artery contains focal fibrous intimal plaques with destruction of elastica interna and narrowing of the lumen. The glomeruli of kidney contain fibrin thrombi and focal necrosis associated with slight proliferation of mesangial and endothelial cells. Renal cortical arteries contain focal fibrous plaques and subendothelial deposits of fibrin. In addition, smooth muscle cells of arteriolar wall are hyperplastic, narrowing the lumen, associated with edema of endothelial cells and subendothelial deposits of fibrin. Electron microscopy reveals deposits of fine granular material similar to basement membrane in glomerular capillaries and extrusions of similar granular material from cytoplasm of endothelial cells of arterioles.

The finding of arteriosclerotic fibrous intimal plaques and vascular damage, as shown by fibrinoid necrosis, fibrin thrombi, and vacuolization of endothelial cells in these rare cases of methionine synthase deficiency, supports the con

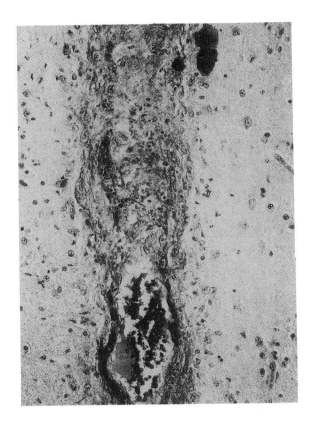

*Figure 8. Arteriole of cerebral cortex is disrupted and surrounded by hemorrhage in methionine synthase deficiency. H&E x75.*

clusion that hyperhomocysteinemia is responsible for rapidly progressive arteriosclerosis by a direct effect of homocysteine on cells and tissues of arterial wall (7,12,13). Because of the rarity of this disease no studies of vascular pathology in heterozygous methionine synthase deficiency have been reported.

As early as 1884 vascular lesions similar to those found in the brain in methionine synthase deficiency were described in cases of pernicious anemia caused by deficiency of vitamin $B_{12}$ (reviewed in 12 and 14). The vascular pathology of vitamin $B_{12}$ deficiency in the brain consists of perivascular hemorrhages, fibrosis, hyalinization and thickening of arteriolar walls by hyperplasia of smooth muscle cells. These vascular changes are sometimes associated with foci of demyelinization and gliosis of adjacent parenchyma. Vitamin

$B_{12}$ deficiency in pernicious anemia leads to prominent hyperhomocysteinemia, supporting the interpretation that homocysteine causes vascular damage and arteriosclerotic plaques by effects on arterial cells and tissues.

## ARTERIOSCLEROSIS IN METHYLENETETRAHYDROFOLATE REDUCTASE DEFICIENCY

Several years after the discovery of hyperhomocysteinemia caused by deficiencies of cystathionine synthase or methionine synthase, a third inherited enzyme deficiency was also shown to lead to homocystinuria and hyperhomocysteinemia (15). In this condition defective remethylation of homocysteine to methionine leads to hyperhomocysteinemia without elevation of plasma cystathionine and with low to normal concentrations of plasma methionine. The first published autopsy findings in a 10-year-old female with methylenetetrahydrofolate reductase deficiency reveals vascular pathology that is strikingly similar to the vascular abnormalities found in the other two enzymatic deficiencies associated with hyperhomocysteinemia (16). Because of this similarity, the vascular lesions are attributed to a toxic effect of homocysteine on cells and tissues of arteries. Essentially identical vascular lesions were subsequently reported in a second case of methylenetetrahydrofolate reductase deficiency (17).

The vascular lesions in hyperhomocysteinemia caused by methylenetetrahydrofolate reductase deficiency consist of fibrous intimal plaques of arteries, thickening of arteriolar walls by smooth muscle cell hyperplasia and swelling and vacuolization of endothelial cells (16,17). The fibrous intimal plaques consist of proliferation of smooth muscle cells with increased deposition of collagen fibrils and splitting and degeneration of elastic interna (17). Focal lesions are also present in aortic wall, consisting of moderate intimal hyperplasia of smooth muscle cells, loss of endothelial cells, and fragmentation and disruption of elastic lamellae (16). In this case multiple recent pulmonary infarcts are associated with thrombosis of pulmonary artery and recent thrombi in pulmonary arterioles and capillaries. Widespread thrombosis also involves superior saggital sinuses, lateral sinuses, and their tributaries in the brain. In the arterioles of brain the lumens are narrowed by thickened hyalinized walls, occasional microthrombi, and swollen vacuolated endothelial cells. Some arterioles contain foci of fibrinoid necrosis, associated with perivascular hemorrhages and foci of demyelinization and neuronal loss in gray matter.

In addition to the vascular changes, the liver and spleen in methylenetetrahydrofolate reductase deficiency contain increased deposits of iron in the form of hemosiderin within splenic macrophages and hepatocytes (16). Similar increased deposition of iron within hepatocytes is observed in experimental animals fed a diet containing excess homocystine (18). Recent observations have suggested that increased iron deposition is associated with increased risk of arteriosclerosis and myocardial infarction in human epidemiological studies (19).

Although the vascular lesions contain no demonstrable lipid or cholesterol deposits, the liver contains extensive fat deposition within hepatocytes in hyperhomocysteinemia secondary to methylenetetrahydrofolate reductase deficiency (16), as well as in cystathionine synthase deficiency (1-3,7,20) and in methionine synthase deficiency (7,13). Electron microscopy of hepatocytes reveals numerous lipid droplets, multivesicular bodies, ferritin and lipofuscin bodies, and abnormal mitochondria (16,20). The smooth endoplasmic reticulum is hyperplastic in cystathionine synthase deficiency (20) but not in methylenetetrahydrofolate reductase deficiency (16). These findings demonstrate a disturbance in lipid metabolism in all three types of hereditary hyperhomocysteinemia.

The abnormalities of mitochondria observed in cystathionine synthase deficiency and in methylenetetrahydrofolate reductase deficiency consist of enlarged and elongated mitochondria with breaks and finger-like projections of outer membranes. Giant mitochondria with irregular, dilated, or bizarre shapes contain enlarged dense bodies of mitochondrial matrix (20). The suggestion that over production of homocysteine is responsible for these abnormalities of mitochondria is supported by the experimental demonstration of similar mitochondrial changes in experimental animals fed large doses of methionine or cholestane triol (21). Homocysteine catalyzes oxidation of low-density lipoprotein in the presence of ferric ions in vitro (22). Cholestane triol is a highly atherogenic cholesterol oxide that is produced by oxidation of low-density lipoprotein within the artery wall. These and other observations led to the proposal of altered mitochondrial function in arteriosclerosis promoted by hyperhomocysteinemia (23).

The finding of accelerated arteriosclerosis in hyperhomocysteinemia caused by methylenetetrahydrofolate reductase deficiency is important independent confirmation of the conclusion that homocysteine produces arteriosclerotic plaques by a direct effect on cells and tissues of artery wall. Regardless of whether the metabolic origin of hyperhomocysteinemia is from failure of cystathionine formation by the transsulfuration pathway or from failure of conversion of homocysteine to methionine by the remethylation pathway, arteriosclerotic plaques and accelerated atherogenesis are observed. The finding of vascular damage, characterized by fibrin deposition, focal necrosis of artery wall, swelling of endothelial cells, and microthrombi suggests a common pathophysiological atherogenic process in all three major types of hereditary hyperhomocysteinemia.

## VASCULAR PATHOLOGY ASSOCIATED WITH MODERATE HYPERHOMOCYSTEINEMIA

The first human study to implicate homocysteine in moderate hyperhomocysteinemia without known enzymatic disorders or homocystinuria was conducted in patients with coronary heart disease (24). Following an oral dose of methionine, the only precursor of homocysteine, the plasma levels of homocystine and homocysteine cysteine disulfide were found to be elevated in coronary heart disease compared with normal controls. Subsequently, numerous studies of patients with cerebrovascular, coronary and peripheral vascular disease have established moderate hyperhomocysteinemia as an independent risk factor for arteriosclerosis, as explained in other chapters. Dietary deficiencies of vitamin $B_6$, folic acid, and faulty absorption of vitamin $B_{12}$ have been implicated in the etiology of moderate hyperhomocysteinemia (25). Population studies have demonstrated that plasma homocysteine correlates with known risk factors for arteriosclerosis, including lack of fruits and vegetables, lack of exercise, abuse of tobacco, age, sex, postmenopausal status, hypertension, and other factors (26). Almost all retrospective studies and most prospective studies have implicated hyperhomocysteinemia as a causative factor in vascular pathology. A recent prospective study of 21,520 men showed that homocysteine levels were significantly higher in 229 men who died of ischemic heart disease compared with 1126 matched controls in a nested case-control study (27). These results help to resolve the uncertainty about the causative role of hyperhomocysteinemia from previous prospective and retrospective studies.

In contrast to cases of hyperhomocysteinemia caused by homozygous deficiencies of enzymes controlling homocysteine metabolism, the vascular pathology of most cases of moderate hyperhomocysteinemia is examined at a later stage in the development of arteriosclerosis. Vascular lesions are at an earlier and more rapidly progressive stage of development in homozygous homocystinuria than in cases of moderate hyperhomocysteinemia without known enzymatic deficiencies. The fibrinoid necrosis, fibrin deposition, microthrombi, and swollen vacuolated endothelial cells that are found in all three major types of homocystinuria are rarely encountered in cases of moderate hyperhomocysteinemia.

No histopathological study has yet been published to document the detailed characteristics and development of arteriosclerotic plaques in cases with moderate hyperhomocysteinemia. Nevertheless, many studies have delineated the evolution and progression of arteriosclerosis in children and young adults in susceptible populations (28). As many as 40% of these susceptible populations have been found to have moderate hyperhomocysteinemia in multiple surveys.

Moreover, moderate hyperhomocysteinemia is more frequent in populations with high risk of coronary heart disease than in those with a low risk (29).

In susceptible populations diffuse and focal intimal thickenings are present in a fraction of infants at birth (28). These early lesions contain abundant extracellular proteoglycan matrix, isolated macrophage foam cells, increased smooth muscle cells and elastic fibers. From the late first decade to early puberty, fatty streaks contain, in addition to the connective tissue components of intimal thickenings of early lesions, macrophage foam cells, lipid laden smooth muscle cells, and extracellular lipid particles. Beginning in late adolescence and continuing into early adulthood, preatheroma and atheroma lesions begin to accumulate a core of extracellular lipid deposits within the musculoelastic layer of developing plaques. Typical fibrous plaques become evident from the middle of the third decade and increase in prominence in later decades. Typical atheromatous complicated plaques are observed in the fourth and later decades. These advanced lesions develop degenerative changes, hemorrhages into plaques, mural thrombi, neovascularization, cholesterol crystals, amorphous protein, and lipid debris (30). Similar advanced atherosclerotic plaques are observed in older cases of homozygous homocystinuria, sometimes associated with typical arteriosclerotic aneurysm (8).

The important question concerning the similarity of arteriosclerotic plaques in cases of homozygous homocystinuria with arteriosclerotic lesions in typical cases of moderate hyperhomocysteinemia has not definitely been resolved. Certainly all cases of typical arteriosclerosis commonly present fibrous and fibrocalcific plaques that are found in children with homocystinuria. In fact, these fibrous plaques are the most typical lesions found in smaller arteries in all cases of generalized arteriosclerosis. Complicated, degenerative atherosclerotic plaques are most common in aorta and larger arteries, but fibrous and fibrocalcific plaques are the predominant lesions even in larger arteries in many cases. Present interpretations suggest that the arteriosclerotic plaques found in homozygous homocystinuria are at an earlier and more rapid stage of development than plaques associated with moderate hyperhomocysteinemia. Since dyslipidemia typically develops in the fourth and later decades in susceptible populations, prominent lipid deposition in atherosclerotic plaques is more characteristic of moderate hyperhomocysteinemia. The slower pace of development of complex atheromas in this circumstance probably favors more lipid deposition and more prominent degenerative changes. The more rapid pace of development of fibrinous, fibrous and fibrocalcific plaques in homozygous homocystinuria favors a more rapid onset of occlusion and thrombosis in the first two decades in homocystinuria.

The incidence of dyslipidemia and hypercholesterolemia in patients with arteriosclerosis varies from about 50% to as low as 15% of cases, depending upon the study population and the definition of dyslipidemia. The occurrence of advanced arteriosclerosis or coronary heart disease without the presence of traditional risk factors is frequent in susceptible populations. An autopsy study of 194 consecutive cases, designed to estimate the frequency of hypercholesterolemia in patients with arteriosclerosis, concluded that only about 15% of cases with the most severe arteriosclerotic plaques had elevated serum cholesterol levels (31). In two thirds of the 122 cases with severe atherosclerosis, the disease developed without evidence of elevated serum cholesterol, diabetes, or hypertension. Other published studies have shown that moderate hyperhomocysteinemia is associated with arteriosclerosis in many cases without traditional risk factors, explaining the results of this autopsy study.

A fraction of cases of moderate hyperhomocysteinemia have been ascribed to heterozygosity for one of the enzymes controlling homocysteine metabolism. Earlier studies of cases of early onset and familial cerebrovascular, peripheral and coronary vascular disease implicated heterozygosity for cystathionine synthase deficiency as a factor in some cases. Elevated plasma homocysteine following oral methionine and enzyme assay of cultured skin fibroblasts were cited as evidence for this interpretation (32). More recent studies utilizing techniques of molecular genetics have failed to confirm these early findings, and the possible role of heterozygosity for cystathionine synthase deficiency in early onset and familial vascular disease remains controversial. No study of vascular pathology in obligate heterozygotes for cystathionine synthase deficiency has yet been reported in the literature.

Numerous studies have implicated genetic abnormalities of methylenetetrahydrofolate reductase in susceptibility to vascular disease, as explained in other chapters. Up to 13% of the population has been estimated to be homozygous for the thermolabile form of this enzyme. The occurrence of moderate hyperhomocysteinemia in homozygotes for this enzyme mutant has been related to dietary intake of folic acid (33). No study of vascular pathology in these cases of mutant alleles for methylenetetrahydrofolate reductase has yet been reported in the literature.


## HYPERHOMOCYSTEINEMIA AND LIPOPROTEINS IN ATHEROGENESIS

The development of arteriosclerotic plaques in homozygous homocystinuria closely parallels the histogenesis of human atherosclerosis. Many of the pathophysiological processes observed in arteries in homocystinuria have been observed in the development of arteriosclerotic plaques in cases of generalized arteriosclerosis. In general, many of the lesions in homozygous homocystinuria are accelerated in the pace of development, according to present interpretations. The prominence of intimal injury, fibrin deposition, and fibrous plaques in childhood in these cases supports this interpretation.

In cases of moderate hyperhomocysteinemia or in cases of arteriosclerosis developing without known abnormalities of homocysteine metabolism, the amount and rapidity of lipid deposition in developing plaques is delayed in onset and more prominent than in homozygous homocystinuria. In homocystinuria in childhood only a few vascular lesions have been observed to contain prominent lipid deposition, and the predominant type of arteriosclerotic plaque is fibrous and fibrocalcific. A possible reason for this observation is that elevation of plasma lipoproteins begins only after puberty and becomes prominent only in the fourth and later decades of life. In moderate hyperhomocysteinemia lipid deposition in the core of developing plaques begins after the early connective tissue changes have occurred in the first two decades of life. Even in later decades, many arteriosclerotic plaques in moderate hyperhomocysteinemia are of the fibrous and fibrocalcific type. Pathologists dissecting these arteries in elderly persons with atherosclerosis know that most of the plaques are very fibrotic and heavily encrusted with calcium deposits. Only in the aorta and larger arteries are soft fibrolipid plaques and atheromas prominent in many of these cases. In arteries of smaller caliber, fibrosis and calcification are more conspicuous, and lipid deposition is less prominent than in larger arteries.

A current view of the pathogenesis of arteriosclerotic plaques in hyperhomocysteinemia emphasizes the relation between low-density lipoprotein (LDL) particles and homocysteine in atherogenesis (11). Human LDL contains homocysteine in greater quantities in cases of atherosclerosis with dyslipidemia than in control cases (34). Homocysteine thiolactone, the reactive anhydride of homocysteine, reacts with LDL particles to produce small dense particles that aggregate and precipitate spontaneously (35). The homocysteine-LDL aggregates are taken up by cultured human macrophages to form foam cells. These observations suggest that development of arteriosclerotic plaques in both homozygous and moderate hyperhomocysteinemia require participation of LDL as a carrier of homocysteine.

According to one possible concept, the LDL-homocysteine aggregates are taken up by vascular macrophages to form foam cells (11). Degradation of these aggregates within these cells leads to release of lipids into developing plaques, accounting for lipid deposition in fatty streaks and atheromas in moderate hyperhomocysteinemia. Degradation of these aggregates also leads to release of homocysteine thiolactone or homocysteine, affecting the viability and growth of surrounding vascular wall cells. Theoretically homocysteine thiolactone released from these aggregates affects oxygen metabolism of arterial cells, leading to accumulation of oxygen free radicals and causing increased oxidative stress. Thus, homocysteine thiolactone may interact with thioretinaco ozonide, converting this complex to thioco, the complex formed from homocysteine thiolactone and cobalamin (11). As a result thioretinaco ozonide, the active site for oxidative phosphorylation, is converted to an inactive form, allowing accumulation of oxygen free radicals. These free radical oxygen species, in turn, are responsible for intimal damage, degeneration of endothelial cells, and deposition of fibrin in the accelerated vascular lesions found in homozygous homocystinuria, according to this view. The abnormalities of mitochondria observed in hyperhomocysteinemia (20,21) support this concept.

Cultured fibroblasts from the skin of children with homozygous cystathionine synthase deficiency and hyperhomocysteinemia produce an aggregated extracellular proteoglycan matrix of reduced solubility containing increased numbers of sulfate groups (36). Biochemical analysis of homocysteine thiolactone metabolism in these cell cultures and in scorbutic guinea pigs disclosed a pathway of oxidation of homocysteine leading to sulfation of proteoglycan matrix (37). Deposition of extracellular sulfated proteoglycans in early arterial plaques in hyperhomocysteinemia is related to increased sulfation and increased production of proteoglycan aggregates by hyperplastic smooth muscle cells.

Many children with homozygous homocystinuria have accelerated growth in childhood, and homocysteine derivatives have growth hormone-like properties in animals, causing release of insulin-like growth factor (38). Cultured smooth muscle cells respond to homocysteine by increased formation of cyclin mRNA, providing a possible explanation for the hyperplasia of smooth muscle cells in early arteriosclerotic plaques (39). Homocysteine also enhances collagen production by hyperplastic smooth muscle cells in culture (40). These findings suggest that the growth-promoting properties of homocysteine account for the hyperplasia of smooth muscle cells, synthesis of increased extracellular matrix, and deposition of collagen observed in early plaques in hyperhomocysteinemia.

The prominent degeneration of elastica interna and fragmentation of elastic fibers found in early plaques is attributable to increased activity of elastase within aorta and arteries in hyperhomocysteinemia (41). Release of elastase from lysosomes is probably related to decreased lysosomal membrane stability because of increased oxygen free radicals in developing plaques. The deposition of calcium salts in fibrous plaques may also be related to abnormalities of calcium transport by mitochondria through calcium channels, as the result of increased oxygen free radicals.

Homocysteine is a prothrombotic substance, enhancing blood coagulation and fibrin formation through effects on platelets, thrombomodulin, protein C, protein S, thromboxane, prostacyclin, and many of the major blood coagulation factors (42). Although many of the observed effects on blood coagulation are only found at high homocysteine concentrations, the binding of lipoprotein(a) to fibrin was demonstrated at concentrations found in moderate hyperhomocysteinemia (43). Human and animal studies have shown that homocysteine increases vascular reactivity by interaction with nitrous oxide to produce s-nitrosohomocysteine (44). The free base of homocysteine thiolactone produces thrombosis, necrosis, angiogenesis, stromal and epithelial hyperplasia in experimental animals, supporting the role of homocysteine in the vascular injury and thrombosis in hyperhomocysteinemia (45).

In advanced degenerative arteriosclerotic plaques the hemorrhage within plaques, acute thrombosis, and incorporation of mural thrombi within complicated plaques are attributable to the injurious and prothrombotic effects of homocysteine. The final results of the pathophysiological effects of homocysteine on arterial cells and tissues are the complex advanced fibrous, fibrocalcific, fibrolipid and atheromatous plaques of advanced human atherosclerosis. These plaques are the culmination of the effects of hyperhomocysteinemia on cells and tissues of arteries in the development of atherosclerosis.

## REFERENCES

1.  Gibson JB, Carson NAJ, Neill DW. Pathological findings in homocystinuria. J Clin Path 1964; 17:427-437.
2.  Carson NAJ, Dent CE, Field CMB, Gaull GE. Homocystinuria. Clinical and pathological review of ten cases. J Pediat 1965; 66:565-583.
3.  Schimke RN, McKusick VA, Huang T, Pollack AD. Homocystinuria. Studies of 20 families with 38 affected members. J Am Med Assoc 1965; 193:711-719.
4.  Carey MC, Donovan DE, Fitzgerald O, McAuley FD. Homocystinuria. I A clinical and pathological study of nine subjects in six families. Am J Med 1968; 45:7-25.
5.  Case Records of the Massachusetts General Hospital. Case 19471. Marked cerebral symptoms following a limp of three months' duration. N Engl J Med 1933; 209:1063-1066.
6.  Shih VE, Efron ML. Pyridoxine-unresponsive homocystinuria. Final diagnosis of MGH case 19471, 1933. N Engl J Med 1970; 283:1206-1208.
7.  McCully KS. Vascular pathology of homocysteinemia: implications for the pathogenesis of arteriosclerosis. Am J Pathol 1969; 56:111-128.
8.  Almgren B, Eriksson I, Hemingsson A, Hillerdal G, Larsson E, Aberg H. Abdominal aortic aneurysm in homocystinuria. Acta Chir Scand 1978; 144:543-548.
9.  Mudd SH, Levy HL, Abeles RH. A derangement in the metabolism of vitamin $B_{12}$ leading to homocystinuria, cystathioninuria and methylmalonic aciduria. Biochem Biophys Res Commun 1969; 35:121-126.
10. McCully KS. Homocystinuria, arteriosclerosis, methylmalonic aciduria, and methyl transferase deficiency: a key case revisited. Nutr Rev 1992; 50:7-12.
11. McCully KS. Homocysteine and vascular disease. Nature Med 1996; 2:386-389.

12. Dayan AD, Ramsey RB. An inborn error of vitamin $B_{12}$ metabolism associated with cellular deficiency of coenzyme forms of the vitamin. Pathological and neurochemical findings in one case. J Neurol Sci 1974; 23:117-128.

13. Baumgartner ER, Wick H, Maurer R, Egli N, Steinman B. Congenital defect in intracellular metabolism resulting in homocystinuria and methylmalonic aciduria. I Case report and histopathology. Helv Paediat Acta 1979; 34:465-482.

14. Erbsloh F. Funikulare Spinalerkrankung. In: Lubarsch OH, Henle F, Rossle R, Eds. Handbuch der speziellen pathologischen anatomie und histologie, Vol. 13 (Nervensystem), part 2B (Erkrankungen des zentralen Nervensystems). Berlin: Springer, 1958:1526-1601.

15. Mudd SH, Uhlendorf BW, Freeman JM, Finkelstein JD, Shih VE. Homocystinuria associated with decreased methylenetetrahydrofolate reductase activity. Biochem Biophys Res Commun 1972; 46:905-912.

16. Kanwar YS, Manaligod JR, Wong PWK. Morphologic studies in a patient with homocystinuria due to 5,10-methylenetetrahydrofolate reductase deficiency. Pediat Res 1976; 10:598-609.

17. Baumgartner ER, Wick H, Ohnacker H, Probst A, Maurer R. Vascular lesions in two patients with congenital homocystinuria due to different defects of remethylation. J Inher Dis 1980; 3:101-103.

18. Klavins JV. Pathology of amino acid excess. I Effects of administration of excessive amounts of sulfur containing amino acids: homocystine. Brit J Exp Pathol 1963; 44:507-515.

19. Salonen JT, Nyyssonen K, Korpela H, Tuomilehto J, Seppanen R, Salonen R. High stored iron levels are associated with excess risk of myocardial infarction in eastern Finnish men. Circulation 1992; 86:803-811.

20. Gaull GE, Schaffner F. Electron microscopic changes in hepatocytes of patients with homocystinuria. Pediat Res 1971; 5:23-32.

21. Matthias D, Becker CH, Riezler R, Kindling PH. Homocysteine induced arteriosclerosis-like alterations of the aorta in normotensive and hypertensive rats following application of high doses of methionine. Atherosclerosis 1996; 122:201-216.

22. Parthasarathy S. Oxidation of LDL by thiol compounds leads to its recognition by the acetyl LDL receptor. Biochim Biophys Acta 1987; 917:337-340.

23. McCully KS. Chemical pathology of homocysteine. I Atherogenesis II Carcinogenesis and homocysteine thiolactone metabolism III Cellular function and aging. Ann Clin Lab Sci 1993; 23:477-493; 1994; 24:27-59, 134-152.

24. Wilcken DEL, Wilcken B. The pathogenesis of coronary artery disease. A possible role for methionine metabolism. J Clin Invest 1976; 57:1079-1082.

25. Selhub J, Jacques PF, Wilson PWF, Rush D, Rosenberg IH. Vitamin status and intake as primary determinants of homocysteinemia in an elderly population. J Am Med Assoc 1993; 270:2693-2698.

26. Nygard O, Vollsett SE, Refsum H et al. Total plasma homocysteine and cardiovascular risk profile. The Hordaland homocysteine study. J Am Med Assoc 1995; 274:1526-1533.

27. Wald NJ, Watt HC, Law MR, Weir DG, McPartlin J, Scott JM. Homocysteine and ischemic heart disease. Results of a prospective study with implications regarding prevention. Arch Intern Med 1998; 158:862-867.

28. Stary HC. Evolution and progression of atherosclerotic lesions in coronary arteries of children and young adults. Arteriosclerosis Suppl 1 1989; 9:1-19-1-32.

29. Alfthan G, Aro A, Gey KF. Plasma homocysteine and cardiovascular disease mortality. Lancet 1997; 349:397.

30. Osborn GR. The Incubation Period of Coronary Thrombosis. London: Butterworths, 1963.

31. McCully KS. Atherosclerosis, serum cholesterol and the homocysteine theory: a retrospective study of 194 consecutive autopsies. Am J Med Sci 1990; 299:217-221.

32. Boers GHJ, Smals AGH, Trijbels FJM et al. Heterozygosity for homocystinuria in premature peripheral and cerebral occlusive arterial disease. N Engl J Med 1985; 313:709-715.

33. Rozen R. Genetic predisposition to hyperhomocysteinemia: deficiency of methylenetetrahydrofolate reductase (MTHFR). Thromb Haemostasis 1997; 78: 523-526.

34. Olszewski AJ, McCully KS. Homocysteine content of lipoproteins in hypercholesterolemia. Atherosclerosis 1991; 88:61-68.

35. Naruszewicz M, Mirkiewicz E, Olszewski AJ, McCully KS. Thiolation of low-density lipoproteins by homocysteine thiolactone causes increased aggregation and altered interaction with cultured macrophages. Nutr Metab Cardiovasc Dis 1994; 4:70-77.

36. McCully KS. Macromolecular basis for homocysteine-induced changes in proteoglycan structure in growth and arteriosclerosis. Am J Pathol 1972; 66:83-95.

37. McCully KS. Homocysteine metabolism in scurvy, growth and arteriosclerosis. Nature 1971; 231:391-392.

38. McCully KS. Homocysteine theory of arteriosclerosis: development and current status. In: Gotto AMJr, Paoletti R, Eds. Atherosclerosis Reviews, Volume 11. New York: Raven, 1983:157-246.

39. Tsai J-C, Perrella MA, Yoshizumi M et al. Promotion of vascular smooth muscle cell growth by homocysteine: a link to atherosclerosis. Proc Natl Acad Sci USA 1994; 91:6369-6373.

40. Majors A, Ehrhart LA, Pezacka EH. Homocysteine as a risk factor for vascular disease. Enhanced collagen production and accumulation by smooth muscle cells. Arterioscler Thromb Vasc Biol 1997; 17:2074-2081.

41. Rolland PH, Friggi A, Barlatier A et al. Hyperhomocysteinemia-induced vascular changes in the minipig. Circulation 1995; 91:1161-1174.

42. D'Angelo A, Selhub J. Homocysteine and thrombotic disease. Blood 1997; 90:1-11.

43. Harpel PC, Chang VT, Borth W. Homocysteine and other sulfhydryl compounds enhance the binding of lipoprotein(a) to fibrin: a potential biochemical link between thrombosis, atherogenesis and sulfhydryl compound metabolism. Proc Natl Acad Sci USA 1992; 89:10193-10197.

44. Stamler JS, Osborne JA, Jaraki O et al. Adverse vascular effects of homocysteine are modulated by endothelium-derived relaxing factor and related oxides of nitrogen. J Clin Invest 1993; 91:308-318.

45. McCully KS, Vezeridis MP. Histopathological effects of homocysteine thiolactone on epithelial and stromal tissues. Exp Molec Pathol 1989; 51:159-170.

# 8. VASCULAR COMPLICATIONS OF HOMOCYSTINURIA: INCIDENCE, CLINICAL PATTERN AND TREATMENT

PAOLO RUBBA, GIOVANNI DI MINNO AND GENEROSO ANDRIA

## SUMMARY

Homocystinuria is a metabolic disease that leads to premature vascular damage. In recent years homocystinuria has been well characterized from a biochemical and genetic standpoint and, at the same time, strategies for therapeutic intervention have been identified and are currently being tested with some success. The metabolic abnormality thought to be responsible for the clinical events is the plasma accumulation and urinary excretion of homocysteine – an amino acid that is not detectable under normal circumstances. There is more than one defect leading to homocystinuria. The best characterized enzyme abnormality responsible for homocystinuria is the deficiency of cystathionine β-synthase (CBS) activity. The clinical picture is characterized by lens dislocation, mental retardation, skeletal abnormalities, and high incidence of cardiovascular events that lead in several instances to premature death. Homocystinuric patients show considerable heterogeneity in their clinical picture. In homocystinuria, thrombophlebitis and pulmonary embolism are the most frequent vascular events, although pulmonary embolism is seldom a cause of death. Thrombosis of large and medium size-arteries such as carotid and renal arteries is often the terminal event. Coronary artery obstruction has also been reported, but heart disease does not represent a prominent feature of this condition.

*K. Robinson (ed.), Homocysteine and Vascular Disease*, 117-133.
© 2000 *Kluwer Academic Publishers. Printed in the Netherlands.*

The mechanism underlying the occurrence of arterial obstructions even in early-treated patients is unknown. It is unlikely that typical atherosclerotic lesions precede thrombus formation in homocystinuric patients of young age. Pathology studies (reviewed by Dr Mc Cully in Chapter 7) rarely show typical atherosclerotic lesions in young homocystinuric patients who succumbed to thrombosis. A more consistent autopsy finding in these patients is arterial dilatation, which has been suggested to precede the thrombotic event. In homocystinuria arterial histological examinations often show medial alterations, fragmentation of the internal elastic lamina and endothelial thickening. Medial thinning is often observed in association with thick intimas. Direct toxicity of homocysteine on endothelial cells, possibly due to oxidative mechanisms, might increase the susceptibility to intimal damage and thrombosis. On the other hand, several abnormalities, commonly occurring in individuals prone to arterial or venous thrombosis have been demonstrated in patients with homozygous CBS deficiency. In keeping with this, enhanced biosynthesis of thromboxane $A_2$, and index of *in vivo* platelet activation has been found in homozygotes.

A retrospective study using a questionnaire failed to demonstrate any excess of clinical events in heterozygotes. Furthermore, no evidence has been provided of coagulation abnormalities in heterozygous CBS deficiency. Other clinical studies have suggested that heterozygosity for CBS deficiency is a risk factor for premature arterial disease; this hypothesis has been formulated on the basis of results from non-invasive ultrasound investigations for vascular diagnosis, which were able to detect vascular abnormalities in the extracoronary arteries, even in the absence of clinical evidence of ischemia.

Supplementation of $B_6$-responsive homocystinuric patients with pyridoxine, improved their clinical picture and reduced the incidence of vascular events (This is reviewed by Boers et al in Chapter 22). This occurred in association with a reduction of circulating homocysteine levels. Management of vascular events in homocystinuric patients should include standard therapeutic procedures, even if not specifically tested for effectiveness and safety, in controlled clinical trials.

Early detection and treatment of homocystinuria is at its beginning. Which methodology is most helpful for the early diagnosis of vascular disease in hyperhomocysteinemia has yet to be defined. A better definition of the type of vascular damage and pattern of evolution of the arterial lesions will improve our understanding of basic mechanisms leading to premature vascular disease in man.

# INTRODUCTION

In recent years much interest has developed on the abnormalities in the metabolism of sulfur-containing amino acids which in the past had attracted the attention of pediatricians only (1) because one metabolic defect along this pathway (2), homocystinuria, has been indicated as a human model to the study of the basic mechanisms leading to atherogenesis and premature vascular disease (3). A better understanding of the mechanisms underlying premature vascular disease might eventually help identify new strategies of cardiovascular prevention in more common clinical conditions and in the population in general. Homocystinuria (1,2) is an inherited metabolic disease involving cysteine and other sulfur-containing amino acids, which leads to premature vascular damage (4-7).

A direct pathogenic role of high levels of circulating homocysteine has been suggested by the observation of similar histologic abnormalities in different errors of sulfur-containing amino acids, in which different intermediate metabolites accumulate — all leading to severe hyperhomocysteinemia and homocystinuria.

They include CBS deficiency, methionine synthase deficiency and methylenetetrahydrofolatereductase MTHFR deficiency.

# VASCULAR COMPLICATIONS IN HOMOZYGOUS CBS DEFICIENCY

There is more than one defect leading to homocystinuria. The best characterized enzyme defect responsible for homocystinuria is the one involving CBS activity. In recent years homozygous CBS deficiency has been well characterized from both a biochemical and a genetic standpoint; at the same time strategies for therapeutic intervention have been identified and are currently being tested with some success. The clinical picture is characterized by lens dislocation, mental deficit, skeletal abnormalities, and high incidence of cardiovascular events that lead in several instances to premature death (1).

The clinical picture is highly variable and the most common disturbance is lens dislocation (8,9). Vascular complications (arterial and/or venous) are the first clinical abnormality in 25-45% of cases.

The metabolic abnormality thought to be responsible for the clinical events is the plasma accumulation and urinary excretion of homocysteine — an amino acid that is absent from urine under normal circumstances. Homocysteine is a highly reactive molecule that tends to form the dipeptide homocystine, resulting from two homocysteine molecules linked by a disulfide bond.

Homocysteine has a key position in the so-called remethylation and transulfuration pathways, which involve several amino acids, including methionine and cysteine, and vitamin cofactors, such as vitamin $B_6$ (pyridoxine), vitamin $B_{12}$ (cyanocobalamin) and folates.

The diagnosis of homocystinuria (1,10) due to homozygosity for CBS deficiency is based on the following criteria: a) presence of homocysteine in the urine b) abnormally low cystathionine ß-synthase activity in cultured skin fibroblasts and/or hypermethioninemia and hyperhomocystinemia with low or undetectable levels of cysteine in the blood. Determination of total plasma homocysteine takes into account that, ex vivo, free homocysteine becomes progressively associated with plasma proteins and, therefore, in stored plasma, probably all homocysteine is protein-bound.

Unfortunately, the diagnosis of homocystinuria is often delayed until the appearance of severe clinical abnormalities (8,9,11).

In homocystinuria, a high incidence has been reported of thrombophlebitis and pulmonary embolism, although pulmonary embolism seldom represents a cause of death. Thrombosis of large and medium sized arteries such as carotid and renal arteries is often the terminal event (4,6,12). Coronary artery obstruction has also been reported (4,6), but heart disease does not represent a prominent feature of this condition (1,10). A case of long-term survival of homocystinuria has been reported recently (13).

Arterial disease of the lower limbs has been demonstrated also in patients in whom the diagnosis had been established early in infancy and treatment started accordingly. In 13 patients with homocystinuria, ankle pressure was estimated by the continuous wave Doppler method in order to detect asymptomatic arterial disease of the lower limbs. Ankle pressure was abnormally low and indicative of obliterating arterial disease of the lower limbs (14) in 3 cases out of fifteen. Four patients out of 13 had wall irregularities in the iliac arteries based on Duplex evaluation. None of them reported previous myocardial infarction, stroke, angina pectoris or intermittent claudication.

## HOMOCYSTINURIA: SPECIFIC FEATURES OF THE VASCULAR DAMAGE

To better understand the relationship between homocystinuria and atherosclerosis it is of interest to compare the features of arterial damage in patients with homocystinuria as compared to those with familial hypercholesterolemia. Familial hypercholesterolemia is a classical human model of premature and extensive atherosclerosis leading to severe cardiovascular disease. In a study published recently, extent and severity as well as hemodynamic impact of carotid atherosclerosis in homocystinuric patients were entirely different from those in patients with homozygotic familial hypercholesterolemic patients, according to the results of quantitative ultrasound imaging and transcranial Doppler evaluations (15). Carotid arteries of the hypercholesterolemic group had higher values for intima-media thickness than either the homocystinuric or control groups. Focal thickenings, suggesting atherosclerotic lesions were found in all the hypercholesterolemic subjects. Increased intima-media thickness is thus a constant feature of severe hypercholesterolemia and involves the common carotid arteries, which, in the general population, are relatively spared from vascular lesions when compared to the carotid bifurcation or to internal carotid arteries. In the hypercholesterolemic patients, severe thickening often led to an increase in the external diameter of common carotid arteries. This finding can be explained by the compensatory enlargement that occurs in human atherosclerotic arteries (16,17).

Patients with homocystinuria due to CBS deficiency had normal intima-media thicknesses. Blood flow velocity in the middle cerebral artery of homocystinuric patients (which was abnormally elevated in familial hypercholesterolemia), did not differ from that found in healthy controls.

The mechanism underlying the arterial obstructions that occur even in early-treated, pyridoxine-responsive patients is unknown (18,19). It is unlikely that typical atherosclerotic lesions precede thrombus formation in homocystinuric patients of young age. This idea is in agreement with the results of pathology studies (4-6,20-23) which rarely show typical atherosclerotic lesions in young homocystinuric patients who succumbed to thrombosis (Table 1). A more consistent autopsy finding in these patients is arterial dilatation, which has been suggested to precede the thrombotic event (4). In the above mentioned study (15) two homocystinuric patients showed an increase in both the external and internal diameter of their common carotid arteries (fig. 1). This finding is consistent with that of arterial dilatations at autopsy. In the future, scanning procedures specifically aiming at diameter measurement in the carotid arteries should be performed in larger series of homocystinuric patients.

In homocystinuria arterial histology examinations often show medial alterations, fragmentation of the internal elastic lamina and endothelial thickening (table 1). Insights into the pathology of homocystinuria are given by Dr Mc Cully in chapter 7. Medial thinning is often observed in association with thick intimas and may help explain why the overall intima-media thickness in the hyperhomocysteinemic group does not differ from that of controls.

A disturbance of extracellular matrix formation in homozygous CBS deficiency is supported by the clinical analogies with Marfan's syndrome, where abnormalities in synthesis, secretion and deposition of matrix have been docu

TABLE 1

| No. | Author (year) | Ref. | GROSS PATHOLOGY | | | HISTOLOGY | | | |
| | | | THROMBI | | | | | | |
| | | | Arteries | Veins | Aneurysm | Intimal thickneming | Abnormal Elastic fibers | Abnormal media | Atheroma |
|---|---|---|---|---|---|---|---|---|---|
| 1 | Gibson (1964) | 20 | + | + | + | + | + | + | + |
| 2 | Carson (1965) | 5 | + | + | - | + | + | + | - |
| 3 | | | | | | | | | |
| 4 | | | | | | | | | |
| 5 | Shimke (1965) | 4 | + | + | + | + | + | + | - |
| 6 | | | | | | | | | |
| 7 | | | | | | | | | |
| 8 | | | | | | | | | |
| 9 | Carey (1968) | 6 | + | - | - | + | - | + | - |
| 10 | McCully (1969) | 21 | + | - | - | + | + | + | - |
| 11 | Hopkins (1969) | 23 | + | + | | - | + | | |
| 12 | Almgren (1969) | 22 | + | - | + | - | + | + | + |

Table 1 : Gross pathology and histology findings in 12 homocystinuric patients who prematurely died of cardiovascular diseases (from ref. 15)

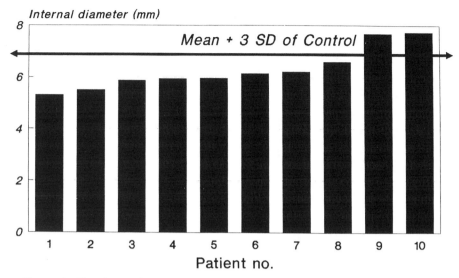

*Figure 1: This figure shows the internal diameters of Common Carotid arteries, as evaluated by B mode ultrasound imaging, in 10 individual patients with homozygous CBS deficiency. In two cases (n .9 and n. 10) this value exceeded 3 standard deviations of the mean of healthy controls of comparable age and gender: this is interpreted as evidence of significant arterial dilatation in these two patients (from ref. 15).*

mented. Furthermore abnormalities in the cross linking of collagen have been demonstrated in CBS deficient patients (24).

At present, B-mode ultrasound is unable to reliably detect the ultrasonic interface between intima and media, i.e. internal elastic lamina, therefore subtle abnormalities in the structure of intima and media go undetected. The relatively frequent finding of high blood pressure levels in severe cases of untreated homocystinuria, in association with the microscopic evidence of alterations in internal elastic lamina and media, leave open the possibility that thrombosis is a consequence of focal intimal damage in the absence of adequate medial support. The frequent occurrence of aneurysmal lesions in homocystinuric patients (4,20,22,25,26) is consistent with the view of a major role of medial damage (27) in this form of premature vascular disease.

Direct toxicity of homocysteine on endothelial cells (7,28), possibly due to oxidative mechanisms (28,29), might increase the susceptibility to intimal damage and thrombosis. However, more recent data indicate that the arterial wall of homocystinuric patients might be protected (30) to a large extent from oxidative damage, possibly by a mechanism that modulates the adverse vascular effects of homocysteine (31). Furthermore, plasma concentrations of homo-

TABLE 2

## Effects of high homocysteine levels on some hemostatic variables

*Homocysteine induces*

*in vitro:*

| | | | |
|---|---|---|---|
| ↑ | RASMC proliferation (Tsai et al. 1994) | | |
| ↑ | Copper-mediated human and bovine EC lysis (Starkebaum et al, 1986) | → | HUVEC viability (De Groot et al, 1983; Blann, 1992) |
| ↑ | LDL oxidation (Parthasarathy et al, 1987) | → | HUVEC adhesion to glass (Wall et al, 1980; Dudman et al, 1981) |
| ↑ | Affinity of Lp(a) for fibrin (Harpel et al. 1992) | → | Heparan sulfate expression (Nishinaga, 1993) |
| ↑ | Platelet-adhesion to EC (De Groot et al, 1983) | → | TM surface expression and activity (Lentz et al, 1991; Hayashi et al, 1992) |
| ↑ | TF production by EC (Fryer et al. 1993) | · | Modulation of t-PA binding to its receptor (Hajjar, 1993) |
| ↑ | FV activity and prothrombin activation in cultured BAEC (Rodgers et al, 1986; Rodgers et al, 1990) | · | Changes is the synthesis of arterial prostacyclin (Panganamala et al, 1986; C ber et al, 1982; Wang et al, 1993) |
| ↑ | TXB₂ production by EC (Graeber et al, 1982) | | |

*ex vivo / in vivo*

| | | | |
|---|---|---|---|
| ↑ | TXB₂ urinary excretion (in CBS homozygous deficiency) (Vesterqvist et al; 1984; Di Minno et al, 1993) | → | AT III levels (Giannini et al, 1975; Maruyama et al, 1977; Palareti et al, 198 |
| ↑ | Patchy loss of arterial EC (Harker et al. 1974; Harker et al. 976) | → | FVII levels (Palareti et al, 1986; Charlot et al. 1982; Mercky et al, 1981) |
| ↑ | SMC proliferation (Harker et al, 1976) | → | Platelet half-life (Harker et al, 1976; Harker et al. 1977) |

EC: endothelial cells; SMC: smooth muscle cells; RASMC: rat aortic smooth muscle cells; HUVEC: human umbilical vein endothelial cells; BAEC: bovine aortic endothelial cells; LDL: density lipoprotein; Lp(a) lipoprotein(a); TF: tissue factor; FV: factor V; FVII: factor VII; t-PA: tissue plasminogen activator; TM: thrombomodulin

*Table 2 : Effects of high homocysteine levels on some hemostatic variables (from ref. 29)*

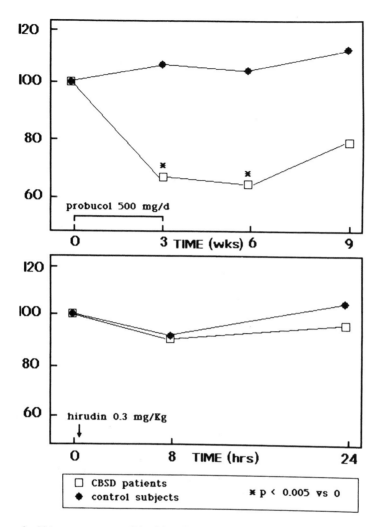

*Figure 2: Urinary excretion (% of baseline values) of 11-dehydro-thromboxane B2 (TXM) following hirudin bolus infusion, 0.3 mg/kg (upper panel) and 3-week oral administration of probucol, 500 mg/day (lower panel), in patients with homozygous CBS deficiency and healthy controls. TXM was determined on urine samples adjusted to pH 4.0-4.5, run on SEP-PAK C18 cartridges, eluted with ethyl acetate, chromatographed on silicic acid columns, and analyzed by radioimmunoassay (for further details see ref. 43)*

cysteine in homocystinuric patients (0.1-0.2 mM) are generally lower than those associated with severe endothelial damage in vitro (31,32). Overall, experimental evidence does not provide consistent support to the hypothesis of enhanced oxidative damage as the basis of vascular abnormalities in homocystinuria due to homozygous CBS deficiency (19,33-37). However recent clinical data collected in homozygous CBS deficiency suggest that further investigation is still needed on the possible relations between oxidative mechanisms and hypercoagulable status in this clinical condition (see below).

Independently of the mechanism leading to vascular damage, there is evidence of endothelial damage in CBS deficiency. The experimental data and findings in vivo are consistent in suggesting impaired vasodilator capacity in affected patients (19, 33, 38, 39, 40). There are also indications that homocysteine might be involved in the hemostatic mechanisms (Table 2), enhancing the proneness to arterial and venous thrombosis (29). Most studies have not reported a consistent or specific effect of homocysteine on circulating coagulation factors. It is possible that homocysteine affects thrombosis mainly through endothelial damage, which in turn leads to disturbances in the coagulation/fibrinolysis systems. Of particular interest is the demonstration that the simultaneous presence of homocystinuria and factor V Leiden are at increased risk of thrombosis (41,42). In addition, patients with homozygous CBS deficiency show several abnormalities that commonly occur in individuals prone to arterial or venous thrombosis. In keeping with this, enhanced biosynthesis of thromboxane (TX) $A_2$—an index of *in vivo* platelet activation--has been demonstrated in homozygotes (33). These individuals have persistently elevated platelet biosynthesis of TX $A_2$ *in vivo*, as reflected by the excretion of its major metabolites, 11-dehydro-$TXB_2$ and 2,3-dinor-$TXB_2$ (fig. 2) We have tested the possibility that such an abnormality may reflect a hypercoagulable state, by infusing a bolus of the specific thrombin inhibitor-- hirudin--to 9 CBS deficient patients. However, a dose of hirudin (0.3 mg/Kg over a 15-min period) that prolonged the activated partial thromboplastin time by 3-4 fold (p<0.001 vs basal) and suppressed the *ex vivo* response of platelets to thrombin for 4-6 hrs, did not affect 11-dehydro-$TXB_2$ excretion in this setting. In contrast, probucol (500 mg/d for 3 wks) did not affect the hypercoagulability indices but lowered by approximately 30% (p <.005) 11-dehydro-$TXB_2$ excretion. A partial reduction in the urinary 11-dehydro-$TXB_2$ excretion (approximately 30%) was also observed in 7 CBSD patients following the supplementation of 600 mg/d of vitamin E for 2 wks (1273$\pm$383 pg/mg creatinine in pre-vitamin E samples vs. 913$\pm$336 after treatment, p <.009). We have therefore concluded that $TXA_2$ biosynthesis in homocystinuria is largely independent of a hypercoagulable state, and is possibly related to mechanisms linking lipid peroxidation to platelet activation (43).

## HETEROZYGOTES FOR CBS DEFICIENCY

A retrospective study using a questionnaire has failed to demonstrate any excess of clinical events in heterozygotes (1); however the sensitivity of questionnaires for clinical events is known to be relatively low. Furthermore, no evidence has been provided of coagulation abnormalities in heterozygous CBS deficiency. Few clinical studies have evaluated whether heterozygosity for CBS deficiency is a risk factor for premature arterial disease (44-46). Evidence has been provided in one study (44) that subjects who are heterozygotes for CBS deficiency have a prevalence of extracoronary flow abnormalities that exceeds that of a healthy control population of comparable age and gender distribution. This finding was obtained using non-invasive ultrasound techniques for vascular diagnosis, which were able to detect arterial flow abnormalities even in the absence of clinical symptoms. The other studies evaluating intima-media thickness of the carotid arteries were negative or weakly positive (45,46). A possible explanation for flow abnormalities without corresponding intima-media thickenings or plaques might be related to a thrombotic nature of most lesions in heterozygotes for CBS deficiency. Further studies by B-mode ultrasound imaging might help investigate with greater accuracy heterozygotes for cystathionine ß-synthase deficiency in order to detect early atherosclerotic or thrombotic lesions.

Heterozygosity for the 844ins68 mutation of the CBS gene, when detected in combination with thermolabile MTHFR (see below), increases by 4-fold the risk of venous and arterial occlusive vascular disease. The high thrombotic risk due to the combination of genetic defects is essentially limited to patients with fasting hyperhomocysteinemia - irrespective of the coexistence of other markers of thrombophilia - and is probably linked to circulating homocysteine levels higher than those of patients with thermolabile MTHFR alone (47).

## OTHER INHERITED METABOLIC DEFECTS LEADING TO SEVERE HYPERHOMOCYSTEINEMIA AND VASCULAR COMPLICATIONS

In recent years it has been suggested (48-50) that some abnormalities in the remethylation pathway might be even more relevant to the occurrence of premature vascular disease (51) than defects in transulfuration.

Homocysteine remethylation is catalyzed by the enzyme methionine synthase, which requires 5-methyltetrahydrofolate as substrate and vitamin $B_{12}$ as cofactor. 5-methyltetrahydrofolate is formed by reduction of 5,10-methylene tetrahydrofolate, through the action of methylenetetrahydrofolate reductase. Deficiencies might lead to a variable degree of elevation in plasma homocysteine concentration. A thermolabile variant of the MTHFR enzyme is characterized by approximately a 50% reduction in its activity as compared to the normal enzyme found in the majority of the population. Both heterozygotes and homozygotes for this variant of MTHFR have an increased concentration of fasting homocysteine; it has been suggested that this genetic mutation is associated with increased risk for cardiovascular events. It has been demonstrated that abnormalities in thermolabile MTHFR account for about one third of cases of hyperhomocysteinemia in vascular patients. A 677 C→T mutation has been demonstrated in the MTHFR gene, and homozygosity for this mutation has been found associated with low specific enzyme activity, thermolability and fasting hyperhomocysteinemia.

Isolated deficiency of the enzyme methionine synthase has also been described in association with hyperhomocysteinemia, megaloblastic anemia and neurological abnormalities. In a few patients association with vascular complication has been reported ( reviewed by Dr Mc Cully in Chapter 7). This disorder has been included among cobalamin disorders and affected patients have been found to respond favorably to high-dose cobalamin treatment (2).

## B-VITAMINS AND HYPERHOMOCYSTEINEMIA

Homozygotes for CBS deficiency show considerable heterogeneity in their clinical picture. This has been related to the presence or absence of responsiveness to pyridoxine treatment, pyridoxine responsive patients having a more benign clinical course (1). In a published series, all patients but one (15) were pyridoxine-responsive, and most had been on treatment for several years. No symptoms of ischemia were reported, but evidence was available of flow-reducing stenoses in lower extremity arterial circulation in three cases. The single homocystinuric patient who was non-responsive to pyridoxine had low middle cerebral artery blood flow velocity and evidence of bilateral arterial obstruction in the lower extremities. It is interesting to note that supplementation with pyridoxine of $B_6$ responsive homocystinuric patients improved the clinical picture and reduced the incidence of vascular events (1). This occurred in association with a reduction of circulating levels of homocysteine. There is evidence of associations between moderate hyperhomocysteinemia and low intake or low plasma concentration of the vitamins involved in the metabolism of sulfur-containing amino acids (10,50,52,53). These associations involve vitamin $B_6$ (pyridoxine), folate and vitamin $B_{12}$ (cyanocobalamin). Case-control studies in patients with cardiovascular disease suggest that, to a large extent, the association between hyperhomocysteinemia and vascular disease is explained by a vitamin deficit (54-59). The evidence is rather consistent, especially with regard to vitamin $B_6$ and folate.

Most likely, the occurrence of both enzymatic defects and vitamin deficiencies combined produces a synergistic effect on cardiovascular risk.

Vitamin $B_6$, $B_{12}$ and folate supplementation can effectively reduce homocysteine concentration in mild (55) and severe hyperhomocysteinemia (60). Effects on cardiovascular events in homocystinuria are described in Chapter 22.

## CONCLUSION

The demonstration of the efficacy of a regimen including pyridoxine, folic acid and intermittent hydroxycobalamin to prevent vascular events in homocystinuria is the current basis of management of affected patients (60). A methionine-restricted diet with supplementation with cystine and betaine is commonly used in the case of pyridoxine non-responsive patients. However its efficacy in preventing vascular complications is not definitely proved (see Boers et al in Chapter 22).

In the primary prevention of cardiovascular events, there is no clear indication for other treatments (anticoagulants, antiplatelet drugs, antioxidants) potentially active on the vascular systems, in view of the uncertainties that still exist about the mechanisms underlying the vascular events in homocystinuric patients. Among new possible interventions, antioxidant supplementation represents the most promising therapeutic development.

After the occurrence of venous or arterial thrombotic events, intervention strategies commonly employed in practice, as far as dosage and scheduling is concerned, should be adopted in homocystinuric patients. Further clinical controlled trials are needed to test the effectiveness and safety of these interventions in patients with homocystinuria due to inherited metabolic defects.

The different type of lesions demonstrated in homocystinuria as compared to hypercholesterolemia are likely to reflect two different mechanisms of arterial damage (3,4,15). Hypercholesterolemia or hyperhomocysteinemia of milder degree are frequent in the population and have both been associated with premature development of cardiovascular disease. In most instances the inherited defect is likely to interact with environmental influences (diet, smoking habits) or with coexisting diseases (diabetes mellitus, hypertension), giving rise to a mixed pattern of stenotic and aneurysmal lesions, with intima-media thickening and/or thrombosis.

While detection and treatment of hypercholesterolemia has already achieved widespread acceptance, early detection and treatment of hyperhomocysteinemia is only beginning. B-mode ultrasound imaging offers adequate means for early detection and follow-up of hypercholesterolemia-related vascular damage. Which method is most helpful for the early diagnosis and follow-up of vascular disease in hyperhomocysteinemia has yet to be defined. A better definition of the type of vascular damage and of the pattern of evolution of the arterial lesions will improve our management of homocystinuric patients and potentially help clarify the basic mechanisms that lead to premature vascular disease in man.

## REFERENCES

1.  Mudd ST, Skovby F, Levy HL, Wilcken B, Pyeritz RE, Andria G, Boers GHJ, Bromberg IL, Cerone R, Fowler B, Grobe H, Schmidt H, Schweitzer L. The natural history of homocystinuria due to cystathionine ß-synthase deficiency. Am J Hum Genet 1985; 37:1-31
2.  Fowler B. Disorders of homocysteine metabolism. J Inher Metab Dis 1997; 20:270-285
3.  Ross R. The pathogenesis of atherosclerosis - An update. New Engl J Med 1986; 314: 488-500
4.  Schimke RN, Mc Kusick VA, Huang T, Pollack AD. Homocystinuria. Studies on 20 families with 38 affected members. J Am Med Ass 1965; 193:711-719
5.  Carson NAJ, Dent CE, Field CMB, Gaull GE. Homocystinuria. Clinical and pathological review of ten cases. J Pediatrics 1965; 66:565-583
6.  Carey MC, Donovan DE, Fitzgerald O, Mc Auley FD. Homocystinuria. I. A clinical and pathological study of nine subjects in six families. Am J Med 1968; 45:7-31
7.  Harker LA, Slichter SJ, Scott R, Ross R. Homocystinemia. Vascular injury and arterial thrombosis. New Engl J Med 1974; 291:537-543
8.  Cruysberg JRM, Boers GHJ, Trijbels JMF, Deutman AF. Delay in diagnosis of homocystinuria: retrospective study of consecutive patients. Br Med J 1996;313:1037-1040
9.  De Franchis R, Sperandeo MP, Sebastio G, Andria G. The Italian Collaborative Study Group on Homocystinuria. Clinical aspects of cystathionine ß-synthase deficiency: how wide is the spectrum? Eur J Pediatr 1998; 157 (suppl 2):S67-S70
10. Ueland PM, Refsum H, Brattström . Plasma homocysteine and cardiovascular disease. In Atherosclerotic cardiovascular disease, hemostasis and endothelial function, Francis RB,Jr ed., Marcel Dekker,Inc, New York, 1992, pg.183-236
11. Isherwood DM. Homocystinuria. Br Med J 1996; 313:1025-1026.
12. Lu CY, Hou JW, Wang PJ, Chiu HH, Wang TR. Homocystinuria presenting as fatal common carotid artery occlusion. Pediatr Neruol 1996; 15:159-162
13. Nugent A, Hadden DR, Carson NAJ. Long-term survival of homocystinuria: the first case. Lancet 1998; 352:624-625
14. Rubba P, Faccenda F, Strisciuglio P, Andria G. Ultrasonographic detection of arterial disease in treated homocystinuria. New Engl J Med 1989; 321:1759-1760
15. Rubba P, Mercuri M, Faccenda F, Iannuzzi A, Irace C, Strisciuglio P, Gnasso A, Tang R, Andria G, Bond GM, Mancini M. Premature carotid atherosclerosis: Does it occur in both

Familial hypercholesterolemia and homocystinuria? Ultrasound assessment of arterial in-tima-media thickness and blood flow velocity. Stroke 1994, 25:943-50

16. Glagov S, Weisenberg E, Zarins CK, Stankunavicius R, Kolettis GJ. Compensatory en-largement of human atherosclerotic coronary arteries. N Engl J Med 1987; 316:1371-1375

17. Tomaki K, Armstrong M, Heistad d. Effects of atherosclerosis on cerebral vessels: hemo-dynamic and morphometric studies. Stroke 1986; 17:1209-1214

18. Newman G, Mitchell JRA. Homocystinuria presenting as multiple arterial occlusions. Quart J Med 1984; 53:251-258

19. Bellamy MR, McDopwell IFW. Putative mechanisms for vascular damage by homocyste-ine. J Inher Metab Dis 1997; 20:307-315

20. Gibson JB, Carson NA, Neill DW. Pathological findings in homocystinuria. J Clin Pathol 1964; 17:427-437

21. Mc Cully K, Vascular pathology of homocysteinemia: implications for the pathogenesis of arteriosclerosis. Am J Pathol 1969; 56:111-128

22. Almgren B, Eriksson I, Hemmingsson A, Hillerdal G, Larsson E, Aberg H. Abdominal aortic aneurism in homocystinuria. Acta Chir Scand 1978; 144:545-548

23. Hopkins I, Townley RRW, Shipman RT. Cerebral thrombosis in a patient with homocys-tinuria. J Pediatrics 1969; 75:1082-1083

24. Lubec B, Fang-Kircher S, Lubec T, Blom HJ, Boers GHJ.Evidence for McKusick's hy-pothesis of deficient collagen cross-linking in patients with homocystinuria. Biochim Bio-phys Acta 1996; 1315:159-162

25. Wicherink-Bol HF, Boers GHJ, Drayer JIM, Rosenbush G. Angiographic findings in ho-mocystinuria. Cardiovasc Intervent Radiol 1983; 6:125-128

26. Vandresse JH, de Saint Hubert E, Evrard P. Homocystinuria and carotid arteriography. Neuroradiology 1978; 17:57-58

27. Powell J. Models of arterial aneurisms: for the investigation of pathogenesis and pharma-cotherapy - a review. Atherosclerosis 1991; 87:93-102

28. Starkebaum G, Harlan JM. Endothelial cell injury due to copper-catalyzed hydrogen per-oxide generation from homocysteine. J Clin Invest 1986; 77:1370-1376

29. Mancini FP, Di Minno G. Hyperhomocysteinemia and thrombosis: the search for a link. Nutr Metab Cardiovasc Dis 1996; 6:168-177

30. Dudman NP, Wilcken DE, Stocker R. Circulating hydrperoxide levels in human hyperho-mocysteinemia. Relevance to development of arteriosclerosis. Arterioscl Thromb 1993; 13:512-516

31. Stamler J, Osborne JA, Jaraki O, Rabbani LE, Mullins M, Singel D, Loscalzo J. Adverse vascular effects of homocysteine are modulated by endothelium-derived relaxing factor and related oxides of nitrogen. J Clin Invest 1993;91:308-318

32. Dudman NPB, Hicks C, Wang J, Wilcken DEL. Human arterial endothelial cell detach-ment in vitro: its promotion by homocysteine and cysteine. Atherosclerosis 1991; 91:77-83

33. Di Minno G, Davì G, Margaglione M, Cirillo F, Grandone E, Ciabattoni G, Catalano I, Strisciuglio P, Andria G, Patrono C, Mancini M. Abnormally high thromboxane biosyn-thesis in homozygous homocystinuria. Evidence for platelet involvement and probucol-sensitive mechanisms. J Clin Invest 1993;92:1400-1406

34. Mansoor MA, Ueland PM, Aarsland A, Svardal AM. Redox status and protein binding of plasma homocysteine and other aminothiols in patients with homocystinuria. Metabolism 1993;42:1481-1485

35. Hirano K, Ogihara T, Miki M, Yasuda H, Tamai H, Kawamura N, Mino M. Homocysteine induces iron-catalyzed lipid peroxidation of low-density lipoprotein that is prevented by alpha-tocopherol. Free Radic Res 1994; 21:267-76

36. Cordoba-Porras A, Sanchez-Quesada JL, Gonzales-Sastre F, Ordonez-LlanosJ, Blanco-Vaca F. Susceptibility of plasma low- and high-density lipoproteins to oxidation in patients with severe hyperhomocysteinemia. J Mol Med 1996;74:771-776

37. Halvorsen B, Brude I, Drevon CA, Nysom J, Ose L, Christiansen EN, Nenseter MS. Effect of homocysteine on copper ion-catalyzed, azo compound-initiated, and mononuclear cell-mediated oxidative modification of low density lipoprotein. J Lipid Res 1996; 37:1591-1600

38. Celermajer DS, Sorensen K, Ryalls M, Robinson J, Thomas O, Leonard JV, Deanfield JE. Impaired endothelial function occurs in the systemic arteries of children with homozygous homocystinuria but not in their heterozygous parents. J Am Coll Cardiol 1993;22:854-858

39. Wang J, Dudman NPB, Wilcken DEL. Effects of homocysteine and related compounds on prostacyclin production by cultured human vascular endothelia cells. Thromb Haemost 1993;70:1047-1052

40. van der Molen EF, Hiipakka MJ, van Lith-Zanders H, Boers GH, van den Heuvel LP, Monnens LA, Blom HJ. Homocysteine metabolism in endothelial cells of a patient homozygous for cystathionine ß-synthase (CS) deficiency. Thromb Haemost 1997;78:827-833

41. Mandel H, Brenner B, Berant M, Rosenberg N, Lanir N, Jakobs C, Fowler B, Seligsohn U. Coexistence of hereditary homocystinuria and factor V Leiden – effect on thrombosis. N Engl J Med 1996; 336:763-768

42. Ridker PM, Hennekens CH, Selhub J, Miletich JP, Malinow MR, Stampfer MJ. Interrelation of hyperhomocyst(e)inemia, factor V Leiden, and risk of future venous thromobembolism. Circulation 1997;95:1777-1782

43. Di Minno G, Davì G, D'Angelo A, Cerbone AM, Coppola A, Viganò D'Angelo S, della Valle P, Mancini FP, Bucciarelli T, Ciabattoni G, Rubba P, Andria G, Patrono C. Platelet activation in homozygous homocystinuria: role of oxidative stress and thrombin. Arterioscl Thromb Vasc Biol, in press

44. Rubba P, Faccenda F, Pauciullo P, Carbone L, Mancini M, Strisciuglio P, Carrozzo R, Sartorio R, Del Giudice E, Andria G. Early signs of vascular disease in homocystinuria: A non-invasive study by ultrasound methods in eight families with cystathionine β-synthase deficiency. Metabolism 1990; 39: 1191-1195

45. Clarke R, Fitzgerald D, O' Brien C, Roche G, Parker RA, Graham I. Hyperhomocysteinemia. A risk factor for extracranial carotid artery atherosclerosis. Ir J Med Sci 1992; 161:61-65

46. de Valk HW, van Eeden MKG, Banga JD, van der Griend R, de Groot E, Haas FJLM, Meuwissen OJAT, Duran M, Smeitink JAM, Poll-The BT, de Klerk JBC, Wittebol-Post D, Rolland M-O. Evaluation of the presence of premature atherosclerosis in adults with heterozygosity for cystathonine ß-synthase deficiency. Stroke 1996; 27:1134-1136

47. de Franchis R, Buoninconti A, Fermo I, Sebastio G, Sperandeo MP, Mazzola G, Cerbone AM, Soriente L, Orefice G, Di Minno G, D'Angelo A, Andria G. Increased thrombotic

risk for patients with associated 844ins68 mutation of the cystanionine ß-synthase (CBS) gene and the 677C->T mutation of the methylenetetrahydrofolate reductase (MTHRF) gene. Am J Hum Gen 1998; 63:A210 (abstract).

48. Kang SS, Passen EL, Ruggie N, Wong PW, Sora H. Thermolabile defect of methylenetet-rahydrofolate reductase in coronary heart disease. Circulation 1993; 88:1463-1469

49. Engbersen AMT, Franken DG, Boers GHJ, Stevens EMB, Trijbels FJM, Blom HJ. Thermolabile 5,10-methylenetetrahydrofolate reductase as a cause of mild hyperhomocysteinemia. Am J Hum Genet 1995; 56:142-150

50. Dudman NPB, Wilcken DEL, Wang J, Lynch JF, Macey D Lundberg P. Disordered Methionine/Homocysteine metabolism in premature vascular disease - Its occurrence, cofactor therapy, and enzymology. Arterioscler Thromb 1993; 13:1253-1260

51. Kluijtmans LAJ, Boers GHJ, Verbruggen B, Trijbels FJM, Novàkovà I, Blom HJ. Homozygous cystathionine ß-synthase deficiency, combined with factor V Leiden or thermolabile methylenetetrahydrofolate reductase in the risk of venous thrombosis. Blood 1998; 91;2015-2018

52. Miller JW, Nadeau MR, Smith D, Selhub J. Vitamin $B_6$ deficiency versus folate deficiency: comparison of responses to methionine loading in rats. Am J Clin Nutr 1994; 59:1033-1039

53. Selhub J, Jacques PF, Wilson PWF, Rush D, Rosenberg IH. Vitamin status and intake as primary determinants of hyperhomocysteinemia in an elderly population. JAMA 1993; 270:2693-2698

54. Boushey CJ, Beresford SAA, Omenn GS, Motulsky AG. A quantitative assessment of plasma homocysteine as a risk factor for vascular disease. Probable benefits of increasing folic acid intake. JAMA 1995; 274:1049-1057

55. Franken D, Boers GHJ, Blom HJ, Trijbels FJM, Kloppenborg PWC. Treatment of mild hyperhomocysteinemia in vascular disease patients. Arterioscler Thromb 1994; 14:465-470

56. Robinson K, Mayer EL, Miller DP. Hyperhomocysteinemia and low pyridoxal phosphate. Common and independent reversible risk factors for coronary artery disease. Circulation 1995; 92:2825-2830

57. Selhub J, Jacques PF, Bostom AG, D'Agostino RB, Wilson PWF, Belanger AJ, O'Leary DH, Wolf PA, Schaefer EJ, Rosenberg IH. Association between plasma homocysteine concentrations and extracranial carotid-artery stenosis. N Engl J Med 1995; 332:286-291

58. Graham IM, Daly LE, Refsum HM, Robinson K, Brattström LE, Ueland PM, Palma-Reis RJ, Boers GHJ, Sheahan RG, Israelsson B, Uiterwall CS, Meleady R, McMaster D, Verhoef P, Witteman J, Rubba P, Bellet H, Wautrecht JC, de Valk HW, Sales Lùis AC, Parrot-Roulaud FM, Soon Tan K, Higgins I, Garcon D, Medrano MJ, Candito M, Evans AE, Andria G. Plasma homocysteine as a risk factor for vascular disease. The European Concerted Action Project. JAMA 1997, 277:1775-1781

59. Robinson K, Arheart K, Refsum H, Brattstrom L, Boers GHJ, Ueland P, Rubba P, Palma-Reis R, Meleady R, Daly L, Witteman J, Graham I, for the European COMAC Group. Low circulating folate and vitamin $B_6$ concentrations. Risk factor for stroke, peripheral vascular disease, and coronary artery diseases. Circulation 1998, 97:437-443

60. Wilcken DEL, Wilcken B. The natural history of vascular disease in homocystinuria and the effects of treatment. J Inher Metab Dis 1997; 20:295-300

# 9. HOMOCYSTEINE AS A RISK FACTOR FOR PERIPHERAL VASCULAR DISEASE

AHMED M. ABOU-ZAMZAM, JR., GREGORY L. MONETA,
JOHN M. PORTER, AND LLOYD M. TAYLOR, JR.

## SUMMARY

Since the observation that patients suffering from homocystinuria had marked and early progression of diffuse atherosclerosis, the association between mildly elevated homocysteine levels and atherosclerosis has been documented. The identification of a large number of people with elevated homocysteine levels due to genetic and/or dietary effects has pushed research to evaluate the question of whether homocysteine is a modifiable risk factor for atherosclerosis. The ability to return elevated homocysteine levels to normal with vitamin therapy has given rise to the possibility of not only secondary prevention, but also primary prevention of atherosclerosis. We will focus on the relationship between homocysteine and peripheral vascular disease.

A clear association between elevated homocysteine and the presence of peripheral vascular disease has been demonstrated by several investigators. In studies excluding patients with standard risk factors (diabetes mellitus, hypertension, elevated lipids) or statistically eliminating these factors, elevated homocysteine has been shown to be an independent risk factor for the presence of peripheral vascular disease. Moreover, the magnitude of the risk appears to be proportional to the elevation in homocysteine and not a threshold effect.

Supported in part by: Grant #RR00234, Clinical Research Centers Branch, NIH and Grant #2R01HL4526705, NIH, NHLBI.

*K. Robinson (ed.), Homocysteine and Vascular Disease, 135-149.*
© 2000 *Kluwer Academic Publishers. Printed in the Netherlands.*

The effect of elevated homocysteine appears to be of a magnitude similar to elevated cholesterol.

With the association established between elevated homocysteine and peripheral vascular disease, the next step was to evaluate whether the elevation of homocysteine could be modified. Several studies have demonstrated that treatment with vitamin $B_6$, folate, or a combination of these can successfully lower homocysteine levels in patients with peripheral vascular disease. Moreover, while the underlying cause of elevated homocysteine is varied (genetic {cystathionine β-synthase mutations, thermolabile methylenetetrahydrofolate reductase}, nutritional), the success of vitamin therapy appears applicable across the board.

A link has also been documented between elevated homocysteine and progression of peripheral vascular disease. A key retrospective study has demonstrated greater progression of peripheral vascular disease in patients with elevated homocysteine levels compared to those with normal levels. Homocysteine elevation has also been shown to adversely affect the outcome of surgical interventions for peripheral vascular disease, as well as to contribute to a higher incidence of vein graft stenosis following lower extremity bypass.

The key question looms ahead: Will the treatment of elevated homocysteine levels retard or even halt the progression of peripheral vascular disease? We are currently involved in a prospective study evaluating the natural history of elevated homocysteine as pertains to peripheral vascular disease, as well as the role of treatment with folate on the progression of peripheral vascular disease. Phase one of this trial has recently been completed which evaluated the effect of elevated homocysteine on the progression of peripheral vascular disease. Over a follow-up period of 37 months, elevated homocysteine did appear to have an adverse effect on progression of lower extremity arterial disease, however this effect did not reach statistical significance. The most important results from this observational phase of the study were the marked increase in both progression of cardiac disease as well as death in patients with elevated homocysteine levels. Phase two of this study is ongoing and includes treatment with either folic acid or placebo with an additional 5 years of observation. Data from this study, and other ongoing prospective studies, will offer more definitive information regarding the potential role of nontoxic vitamin therapy in the treatment of peripheral vascular disease.

INTRODUCTION

Elevated plasma homocysteine is now an established risk factor for peripheral vascular disease (PVD, herein used to describe lower extremity ischemia ranging from claudication to gangrene). Initial studies showed an association between elevated homocysteine levels and the presence of PVD. Cross-sectional studies showed that elevated homocysteine was an *independent* risk factor for PVD. The prospect of lowering homocysteine levels with vitamin therapy has been explored. Several studies have documented the ability to reduce levels with vitamin $B_6$ or folate either alone or in combination. Evidence from retrospective studies has demonstrated more severe disease progression in patients with elevated homocysteine compared to those with normal levels. A worse outcome following vascular procedures in patients with elevated homocysteine compared to those with normal homocysteine levels has also been suggested.

In this chapter we will review the literature linking elevated plasma homocysteine levels and PVD and present the data that exists on vitamin therapy, as well as the results of the first phase of our ongoing prospective study on homocysteine in PVD. The critical clinical question - whether lowering homocysteine levels will favorably modify PVD progression remains unanswered. An ongoing, randomized, prospective, double-blind, placebo-controlled study evaluating homocysteine and PVD will produce data regarding therapeutic intervention with folate and its effect on PVD in patients with elevated homocysteine levels in a few years.

## ASSOCIATION BETWEEN ELEVATED HOMOCYSTEINE AND PERIPHERAL VASCULAR DISEASE

In 1985 Boers et al. evaluated homocysteine levels in 75 patients with early onset atherosclerosis.[1] This group included 25 patients with severe PVD present before the age of 50 in the absence of diabetes mellitus, hyperlipidemia, or hypertension. All patients had angiographic documentation of disease. Seven of the 25 (28%) had abnormally elevated homocysteine levels (> 2 standard deviations above the mean for normal controls) following a methionine loading test (PML). These patients were also shown to be heterozygous for cystathionine β-synthase (CBS) deficiency by skin fibroblast culture. Given the estimated prevalence of CBS heterozygosity in the general population of 1:70, the 28% prevalence in patients with PVD suggested that patients with heterozygosity for CBS and elevated homocysteine were at an increased risk for PVD.

Brattström et al., in 1989 reported on 72 patients with early-onset peripheral and/or cerebrovascular disease.[2] Patients were all less than 55 years old and lacked diabetes or renal disease. The study included 37 patients with aortoiliac disease who had previously undergone aortoiliac bypass. Homocysteine levels were assessed by basal homocysteine and PML. Homocysteine levels were elevated (>2 s.d.) in 32% of patients compared to 4% (when measured as basal) and 2% (when measured by PML) of controls. Multivariate analysis revealed no effect on homocysteine levels by age, hypertension, tobacco, or cholesterol, thereby implicating homocysteine as an independent risk factor for PVD.

Also in 1989, Malinow et al. reported on homocysteine levels in patients with PVD and cerebrovascular disease.[3] Basal levels of homocysteine were analyzed using high performance liquid chromatography (HPLC) in 47 patients and 103 controls. Unlike the report by Brattström, et al., this report included typical vascular patients with a mean age of 70 years. The patients included 32 patients with iliofemoral disease and 8 with aortic disease. Patients, when compared to age-matched controls, had significantly higher homocysteine. The 47 patients included 22 with elevated (>2 s.d. above mean) homocysteine, and 25 with normal homocysteine. When these two groups were compared, there were no significant differences in age, cholesterol, tobacco use, or the presence of diabetes. The authors concluded that elevated homocysteine was an independent risk factor for peripheral arterial occlusive disease (including both PVD and cerebrovascular disease).

Clarke et al., in 1991 evaluated hyperhomocysteinemia as a risk factor for premature vascular disease.[4] This group of 123 patients included 25 patients with PVD (all with intermittent claudication (IC)). Seven of the patients with PVD (28%) had hyperhomocysteinemia (defined as a level differentiating heterozygous CBS from normal controls). The lower 95% confidence level of the adjusted odds ratio for all types of vascular disease among patients with hyperhomocysteinemia was significant at 3.3. The unadjusted odds ratio for PVD among patients with hyperhomocysteinemia was 22.3. However, when adjusted for other risk factors, the lower 95% confidence level of the odds ratio was 0.4. With regard to PVD, this study supported the findings of Brattström, et al.,[2] with the increased incidence of elevated homocysteine in patients with PVD, but could not clearly support the status of hyperhomocysteinemia as an independent risk factor for PVD.

Greater support for the role of elevated homocysteine as a risk factor for PVD came from a study by Molgaard et al.[5] This study was the first to assess only patients with isolated PVD. In this study, 78 patients (45-69 years old) with IC were compared with 98 healthy, age-matched controls. All patients had IC confirmed by treadmill testing. Twenty-five of the patients had undergone prior surgery for IC. Basal homocysteine levels were determined by HPLC and elevation was defined as greater than 2 standard deviations above the control mean. Overall, the incidence of elevated homocysteine was 23%. This elevation was independent of smoking, elevated cholesterol, hypertension, diabetes, and age. Interestingly, the elevated homocysteine was mainly confined to patients with low folate. The importance of this study was its limitation to patients with objectively documented PVD, and that it included patients of all ages.

Aronson et al. subsequently published a similar study evaluating 80 patients with PVD presenting prior to the age of 45.[6] These patients were identified by a retrospective review and returned for homocysteine evaluation by PML 4-14 years later. All patients had undergone surgery. The PML was abnormal in 19%, while $B_6$, $B_{12}$, and folate levels were normal. Atherosclerotic risk factors did not differ between the groups with elevated and normal homocysteine. This was presented as supportive evidence of the independent association of elevated homocysteine with PVD.

Bergmark et al. in 1993 published a report on 58 patients who had undergone operations for PVD prior to the age of 50.[7] Subjects were examined 0-11 years after surgery for determination of homocysteine levels. Twenty-eight percent had elevated (>2 s.d.) homocysteine compared to controls. Interestingly, patients with multilevel disease (suprainguinal and infrainguinal) had the highest levels of homocysteine. This study provided more support for the role of hyperhomocysteinemia as a risk factor in PVD and suggested a direct relationship between the magnitude of elevation and the extent of disease.

Van den Berg et al. subsequently supported the relationship between the magnitude of homocysteine elevation and the severity of PVD.[8] This study evaluated 171 patients presenting with their first symptoms of PVD prior to age 55. Homocysteine was measured at basal levels and PML. All patients underwent angiography to document lower extremity disease. By multivariate analysis, the extent of lower extremity disease was weakly correlated to basal homocysteine levels, but strongly correlated with PML. The prevalence of multilevel disease was significantly increased in patients with homocysteine levels in the upper quartile, suggesting a direct relation between actual homocysteine level and the extent of PVD.

An important prospective, case-control study evaluating homocysteine in patients with PVD was published by Cheng et al. in 1997.[9] This study included 100 patients (mean age 67 years) with PVD (ranging from IC to ischemic gangrene) and 100 controls. The incidence of elevated (>90th %) homocysteine was 27%. Multivariate analysis demonstrated elevated homocysteine to be an independent risk factor for the presence of PVD with an odds ratio of 3.74. This study added to the already large database supporting elevated homocysteine as a risk factor for PVD but was important for its prospective design.

The European Concerted Action Project was a large, case-control, cross-sectional analysis of plasma homocysteine as a risk factor for all types of vascular disease.[10] Patients were identified on the basis of having symptomatic vascular disease before the age of 60 in the absence of diabetes, renal dysfunction, or a recent myocardial infarction. Overall, 750 patients were identified and 800 controls were chosen. One hundred fifty-six of these patients had PVD with symptoms of IC confirmed by either noninvasive testing or angiography. All patients had evaluation of homocysteine at baseline and PML. The relative risk for vascular disease for patients with homocysteine in the top 1/5 compared to those with levels in the bottom 4/5 was 2.2. This risk was independent of other risk factors and appeared dose-related. For PVD the analogous relative risk was 1.7. An important observation of this study was that the additional evaluation of PML along with basal homocysteine identified an additional 27% of patients potentially at risk.

Boushey et al. used a meta-analysis to determine a quantitative assessment of plasma homocysteine as a risk factor for vascular disease.[11] This revealed a strong association between elevated homocysteine and the presence of PVD. The odds ratio for the presence of PVD in patients with elevated homocysteine was 6.8 (2.9-15.8). Interestingly, this calculated odds ratio was significantly greater than that for CAD (1.8) and CVD (2.5).

A large body of evidence clearly implicates elevated levels of homocysteine in the development of PVD. Based on studies which include retrospective, cross-sectional, and prospective designs, certain conclusions can be reached: 1) The incidence of elevated homocysteine is higher in patients with PVD (19%-47%) than in the general population (2-4%). 2) The relative risk of PVD in patients with elevated homocysteine ranges from 1.7-6.8. 3) An elevated homocysteine is an independent risk factor for PVD of the same magnitude as conventional risk factors (tobacco, cholesterol). 4) The degree of PVD appears to be directly related to the degree of homocysteine elevation. 5) The increased risk is present for patients of all ages, both genders and of multiple nationalities. 6) The increased risk is present regardless of whether homocysteine is measured as random, fasting, or following a methionine load.

## THE ROLE OF $B_6$, $B_{12}$, AND FOLATE IN PATIENTS WITH PVD AND ELEVATED HOMOCYSTEINE

With the identification of elevated homocysteine as a risk factor for peripheral vascular disease, the role of abnormal vitamin levels in patients with PVD is a logical field of research. Brattström, et al., in their evaluation of patients with cerebrovascular disease and PVD found that there was a negative correlation between homocysteine levels and folate as well as vitamin $B_{12}$.[2] Clarke, et al. found mean folate levels to be lower in patients with hyperhomocysteinemia than in controls, and they also documented an inverse relation between homocysteine and both vitamin $B_{12}$ and folate.[4]

The finding of an inverse relation between folate and homocysteine was again confirmed by Molgaard, et al.[5] In their study of 78 patients with IC, elevated homocysteine was mainly confined to those patients with low levels of plasma folate. Bergmark, et al. also found an inverse relation between homocysteine and folate, as well as homocysteine and vitamin $B_{12}$.[7]

The relationship between vitamin levels and PVD was addressed in the first of 2 reports from the European Concerted Action Project in 1997.[10] In this large group of patients, those taking vitamins containing $B_6$, $B_{12}$ or folate had a relative risk for all types of vascular disease of 0.38. There was an inverse relationship between homocysteine (measured as basal homocysteine and PML) and plasma levels of folate, vitamin $B_6$, and vitamin $B_{12}$. The relative risk for PVD was not specified. The interaction between folate and vitamin $B_6$ concentrations and vascular disease was reported separately in 1998.[12] A folate level below the 10th percentile was more common in vascular cases than in controls. This was partly explained by elevated homocysteine. A vitamin $B_6$ level below the 20th percentile was an independent risk factor for vascular disease irrespective of homocysteine level. Indeed, numerous other studies have evaluated vitamin levels in patients with PVD and elevated homocysteine levels and have found a negative relationship between homocysteine levels and plasma levels of some or all of the vitamins evaluated (folate, $B_6$, $B_{12}$).[9-14]

While the association of low vitamin levels with elevated homocysteine is clear in patients with PVD, the underlying etiology of these low vitamin levels is not clear. To address this issue, Selhub, et al. in 1993 presented a cross-sectional analysis of homocysteine, vitamin levels, and vitamin intake in elderly patients in the Framingham study.[15] The prevalence of hyperhomocysteinemia (>95th %) was 19%. Total homocysteine appeared to correlate positively with age. There was a strong inverse association between homocysteine and folate levels. Homocysteine also demonstrated inverse associations with plasma vitamin $B_{12}$ and $B_6$. Similar inverse associations were seen between homocysteine and dietary intake of folate and $B_6$. These authors estimated that B vitamin deficiencies may account for up to 67% of the elevated homocysteine seen in elderly people.

The primary factor leading to elevated homocysteine continues to be debated. The primary genetic defects are heterozygous CBS deficiency and thermolabile methylenetetrahydrofolate reductase. The primacy of genetic defects in the etiology of elevated homocysteine levels has been stressed by Kang and Wong.[14] These authors cite the observation that enzyme defects have a combined prevalence of 6% in the general population which coincides with the prevalence of hyperhomocysteinemia. A more moderate view remains that both genetic factors and dietary factors may act alone or in concert to cause elevated homocysteine levels.[16-18]

The role of homocysteine-lowering therapy with vitamin treatment has been evaluated in a few patients with PVD. Brattström, et al. examined the effects of pyridoxine and folic acid treatment on patients with cerebrovascular and aortoiliac disease.[2] Twenty-one patients with hyperhomocysteinemia were recalled one year after initial evaluation. Twenty (20/21) had persistent hyperhomocysteinemia. The one patient with normalization had been treated with folic acid for celiac disease. The remaining 20 patients were treated with vitamin $B_6$ (240 mg/day) for 2 weeks, and then vitamin $B_6$ and folate (10 mg/day) for an additional 2 weeks. Therapy lead to a mean reduction of homocysteine of 53%.

Franken, et al. in 1994 presented 421 patients with premature cerebrovascular disease or PVD.[19] This study included 131 patients with IC or renovascular hypertension. One-third of these patients with PVD had mild hyperhomocysteinemia (>2 s.d.) documented by post-methionine load. The effect of homocysteine-lowering treatment was assessed retrospectively in 82 of the 421 patients. Patients were treated with vitamin $B_6$ (250 mg/day) for 6 weeks, followed by vitamin $B_6$, folate (5 mg/day), betaine (6 gm/day) or some combination of these three treatments for an additional 6 weeks. After the initial 6 weeks of treatment, 56% of the patients had normal homocysteine levels, and after 12 weeks 95% had normalized their homocysteine levels.

Van den Berg, et al. published similar results in a group of 72 young patients (<50 years old) with mild hyperhomocysteinemia and atherosclerosis.[13] This group included 36 patients with PVD (ranging from IC to gangrene). All patients had normal baseline levels of folate, vitamin $B_6$ and vitamin $B_{12}$. A prospective evaluation of the response to homocysteine lowering therapy was performed. Patients received 6 weeks of vitamin $B_6$ (250 mg/day) and folate (5 mg/day) leading to normalization of homocysteine in 92% when measured by PML and 91% when measured as basal homocysteine. An additional 6 weeks of therapy (with betaine added in some patients) lead to normalization of homocysteine (measured by PML) in all patients. This same group reported endothelial dysfunction with elevated von Willebrand factor and elevated thrombomodulin in 18 patients with mild hyperhomocysteinemia.[20] Treatment with folate (5 mg/day) and pyridoxine (250 mg/day) was carried out for one year. All patients had normalization of homocysteine at one year with decreased von Willebrand factor and thrombomodulin. Interestingly, these surrogate measures of endothelial function did not normalize, despite normalization of homocysteine levels.

Boushey, et al., in their meta-analysis, estimated that increased folic acid intake by as little as 400 micrograms/day (as from a vitamin supplement) would decrease basal homocysteine levels by about 6 $\mu$mol/L.[11] These authors felt that since a 5 $\mu$mol/L increase in basal homocysteine has as much effect on coronary artery risk as much as a 20 mg/dL increase in cholesterol, the influence of folic acid therapy on primary and secondary prevention of atherosclerosis with folic acid could be dramatic.

## CORRELATION OF HYPERHOMOCYSTEINEMIA WITH DISEASE PROGRESSION AND OUTCOME

The above studies have demonstrated elevated homocysteine in 19-47% of patients with peripheral vascular disease. Therapy with folate and/or vitamin $B_6$ has been shown to successfully reduce homocysteine to normal levels in virtually all patients. An extension of this line of investigation is the effect of elevated homocysteine on the progression of PVD.

Taylor et al. in 1991 published a series of 214 patients with symptomatic lower extremity and/or cerebrovascular disease.[21] This retrospective series is one of the few that has documented disease progression in patients with hyperhomocysteinemia. Basal homocysteine levels were elevated (>2 s.d.) in 39% of the patients. At a mean follow-up of 54 months, patients with elevated homocysteine were more likely to have clinical progression of lower extremity disease than those with normal homocysteine levels (89% vs. 72%). Over a mean follow-up of 29 months, patients with elevated homocysteine were more likely to have disease progression as determined in the vascular laboratory (52% vs. 33%). The patients with elevated homocysteine were also noted to have more rapid progression of lower extremity disease, as well as greater and more rapid progression of coronary disease. Interestingly, progression of cerebrovascular disease did not appear to be influenced by homocysteine.

The effect of elevated homocysteine on the results of vascular intervention are also poorly characterized but of great importance. Currie et al. in 1996 evaluated 66 patients who underwent angioplasty or vascular surgery for lower extremity ischemia.[22] Forty-one young patients (under 45 years old) were matched with 25 older patients. Basal homocysteine was measured by HPLC. Elevated homocysteine (>95th %) was seen in 19% of patients. Multivariate analysis identified young age, diabetes, and elevated homocysteine as independent risk factors for failure of vascular procedures.

A similar relationship between elevated homocysteine and failure following surgical intervention was noted by Irvine et al.[23] In this study, homocysteine was found to be an independent risk factor for the development of vein graft stenosis following lower extremity bypass. Using a case-control study design, 19 patients with vein graft stenoses and 19 controls were matched for age, sex, diabetes, tobacco, and time from surgery. Patients with vein graft stenosis had significantly higher homocysteine than controls, suggesting that elevated homocysteine may lead to vein graft stenosis.

Table 1. Nonfatal Progression of Atherosclerosis

| Parameter | Group | % with progression after 3 yrs* | p ** |
|---|---|---|---|
| CAD | highest 20%Hcy | 80% | 0.0068 |
| | lowest 20% Hcy | 39% | |
| CVD | highest 20%Hcy | 11% | 0.659 |
| | lowest 20%Hcy | 9% | |
| LED | highest 20%Hcy | 15% | 0.31 |
| | lowest 20%Hcy | 7% | |
| Stroke | highest 20%Hcy | 9% | 0.279 |
| | lowest 20%Hcy | 2% | |
| MI | highest 20%Hcy | 11% | 0.454 |
| | lowest 20%Hcy | 5% | |
| Worse ischemia | highest 20%Hcy | 15% | 0.171 |
| | lowest 20%Hcy | 3% | |

* life table method, ** probability by log rank test, Hcy - homocysteine, CAD - coronary artery disease, CVD - cerebrovascular disease, LED - lower extremity disease, MI - myocardial infarction, Worse ischemia - increase in severity of lower extremity ischemia, highest 20% Hcy - 1/5 of subjects with highest Hcy levels (17.9 - 64.1 µmol/L), lowest 20% Hcy - 1/5 of subjects with lowest Hcy levels (5.6 - 9.3 µmol/L), (Used with permission from Taylor, et al.[24])

## PROSPECTIVE EVALUATION OF HOMOCYSTEINE AND PROGRESSION OF PERIPHERAL VASCULAR DISEASE

To definitively answer the question of whether folate therapy can prevent the progression of peripheral vascular disease, the results of prospective, randomized studies must be awaited. We are currently engaged in such a study evaluating the influence of homocysteine on the progression of cerebrovascular and peripheral vascular disease (the Homocysteine and Progression of Atherosclerosis Study {HPAS}). Four-hundred and eight subjects were initially recruited, with 351 remaining available for follow-up. Vascular disease was defined as vascular laboratory evidence of lower extremity disease (85%), cerebrovascular disease (CVD, 35%), or both (25%). Progression of disease was documented by serial noninvasive peripheral arterial vascular laboratory exams, vascular laboratory carotid duplex exams, and clinical exams every 6 months. Plasma homo cysteine was measured by high performance liquid chromatogrphy (HPLC) at enrollment and every 6 months. Primary endpoints were defined as death, or disease progression (ankle-brachial index decrease >0.15, or cerebrovascular exam increase by one category according to the University of Washington criteria). Secondary endpoints were clinical progression of CVD, PVD, or coronary artery disease (CAD).

The first phase of HPAS was a 3 year observational study which has now been completed.[24] At a mean follow-up of 37 months, several important observations have been made. The mean homocysteine level of all patients was at the cutoff of the 95th percentile for normal controls in our lab (14 µmol/L). Homocysteine showed an inverse association with folate, vitamin $B_6$, and vitamin $B_{12}$ levels. Patients with homocysteine levels above 14 had a greater risk of death, death from CAD, and clinical progression of CAD at 3 years compared to patients with homocysteine < 14 µmol/L. Each 1.0 µmol/L increase in homocysteine conferred a 3.3% increase in the risk of death from any cause at 3 years, and a 5.6% increase in the risk of cardiovascular death at 3 years.

Both vascular laboratory evidence of progression and clinical progression of lower extremity disease were worse in patients in the upper 20th percentile of homocysteine compared to those in the lower 20th percentile, but did not reach statistical significance (Table 1). Interestingly, clinical and laboratory progression of CVD appeared unaffected by homocysteine level. Nonfatal clinical progression of CAD was significantly worse in patients with homocysteine in the upper 20th percentile, compared to those in the lower 20th percentile.

Multivariate analysis determined the relative risk of death associated with vascular lab progression of disease was 1.58 (Table 2). Elevated homocysteine (>95th%) had a marginal effect on the risk of death. However, when stratified by levels of homocysteine, there was a clear influence on death (Table 3). Homocysteine in the highest quintile conferred a relative risk of death of 3.13 compared to the lowest quintile. There was a nearly linear relationship between homocysteine and the relative risk of cardiovascular death (Figure 1). Decreased levels of folate, vitamin $B_6$, and vitamin $B_{12}$ were associated with an increased risk of death, but this effect was never more than that seen due to elevated homocysteine.

These results document in prospective, blinded fashion the significant effect of elevated homocysteine on cardiovascular mortality. An effect of elevated homocysteine on the progression of lower extremity disease is suggested but not proven. The lack of statistical significance may be due to the relatively short follow-up (37 months), or possibly the censoring effect of early death. This latter suggestion is supported by the increased risk of death conferred by vascular lab progression of PVD.

Phase two of HPAS is a randomized, double-blind, placebo-controlled treatment phase and is ongoing. During this portion of the study, patients will be

Table 2. Relative Risk of Death* Associated with Various Atherosclerosis Risk Factors

| Factor | Relative Risk of Death | 95% C.I. | p ** |
|---|---|---|---|
| VL Progression | 1.58 | 1.17 - 2.19 | 0.003 |
| Elevated Hcy | 1.30 | 0.96 - 1.46 | 0.088 |
| Hypertension | 1.47 | 1.05 - 2.12 | 0.024 |
| Age | 1.03 | 1.00 - 1.07 | 0.049 |
| Smoking | 1.001 | 1.00 - 1.002 | 0.043 |

* significant risk factors influencing time to death in a Cox proportional hazards model which originally considered age, gender, diabetes, cholesterol, smoking, hypertension, CAD, LED, CVD, vascular laboratory progression of CVD and/or LED, creatinine, levels of folate, $B_{12}$, $B_6$, and plasma Hcy. Insignificant variables were eliminated in sequential fashion to determine the relative risk of those remaining significant.
** probability by likelihood ratio testing, Hcy - homocysteine, Elevated Hcy - plasma Hcy > 14 $\mu$mol/L, Age - Relative risk due to increasing age in yearly increments over age 40 yrs, Smoking - Relative risk due to each mg/ml increase in plasma cotinine over 150 mg/ml, VL Progression - Relative risk due to occurrence of progression of lower extremity or carotid artery disease by vascular laboratory testing, (Used with permission from Taylor, et al.[24])

given daily folate (4 mg/day) or placebo. These patients will undergo clinical and vascular laboratory follow-up every 6 months for five years. The results of this second phase prove to be important and will have significant ramifications for the treatment of patients not only with peripheral vascular disease, but also cerebrovascular and coronary artery disease.

CONCLUSIONS

There is a clear association between elevated homocysteine and the presence of peripheral vascular disease. This relationship appear to be independent of any traditional risk factors (diabetes, smoking, hypertension, lipid abnormalities) and is present in 20-50% of patients with peripheral vascular disease. There appears to be an inverse relationship between homocysteine and levels of folate, vitamin $B_6$ and vitamin $B_{12}$. Treatment with folic acid and/or vitamin $B_6$ reliably and quickly (4-6 weeks) reduces elevated homocysteine levels to normal with no appreciable side effects.

Table 3. Relative Risk of Death* Associated with Increasing Levels of Plasma Homocysteine

| Homocysteine group | Relative Risk | 95% C.I. | p ** |
|---|---|---|---|
| elevated Hcy vs nl Hcy | 1.30 | 0.96 - 1.46 | 0.088 |
| highest 33% Hcy vs lowest 33% Hcy | 1.61 | 1.04 - 2.56 | 0.029 |
| highest 25% Hcy vs lowest 25% Hcy | 2.02 | 1.23 - 3.51 | 0.005 |
| highest 20% Hcy vs lowest 20% Hcy | 3.13 | 1.69 - 6.64 | 0.0001 |

* influence of plasma Hcy levels on time to death in a Cox proportional hazards model which included age, smoking, hypertension, and vascular laboratory progression of disease.
** probability by likelihood ratio testing
Hcy - homocysteine
highest 33% Hcy - 1/3 of subjects with highest Hcy levels (14.9 - 64.1 μmol/L)
lowest 33% Hcy - 1/3 of subjects with lowest Hcy levels (5.6 10.6 μmol/L)
highest 25% Hcy - 1/4 of subjects with highest Hcy levels (16.7 - 64.1 μmol/L)
lowest 25% Hcy - 1/4 of subjects with lowest Hcy levels (5.6 - 9.8 μmol/L)
highest 20% Hcy - 1/5 of subjects with highest Hcy levels (17.9 - 64.1 μmol/L)
lowest 20% Hcy - 1/5 of subjects with lowest Hcy levels (5.6 - 9.3 μmol/L)
(Used with permission from Taylor, et al.[24])

   While elevated homocysteine is associated with peripheral vascular disease, its effect on the progression of PVD remains largely undocumented. Retrospective studies have suggested that elevated homocysteine is a risk factor for the progression of peripheral vascular disease, as well as the failure of vascular procedures. Large, prospective trials are currently underway to evaluate the role of folic acid and vitamin B$_6$ therapy in secondary prevention of all forms of vascular disease, including peripheral vascular disease.
   The Homocysteine and Progression of Atherosclerosis Study is ongoing to provide some important answers. Phase one of has shown that coronary artery disease and death are strongly influenced this study by elevated homocysteine. A trend toward more rapid progression of PVD was seen in patients with elevated homocysteine, but statistical significance was not reached. Prospective information is being accumulated in phase two of HPAS to evaluate the effects of folate therapy on patients with PVD and will be available in several years.

## RELATIVE RISK OF DEATH FROM CARDIOVASCULAR DISEASE WITH INCREASING HOMOCYSTEINE

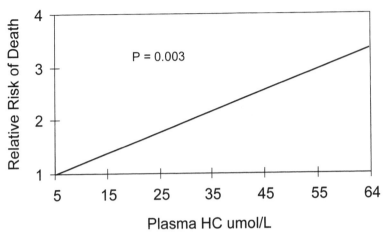

*Figure 1. Increasing relative risk of death from cardiovascular disease associated with increasing levels of plasma homocysteine (in μmol/L). Brackets indicate 95% C.I. (Used with permission from Taylor, et al.[24])*

REFERENCES

1. Boers GHJ, Smals AGH, Trijbels FJM, et al. Heterozygosity for homocystinuria in premature peripheral and cerebral occlusive arterial disease. N Engl J Med 1985;313:709-15.

2. Brattström L, Israelsson B, Norrving B, et Impaired homocysteine metabolism in early-onset cerebral and peripheral occlusive arterial disease: effects of pyridoxine and folic acid treatment. Atherosclerosis 1990;80:51-60.

3. Malinow MR, Kang SS, Taylor LM, et al. Prevalence of hyperhomocyst(e)inemia in patients with peripheral arterial occlusive disease. Circulation 1989;79:1180-88.

4. Clarke R, Daly L, Robinson K, et al. Hyperhomocysteinemia: an independent risk factor for vascular disease. N Engl J Med 1991;324:1149-55.

5. Molgaard J, Malinow MR, Lassvik C, Holm AC, Upson B, Olsson AG. Hyperhomocyst(e)inemia: an independent risk factor for IC. J Int Med 1992;231:273-9.

6. Aronson DC, Onkenhout W, Raben AMTJ, Oudenhoven LFIJ, Brommer EJP, vanBockel JH. Impaired homocysteine metabolism: a risk factor in young adults with atherosclerotic arterial occlusive disease of the leg. Br J Surg 1994;81:1114-8.

7. Bergmark C, Mansoor MA, Swedenborg J, deFaire U, Svardal AM, Ueland PM. Hyperhomocysteinemia in patients operated for lower extremity ischemia below the age of 50 - effect of smoking and extent of disease. Eur J Vasc Surg 1993;7:391-6.

8.  Van den Berg M, Stehouwer CDA, Bierdrager E, Rauwerda JA. Plasma homocysteine and severity of atherosclerosis in young patients with lower-limb atherosclerotic disease. Arterioscler Thromb Vasc Biol 1996;16:165-71.

9.  Cheng SWK, Ting ACW, Wong J. Fasting total plasma homocysteine and atherosclerotic peripheral vascular disease. Ann Vasc Surg 1997;11:217-23.

10. Graham IM, Daly LE, Refsum HM, et Plasma homocysteine as a risk factor for vascular disease. JAMA 1997;277:1775-81.

11. Boushey CJ, Beresford SAA, Omenn GS, Motulsky AG. A quantitative assessment of plasma homocysteine as a risk factor for vascular disease: probable benefits of increasing folic acid intakes. JAMA 1995;274:1049-1057.

12. Robinson K, Arheart K, Refsum H, et al. Low circulating folate and vitamin $B_6$ concentrations: risk factors for stroke, peripheral vascular disease, and coronary artery disease. Circulation 1998;97:437-43.

13. Van den Berg M, Franken DG, Boers GHJ, et al. Combined vitamin $B_6$ plus folic acid therapy in young patients with arteriosclerosis and hyperhomocysteinemia. J Vasc Surg 1994;20:933-40.

14. Kang SS, Wong PWK. Genetic and nongenetic factors for moderate hyperhomocyst(e)inemia. Atherosclerosis 1996;119:135-8.

15. Selhub J, Jacques PF, Wilson PWF, Rush D, Rosenberg IH. Vitamin status and intake as primary determinants of homocysteinemia in an elderly population. JAMA 1993;270:2693-8.

16. Welch GN, Loscalzo J. Homocysteine and atherothrombosis. N Engl J Med 1998;338:1042-50.

17. Taylor LM Jr, Porter JM. Elevated plasma homocysteine as a risk factor for atherosclerosis. Sem Vasc Surg 1993;6:36-45.

18. Nehler MR, Taylor LM Jr, Porter JM. Homocysteinemia as a risk factor for atherosclerosis: a review. Cardiovasc Surg 1997;5:559-567.

19. Franken DG, Boers GHJ, Blom HJ, Trijbels FJM, Kloppenborg PWC. Treatment of mild hyperhomocysteinemia in vascular disease patients. Arterioscler Thromb 1994;14:465-70.

20. Van den Berg M, Boers GHJ, Franken DG, et al. Hyperhomocysteinemia and endothelial dysfunction in young patients with peripheral arterial occlusive disease. Eur J Clin Invest 1995;25:176-81.

21. Taylor LM Jr, DeFrang RD, Harris EJ Jr, Porter JM. The association of elevated plasma homocyst(e)ine with progression of symptomatic peripheral arterial disease. J Vasc Surg 1991;13:128-36.

22. Currie IC, Wilson YG, Scott J, et al. Homocysteine: an independent risk factor for the failure of vascular intervention. Br J Surg 1996;83:1238-41.

23. Irvine C, Wilson Y, Currie I, et al. Hyperhomocysteinemia: a risk factor for vein graft stenosis. Br J Surg 1996;83:556.

24. Taylor LM Jr, Moneta GL, Sexton GJ, Schuff RA, Porter JM, and the HPAS Investigators. Prospective blinded study of the relationship between plasma homocysteine and progression of symptomatic peripheral arterial disease. J Vasc Surg 1999;29:8-21.

# 10. HOMOCYSTEINE AS A RISK FACTOR FOR CEREBROVASCULAR DISEASE AND STROKE

IVAN J PERRY

## SUMMARY

The balance of evidence from observational studies suggests that elevated homocysteine levels are associated with increased risk of carotid artery disease and stroke. There are also preliminary data linking hyperhomocysteinemia with cognitive decline in the elderly and specifically with vascular and non-vascular dementia. However, much of the current data are based on cross-sectional and case control study designs that are susceptible to selection and measurement bias. There are additional concerns regarding unmeasured and residual confounding due to a range of factors associated with hyperhomocysteinemia, including an atherogenic diet and cigarette smoking. There is a paucity of good prospective data. Moreover, homozygosity for a defective thermolabile variant of MTHFR, a common genetic polymorphism which results in hyper-homocysteinemia, has not been consistently linked with stroke or other vascular disease. There is a need for additional prospective studies with sufficient power to characterise the form of the association between homocysteine concentrations and cerebrovascular disease risk, whether linear or threshold, and to study the independent effects of homocysteine concentrations in analyses adjusted for additional dietary exposures such as vitamin $B_6$ and established stroke risk factors, such as smoking and hypertension. Given the extent to which dietary exposures are intercorrelated and are measured with varying but generally limited reliability, this poses a

*K. Robinson (ed.), Homocysteine and Vascular Disease, 151-172.*
© 2000 *Kluwer Academic Publishers. Printed in the Netherlands.*

major challenge for observational epidemiology. Folate supplementation effectively lowers homocysteine levels, regardless of the origin of hyperhomocysteinemia. Ultimately, the case for a causal role for elevated homocysteine concentrations in cerebrovascular disease and related conditions will depend on the findings from randomized controlled trials of the effect of folate supplementation in the primary and secondary prevention of vascular end-points. A number of such trials are ongoing at present. It is likely that the data from these trials will show, at best, a modest independent effect of homocysteine on risk of cerebrovascular disease. However, given the high prevalence of hyperhomocysteinemia in apparently well nourished populations and the tendency for homocysteine concentrations to increase with age, modest effects on cerebrovascular disease risk will have profound implications for public health.

## INTRODUCTION

It is now almost three decades since McCully first linked elevated plasma homocysteine concentrations with vascular disease on the basis of clinical observations in patients with homocystinuria[1]. Homocystinuria results from one of several rare genetic disorders of enzymes involved in homocysteine metabolism. It is characterized by markedly elevated concentrations of homocysteine in plasma and high risk of atherothrombotic events, including myocardial infarction and stroke in early adolescence and even in childhood[2]. It is estimated that approximately 50% of patients with untreated homocystinuria will have a major vascular event before the age of 30 years[2]. A plethora of pathophysiological mechanisms linking hyperhomocysteinemia with atherothrombotic vascular disease have been proposed on the basis of studies in humans and in animal models, reviewed in reference 3 and in chapters 7 and 19-21[3].

In recent years it has emerged that moderately elevated plasma homocysteine concentrations are common in the general population[9,5] and that moderate hyperhomocysteinemia may also be a risk factor for vascular disease, including peripheral[7] vascular disease, ischemic heart disease and stroke[6]. Hyperhomocysteinemia has also been linked with deep venous thrombosis[7], vascular disease in systemic lupus erythematosus[8] and tentatively with a number of other conditions including dementia[9,10] and pre-eclampsia[11,12]. Moderate hyperhomocysteinemia reflects less critical genetic defects combined with deficiency of nutritional co-factors required for homocysteine metabolism, folate, vitamin $B_{12}$ and vitamin $B_6$[4,13]. Folate intake is the key nutritional determinant of homocysteine concentrations in the general population and it appears that dietary supplementation, at modest dose levels (circa 400µg folate daily), effectively lowers homocysteine concentrations, regardless of the origin of hyperhomocysteinemia[6]. Thus, the putative link between total homocysteine concentrations in blood and vascular disease end-points has clear and important implications for basic laboratory science, clinical practice and public health.

As we approach the 30th anniversary of McCully's classic paper it may now be timely to consider the current status of this hypothesis. Specifically, this review will consider the evidence from observational studies linking raized homocysteine concentrations to risk of cerebrovascular disease and stroke. Associations between homocysteine and established stroke risk factors will be addressed, with particular reference to the data on smoking and blood pressure. The potential role of hyperhomocysteinemia in vascular and non vascular dementia and in related neuropsychiatric disorders in the elderly will be briefly considered. The metabolism of homocysteine, which is critical to understanding the genetic and environmental determinants of hyperhomocysteinemia is addressed in detail in Chapter 3. Suggested pathophysiological mechanisms linking hyperhomocysteinemia with arteriosclerotic vascular disease are reviewed in (Chapters 19-21).

## HOMOCYSTEINE AND ESTABLISHED CVD RISK FACTORS

Elevated homocysteine levels are associated with declining renal function and, to a variable degree, with established risk factors for cardiovascular disease including increasing age, male sex, cigarette smoking, high blood pressure, elevated cholesterol levels and lack of exercise[14,15]. The age-related increase in homocysteine levels, which is most marked in the oldest age groups[4,14], may be linked in part to renal impairment. It is hypothesized that the sex differences are due to the fact that more than 75% of homocysteine production occurs by demethylation of methionine in direct conjunction with creatine-creatinine synthesis which is a function of muscle mass and is higher in men than in women[15]. A homocysteine lowering effect of oestrogen has also been suggested[16]. Studies examining differences in homocysteine levels before and after the menopause and in women using or not using oestrogen containing oral contraceptives are[17] discussed in chapter 13.

### Homocysteine and cigarette smoking

In the Hordaland Study, associations between homocysteine concentrations and key stroke risk factors, including cigarette smoking, physical inactivity and blood pressure have been examined with considerable power. In contrast to the findings in some earlier, relatively small, studies[17], homocysteine levels were consistently higher in smokers than in non-smokers and increased steadily with the number of cigarette smoked in men and women and in younger and older age groups. The dose response relation between homocysteine and cigarette smoking was strongest in the oldest age group (65-67 years) and in women. In multivariate analysis, homocysteine increased by an average of 1% in women and by 0.6% in men for each cigarette smoked per day[15]. While the mechanism whereby smoking increases homocysteine concentrations has not been clarified, dietary folate intake is likely to be lower in smokers than non-smokers[18] and cigarette smoking may interfere with the synthesis of vitamin $B_6$[19].

## Homocysteine and blood pressure

It would seem reasonable to predict an association between homocysteine and blood pressure in the general population, given the well described associations between hyperhomocysteinemia and renal impairment[14] and the postulated effects of homocysteine on vascular endothelial function and proliferation of vascular smooth muscle cells[3]. Few studies have addressed this question directly with adequate power. In the Hordaland Study, a significant positive association with blood pressure was observed[15]. However this association was weak and was confined to younger men and women (40-42 age group). In this study, homocysteine was not significantly associated with blood pressure in a sub-group of 1386 men and 1932 women aged 65 to 74 years. Similarly, in data from the UK National Diet and Nutrition Survey, homocysteine was only weakly associated with blood pressure in a group of 972 people aged 65 years and over[20]. Dalery and colleagues determined plasma levels of homocysteine in 584 healthy French Canadian subjects (380 men and 204 women) and in 150 subjects (123 men and 27 women) with angiographically documented coronary artery disease (age < 60 years). No significant correlation was found between plasma homocysteine levels and the presence of hypertension in healthy subjects or in patients with coronary artery disease[21]. By contrast, in a small case-control study involving less than 400 older adults, Sutton-Tyrrell and colleagues found that fasting homocysteine was significantly associated with isolated systolic hypertension[22]. Of course, weak or inconsistent associations between homocysteine and blood pressure may simply reflect measurement error or the limited reliability with which homocysteine and blood pressure are measured. In the Hordaland study for instance, measurements of homocysteine concentrations were obtained from non-fasting samples and the blood pressure data were based on the second of three measurements. Aside from the error in blood pressure measurement, it is estimated that studies based on single homocysteine measurements underestimate the magnitude of risk associations with disease by 10-15%, given the degree of within subject relative to between subject variation in homocysteine measurements[23].

Given the putative pathophysiological mechanisms linking hyperhomocysteinemia with vascular disease, there is a clear need for additional studies of the relation between homocysteine and blood pressure. Good data on the effect of folate supplementation on blood pressure would be of particular interest. In a recent paper, Nakata and colleagues have described lower blood pressure in a group of patients with the common V allele of the MTHFR gene relative to those without this mutation[24]. The latter mutation, which is associated with a defective thermolabile variant of MTHFR, is an important cause of hyperhomocysteinemia in the general population[25]. It has not been consistently found to be associated with stroke or with other manifestations of cardiovascular disease[26,27]. Clearly, this intriguing finding of lower blood pressure in association with an important genetic cause of hyperhomocysteinemia requires replication in other populations. If confirmed, it raises important questions about the postulated adverse effects of mild hyperhomocysteinemia and it may help clarify the interpretation of the negative gene association studies in this area.

## Homocysteine and markers for the insulin resistance syndrome

Associations between homocysteine, obesity and diabetes have received remarkably little direct attention despite the importance of the latter factors in the development of cardiovascular disease, including stroke. Earlier investigations of these associations were largely confined to relatively small case control studies in which the focus was on the link between homocysteine and major vascular disease end points. No significant associations between homocysteine and either obesity or diabetes were identified in these studies but most lacked power to address associations between homocysteine and established risk factors[17]. Unfortunately, in the Hordaland study, data on measures of obesity and glucose tolerance were not available[15]. In a recent study, Araki and colleagues compared homocysteine levels in diabetic patients with and without macroangiopathy and in a group of 57 non-diabetic control subjects. Homocysteine levels were highest in diabetics with macroangiopathy, intermediate in those without macro angiopathy and lowest in the control group. However, the differences in homocysteine levels between diabetics without macro angiopathy (the group of major interest) and controls were small and were significant only in women[28]. In a further small study, it was reported that type 2 diabetes patients with complications had higher basal homocysteine values than diabetics without complications[29]. In this study diabetics with elevated homocysteine levels had significantly higher diastolic blood pressure and mean arterial pressure and higher plasma folate values were associated with lower systolic blood pressure and mean arterial pressure. While these finding on homocysteine and nutritional determinants in diabetes are interesting, the question of confounding due to renal impairment needs to be addressed in detail.

Physical activity levels are important predictors of insulin resistance and type 2 diabetes. In the Hordaland study, homocysteine concentrations increased in a graded fashion with increasing heart rate and decreased with increasing reported exercise levels[15]. Thus on the basis of these observations, one would anticipate an association between hyperhomocysteinemia and insulin resistance together with other manifestations of the metabolic (insulin resistance) syndrome. There is, in fact, preliminary evidence that hyperhomocysteinemia is associated with insulin resistance[30]. If confirmed, this observation may have implications for the increased risk of vascular disease associated with the insulin resistance syndrome. However, it also raises the spectre of residual confounding, due to lifestyle related predictors of insulin resistance, in the existing data linking raized homocysteine with vascular disease endpoints.

**Significance of associations with established risk factors**

These associations between hyperhomocysteinemia and established vascular risk factors are likely to reflect, at least in part, links with common underlying dietary and life-style factors, in particular a diet high in saturated fat with inadequate folate intake from fruit and vegetables combined with smoking and physical inactivity. Given this background of multiple inter-correlated dietary and lifestyle factors, measured with variable reliability, it is clear that the question of independent effects of homocysteine concentrations on vascular disease risk, including stroke, must be approached with considerable caution[31]. In the Hordaland Study, for example, sex, age, folate intake, smoking status and coffee consumption were the strongest determinants of plasma homocysteine concentration in multivariate analysis[32]. The combined effect of the latter three factors was considerably larger than the effects from each factor alone. A lifestyle profile characterized by low folate intakes, smoking and coffee consumption was associated with pronounced skewness of the homocysteine distribution towards higher values[32].

The association of homocysteine with renal impairment[14] is of particular relevance to the interpretation of retrospective case control and cross-sectional studies of homocysteine and stroke as in most of these studies the data were not adjusted for serum creatinine or other measures of renal impairment.

## HOMOCYSTEINE AND RISK OF STROKE

Early studies of homocysteine and vascular end points used methionine loading to stress the metabolic pathways responsible for homocysteine degradation. With the development in the 1980's of analytical methods which measure both free and protein bound homocysteine fractions in plasma, it became feasible to measure basal homocysteine levels[34]. In epidemiological studies, it appears that basal fasting (or non-fasting) homocysteine measurements are of broadly similar reliability* to post-methionine load measurements. There is evidence however that a different group of individuals will be identified as at high risk, i.e. hyperhomocysteinemic depending on whether fasting or post-load measurements are used[35].

Associations between homocysteine concentrations and related markers of abnormal methionine metabolism and risk of stroke have been studied for over a decade (Table I). Boushey and colleagues have reported on a meta-analysis of 27 observational studies, published before 1994, relating homocysteine to atherosclerotic vascular disease of which 11 studies addressed the association between homocysteine and risk of stroke. Nine case control studies provided support for the hypothesis that homocysteine is an independent risk factor for stroke while two prospective studies were negative. The summary odds ratio for cerebrovascular disease in persons with elevated homocysteine levels, (generally defined as above the 95th percentile for the control group or above 2SD of the control mean) was 2.5 (95% CI, 2.0 to 3.0). In six studies with fasting blood samples, the summary odds ratio for a 5 umol/L increment in homocysteine (approximately one SD from the mean level in the normal population) was 1.9 (95% CI, 1.6 to 2.3), i.e. an approximate two-fold increase in risk. This association was of broadly similar magnitude to that seen between fasting homocysteine levels and risk of coronary heart disease in this meta-analysis.

Clearly the data from a meta-analysis of observational studies of variable design and methodological rigor with variable and often inadequate adjustment for potential confounders must be interpreted cautiously. In this meta-analysis the study design of seven of the nine case control studies was categorized as "other case control". This "other case control" study category includes a high proportion of small studies based on controls recruited from either ill-defined screening exercises or volunteer samples. In a number of these smaller case control studies, the method of recruitment of cases is also ill defined. The Boushey meta-analysis includes data from the European Concerted Action project which had been presented in abstract

---

* Defined in terms of the ratio of random within subject to between subject variation. A critical determinant of study power.

*Table I: Observational studies of homocysteine and risk of stroke. [77]*

| First Author | Year | No. of Cases/Controls | Age. y | Study design | Support for Hcy as risk factor |
|---|---|---|---|---|---|
| *Brattstrom[68] | 1984 | 19/17 | 34-63 | Other Case-control | YES |
| *Boers[69] | 1985 | 25/40 | <50 | Other case-control | YES |
| *Araki[70] | 1989 | 90/45 | 39-79 | Hospital case-control | YES |
| *Brattstrom[71] | 1990 | 18/46 | 24-63 | Other case-control | YES |
| *Coull[72] | 1990 | 41/31 | 67/61 | Other case-control | YES |
| *Clarke[73] | 1991 | 38/27 | <55 | Other case-control | YES |
| *Brattstrom[74] | 1992 | 70/66 | 38-72 | Population case-control | YES |
| *Dudman[75] | 1993 | 51/56 | <61 | Other case-control | |
| *Graham and Daly ** | 1994 | 214/810 | <55 | Other case-control | YES |
| *Alfthan[37] | 1994 | 74/269M | 40-60 | Nested case-control | NO |
| *Verhoef[38] | 1994 | 109/427 M | 60 | Nested case-control | NO |
| Perry[39] | 1995 | 107/118 | 40-59 | Nested case-control | YES |
| Botts **[41] | 1997 | 120/630 | >60 | Nested case-control | EQUIVOCAL |
| Graham[35] | 1997 | 750/800 | <60 | Other case-control | YES |

* Included in Boushey meta-analysis        ** Abstract

form in 1994. This study contributed 214 of the total of 566 stroke cases included in the meta analysis. Even in this carefully conducted study, less than one half of controls were recruited from random community samples and one sixth were hospital employees. The potential for selection bias due to volunteer controls or those recruited from work place settings should not be under estimated. Given the evidence that homocysteine levels increase post stroke[36], and the fact that the two prospective studies included in this meta-analysis, based on a nested case control design, were negative[37,38], it is clear that the summary estimates of the effect of homocysteine concentrations on stroke risk must be regarded as tentative. The lack of small negative studies in this meta-analysis raises additional concerns regarding publication bias. Although one assumes that the authors made strenuous efforts to identify unpublished work, this issue was not addressed directly in their paper.

## European Concerted Action Project

Data from the European Concerted Action Project study of homocysteine and risk of atherosclerotic vascular disease were published in full in 1997[35]. As one would expect, the findings from this large case-control study involving a total of 750 cases of atherosclerotic vascular disease (cardiac, cerebral and peripheral) and 800 controls of both sexes, younger than 60 years, are largely consistent with the earlier meta-analysis to which it had made a substantial contribution. The relative risk of stroke was increased more than two-fold in the top fifth of both the fasting and post-load total homocysteine distribution, relative to the bottom four-fifths with minimal attenuation on adjustment for major established risk factors. There was also evidence of a modest dose response relation between total homocysteine level and risk of vascular disease including stroke across the distribution of homocysteine. The level of vascular disease risk in the upper quintile of homocysteine was equivalent to that associated with hypercholesterolemia or cigarette smoking and interaction effects were noted with risk amplified in the presence of either cigarette smoking or hypertension[35].

## Recent prospective studies

The association between serum homocysteine concentration (non-fasting) and stroke was examined in a nested case-control study within the British Regional Heart Study cohort[39,40]. During an average of 12.8 years follow-up in the cohort, which is based on a representative sample of over 7000 middle-aged British men, there were 141 incident cases of stroke. Serum homocysteine was measured in 107 cases and 118 controls, the latter chosen from men who were without a history of stroke at screening and who did not develop a stroke or myocardial infarction during follow-up. Levels of homocysteine were significantly higher in cases than controls and there was a graded increase in the relative risk (odds ratio) of stroke in the 2nd, 3rd and 4th quarters of homocysteine (OR 1.3, 1.9, 2.8; trend p = 0.005) relative to the first quarter. In these data, contrary to what one might have anticipated from the Hordaland study findings, adjustment for a wide range of potential confounders, including serum creatinine, did not attenuate the association. In a subgroup analysis, confined to men without clinically detectable evidence of coronary heart disease at baseline (67 cases and 112 controls), the risk of stroke was also significantly increased in the fourth quarter of homocysteine relative to the first, odds ratio 2.5 (95% C.I. 1.1 to 6.1). These data are consistent with a graded relation between homocysteine and risk of stroke without an obvious threshold. However, the possibility of confounding due to specific dietary exposures, or markers of such exposures, which were not measured in this study must be considered.

Bots and colleagues have reported the findings on homocysteine and risk of cardiovascular disease in the Rotterdam Cohort[41]. In this elderly cohort there was a non-linear rather than a graded association between homocysteine (non-fasting) and major cardiovascular disease events, with a sharp increase in risk in the upper quintile of the distribution. The relative risk of stroke, adjusted for age and sex, in the upper quintile of homocysteine relative to the rest of the distribution was 2.1 (95% CI, 1.3 to 3.5) and the corresponding risk for myocardial infarction was 1.7 (95% CI, 1.0 to 2.9). These associations were attenuated and were non-significant on adjustment for additional cardiovascular risk factors. However stronger associations were observed in hypertensives and in current smokers[41]. The latter finding, which suggests an interaction between homocysteine and established stroke risk factors is consistent with the data from Graham and colleagues[35] and other studies[39].

## Homocysteine and carotid artery disease

Additional support for the homocysteine stroke hypothesis is provided by cross sectional studies, showing independent associations between homocysteine concentrations and carotid atherosclerosis[42,43,44,45,46]. In a study of 25 obligate heterozygotes for cystathionine β-synthase deficiency and 21 controls, Clarke and colleagues described elevated post methionine load homocysteine concentrations in subjects with asymptomatic carotid artery atherosclerosis on the basis of duplex ultrasound examination[42]. In the Atherosclerosis Risk in Communities (ARIC) study, the odds ratio for having a thickened carotid artery wall, as measured by B-mode ultrasound, was increased over three-fold among subjects in the top quintile of plasma homocysteine levels compared with those in the bottom quintile. This association was independent of a wide range of established cardiovascular disease risk factors, including age, waist-hip ratio, smoking and systolic blood pressure[43]. In a study of 1041 elderly participants in the Framingham Heart Study, Selhub and colleagues observed a significant association between plasma homocysteine and the prevalence of significant extracranial carotid artery stenosis in men and a similar, although weaker, association in women[44]. In this study the association between homocysteine and carotid artery disease was linear with abnormal findings at homocysteine concentrations regarded as within the normal range. Plasma concentrations of folate and pyridoxal-5'-phosphate and the level of dietary folate intake were inversely associated with carotid artery stenosis after adjustment for age, sex and other risk factors. Homocysteine and plasma folate predicted significant extracranial carotid artery stenosis independently of each other and the association with plasma pyridoxal-5'-phosphate was of borderline significance in regression models which included plasma homocysteine concentration.

Clearly, in these studies showing continuous associations between homocysteine and carotid atherosclerosis, there was less potential for bias due to event related dietary change or renal impairment than in cross sectional or conventional case control studies with symptomatic disease as the end point.

None the less, concerns about the confounding remain. For instance in both the ARIC study[43] and the Framingham Study of homocysteine and carotid artery stenosis[44], the data were not adjusted for serum creatinine or other measures of renal impairment. Moreover, there is growing evidence that atherosclerotic vascular disease is an inflammatory process[47,48]. It has been suggested that the inflammatory process, associated with vascular disease might result in an increased demand for folic acid with secondary elevation of homocysteine concentrations[49]. Although this suggestion must be regarded as speculative, it further emphasises the need to interpret data from cross sectional observational studies with caution.

## Folate/B vitamins and stroke

As folate intake is a key determinant of homocysteine levels in the general population[4] one would expect to find evidence of an association between serum folate levels and vascular risk. In prospective data from the US National Health and Nutrition Examination survey, a serum folate level $\leq 9.2$ nmol/L was associated with an over 3-fold increased risk of ischemic stroke in Black Americans, independent of major risk factors[50]. By contrast however, no association between folate levels and stroke risk was seen in White

Americans[50]. In a further paper from the European Concerted Action Project, it was reported that lower concentrations of both red cell folate and vitamin $B_6$ were associated with increased risk of vascular disease[51]. The association with folate was explained in part by increased homocysteine levels. In contrast, however, the relation between vitamin $B_6$ and atherosclerosis was independent of homocysteine levels, both before and after methionine loading[51]. The apparent independent effects of vitamin $B_6$ in this study emphasises the need for caution in ascribing independent effects of homocysteine on vascular disease. This concern has been further augmented by the recent prospective data from the ARIC study on the incidence of coronary heart disease in relation to levels of fasting total homocysteine and B vitamins[52]. In the latter study, plasma pyridoxal- 5 - phosphate but not plasma homocysteine was associated with CHD events in multivariate analysis. It is ironic that McCully in his seminal 1969 paper alluded to a earlier 1949 paper describing arteriosclerotic lesions in pyridoxine deficient monkeys[1]. The apparent independence of vitamin $B_6$ of homocysteine concentrations in studies of cardiovascular disease risk may simply reflect the precision or reliability with which this vitamin is measured in plasma or bias due to inclusion of users of multi-vitamin supplements in these observational studies. It is clear however that studies of mechanisms whereby vitamin $B_6$ might protect against atherosclerotic vascular disease, including stroke, are now warranted.

## HOMOCYSTEINE AND DEMENTIA

In clinical studies, deficiencies of both vitamin $B_{12}$ and folate have long been associated with neuropsychiatric disorders in the elderly, including depression and dementia[9,10,53,54,55,56]. There is now considerable evidence from population studies that nutritional deficiencies relating to hyperhomocysteinemia are widespread in the elderly[4] and that such deficiencies may contribute to cognitive decline in this age group[57]. Selhub and colleagues measured plasma homocysteine levels together with dietary intakes and blood levels of vitamin $B_{12}$, $B_6$ and folate in 1160 surviving elderly members of the Framingham Cohort Study. As expected, strong inverse associations between homocysteine concentrations and plasma concentrations of folate, vitamin $B_{12}$ and vitamin $B_6$ were observed and 29% of this relatively affluent population had homocysteine levels in excess of 14 µmol/l, above the 90th percentile in the US physicians' study[4]. In a survey of nutritional status and cognitive function in 260 elderly subjects, aged 60 – 94 years and living in the community, Goodwin and colleagues reported a significant relationship between abstract thinking ability and memory and low levels of folate intake[57].

Given this background and the consistent associations between hyperhomo-cysteinemia and cardiovascular disease in cross sectional studies, it is unsurprising that raized homocysteine levels have been found in patients with vascular dementia and in patients with other neuro-psychiatric disorders, including depression and Alzheimer's Disease. Vascular and non-vascular dementia and depression often co-exist in the elderly and are not reliably delineated from each other. One would also predict that homocysteine levels would be inversely associated with measures of cognitive function in the elderly. However, as with vascular disease generally, the question of whether hyperhomocysteine-mia is a cause or a consequence of vascular and non-vascular dementia, or simply a sensitive marker for underlying causal nutritional deficiencies, remains unclear.

Nilsson and colleagues have reported on measurements of total plasma homocysteine, serum $B_{12}$, and blood folate concentrations in a consecutive series of 510 psycho-geriatric patients and 163 controls[53]. The group of psycho-geriatric patients included 295 individuals with different forms of dementia, including Alzheimer's disease, vascular dementia and non-specified dementia and 215 patients with non-organic mental disorders, including confusional states and depression. Almost all of the different diagnostic groups of demented and non-demented patients exhibited significantly increased plasma homocysteine concentrations compared with control subjects. Significantly decreased blood folate concentrations were mainly found in the different diagnostic groups of demented patients but not in patients with non-organic mental disorders. Serum cobalamin levels were similar in patients and controls. The differences in homocysteine concentrations between controls and patients were substantial and were sustained in analyses confined to subjects with cobalamin and folate levels above the 20$^{th}$ percentile of the control group. The cross-sectional design of this and similar studies obviously precludes causal inference. The detailed findings on concentrations of vitamins in blood and serum in different sub-groups in this study are particularly difficult to interpret given that the data are based on patients referred to a specialist unit, with exclusion of a substantial number of those receiving vitamin supplements.

Joosten and colleagues measured serum folate, vitamin $B_{12}$, serum methylmalonic acid (MMA, a marker for vitamin $B_{12}$ deficiency) and total homocysteine in 52 patients with Alzheimer's disease, 50 non-demented hospitalized controls and 49 healthy elderly subjects living at home[54]. Although serum vitamin $B_{12}$ and folate levels were similar in patients with Alzheimer's disease, hospitalized controls and subjects living at home, patients with Alzheimer's disease had the highest serum methylmalonic acid and total homocysteine levels. The latter (MMA and homocysteine concentrations) were highest in patients with Alzheimer's disease, intermediate in the hospitalized controls and lowest in the community controls. The trend across the 3 groups was stronger for homocysteine than for MMA, with significant differences between Alzheimer's disease patients and hospitalized controls as well as between patients and healthy controls. On the most parsimonious interpretation, these findings (and those of Nilsson et al)[53] suggest that elevated homocysteine concentrations are simply a better marker for folate and B$_{12}$ deficiency than serum concentrations of these vitamins.

McCaddon and colleagues in a small but carefully conducted case control study, have reported substantially higher homocysteine levels a group of 30 patients with Alzheimer's disease, relative to 30 age-matched control subjects, median homocysteine (interquartile range ) 21.9 μmol/L (17.2-28) versus 12.2 μmol/L (9.5-16.6). This difference was independent of serum retinol binding protein, which is regarded as a sensitive marker of nutritional deficiency. In the small group of 30 patients, both serum homocysteine and cobalamin concentrations were significant predictors of cognitive scores in multiple regression analyses, that included adjustment for gender, age, folate, smoking and hypertension[10]. Similarly, in the Normative Ageing study, significant inverse associations were observed between homocysteine concentrations and specific measures of cognitive function, independent of folate and B$_{12}$ status[58]. However, as in studies of cardiovascular disease end-points, these independent associations of higher plasma homocysteine with cognitive dysfunction and with specific forms of dementia must be interpreted cautiously given the perennial problem of variable measurement reliability of the relevant nutritional exposures.

In a recent case-control study, involving 164 patients, aged 55 years or older, with a clinical diagnosis of dementia of Alzheimer type (including 76 patients with histologically confirmed Alzheimer disease) and 108 controls, Clarke and colleagues examined the association of Alzheimer disease with blood levels of homocysteine, folate and vitamin B$_{12}$[56]. Serum homocysteine levels were significantly higher and serum folate and vitamin B$_{12}$ levels were lower in patients Alzheimer disease (including the histologically confirmed group) than in controls. The odds ratio of confirmed Alzheimer disease associated with a homocysteine level in the top third ($\geq$ 14 μmol/L) compared with the bottom third ($\leq$ 11 μmol/L) of the control distribution was 4.5 (95% confidence interval, 2.2-9.2), after adjustment for age, sex, social class, cigarette smoking, and apolipoprotein E epsilon4. The corresponding odds ratio for the lower third compared with the upper third of serum folate distribution was 3.3 (95% confidence interval, 1.8-6.3) and of vitamin B$_{12}$ distribution was 4.3 (95% confidence interval, 2.1-8.8). The mean homocysteine levels were unaltered by duration of symptoms before enrollment and were stable for several years afterward. In a 3-year follow-up of the cases, radiological evidence of disease progression was greater among those with higher homocysteine levels at entry. The findings from this study provide some evidence that raized homocysteine levels in Alzheimers disease are not simply a consequence of disease and they should provide a stimulus for prospective studies (and trials) addressing the relation between homocysteine concentrations and cognitive decline in the elderly.

## Biological mechanisms

The lack of prospective data and of evidence of reversibility has not of course precluded speculation on biological mechanisms linking hyperhomocysteinemia with cognitive decline. It is suggested that hyperhomocysteinemia may be linked to the excitatory amino acid hypothesis of neuro-psychiatric disorders. Homocysteine is a precursor for homocysteic and homocysteine sulfinic acid, which are postulated to have a potent excitatory and toxic effect on the central nervous system, acting as endogenous NMDA receptor[9,55]. There is also evidence that homocysteine may have neurotoxic effects as a result of inhibition of methylation reactions that are regarded as central to the biochemical basis of several neuro-psychiatric disorders[55].

## CONCLUSIONS

Publication of the findings from a further meta-analysis of homocysteine and risk of cardiovascular disease (including cerebrovascular disease) is imminent (R Clarke. Personal communication). It is clear however that a causal link between elevated homocysteine concentrations and cerebrovascular disease has not yet been established. The inconsistent findings from prospective studies of homocysteine and stroke[37-39,41] (and other CVD endpoints[59,60-62,37-39,53]) does not augur well for the hypothesis. In extenuation, the problem of measurement imprecision of both homocysteine and vascular endpoints should be considered. In particular, it should be noted that the prospective studies have largely relied on homocysteine measurements from serum and plasma samples stored for prolonged periods under different conditions. However, the central concern in the existing data is that moderately elevated homocysteine concentrations may be a consequence rather than a cause of atheromatous vascular disease. Even in the positive prospective studies of homocysteine and risk of stroke, the possibility that homocysteine is simply a marker for more extensive sub-clinical disease, or for other dietary or lifestyle exposures related to vascular disease risk, cannot be entirely discounted. There is the additional concern that homozygosity for a defective thermolabile variant of MTHFR, a common genetic polymorphism which results in hyperhomocysteinemia, has not been consistently linked with cardiovascular disease end-points[26,27]. Although the importance of gene markers will vary depending on relevant environmental exposures, diet in this instance, the findings from gene association studies conducted to-date are distinctly unimpressive. Work on pathophysiological mechanisms provides at best a limited basis for causal inference. Unfortunately in this instance, the biological plausibility of the homocysteine-vascular disease hypothesis rests partially on studies that have used un-physiologically high doses of homocysteine[49]. Finally and crucially, we lack data from randomized controlled trials showing that homocysteine lowering interventions prevent vascular end points.

**Further work**

Kuller and Evans have suggested that case-control studies should be abandoned in future studies of homocysteine, vitamins and disease[49]. Indeed it is unlikely that the hypothesis linking raized homocysteine concentrations with risk of stroke will be substantially advanced or disproved by further cohort studies unless based on more reliable measures of all the relevant dietary exposures, including vitamin $B_6$. Ultimately, data from randomized controlled trials of homocysteine lowering interventions will resolve the issue of whether raized homocysteine concentrations are an important, modifiable risk factor for cerebrovascular disease and stroke and other manifestations of cardiovascular disease. Ideally, these trials will need to be large enough to detect both effects of lowering homocysteine concentrations and putative additional independent effects of B vitamins on vascular endpoints. A number of large-scale trials addressing this hypothesis are ongoing at present and are summarized in Chapter 23. Pending the results of these studies there is a need for secondary prevention studies, including studies of patients with established cerebrovascular disease. The latter are likely to be feasible with smaller sample sizes and shorter follow-up. Studies of the effect of homocysteine-lowering interventions on cognitive decline in the elderly will pose a key test of the homocysteine hypothesis and should receive high priority, as should studies of homocysteine lowering therapy in high risk states such as, Type 2 diabetes[63], and systemic lupus erythematosus[8]. Further work on the putative link between hyperhomocysteinemia and preeclampsia is warranted[11,12]. Preeclampsia is a multisystem disorder, characterized by profound vascular endothelial dysfunction, similar to that seen in atheroma[64]. The apparent increased risk of this condition seen in women with hyperhomocysteinemia provides significant support for the general homocysteine vascular disease hypothesis and this specific hypothesis should be readily testable in randomized controlled trials.

It is unlikely that the data from primary and secondary prevention trials will show more than a modest independent effect of homocysteine on risk of stroke and other vascular disease end-points. However, given the high prevalence of hyperhomocysteinemia in apparently well nourished populations and the tendency for homocysteine concentrations to increase with age, modest effects on stroke risk will have profound implications for public health[65]. On a more general but related issue, there is a need for intervention studies to address food based hypotheses, in particular the role of fruit and vegetables[66] (and possibly nuts[67]) in stroke prevention. From the public health perspective, the primary goal of research in this area is to identify modifiable nutritional determinants of cardiovascular disease risk, whether acting via raized homocysteine concentrations or through other mechanisms. The current uncertain status of the homocysteine vascular disease hypothesis highlights the limitations of observational epidemiology and of laboratory and clinical observations considered in isolation. The prize of clarifying the role of common nutritional deficiencies in the aetiology of cardiovascular disease with the attendant possibilities of prevention at the individual and population level will depend on continued collaboration between laboratory, clinical and population science disciplines.

## REFERENCES

1. McCully KS. Vascular pathology of homocysteinemia: implications for the pathogenesis of atherosclerosis. Am JPathol 1969;56: 111 -28.

2. Mudd SH, Skovby F, Levy HL, Pettigrew KD, Wilcken B, Pyeritz RE, et al. The natural history of homocystinuria due to cystathionine beta- synthase deficiency.AmJHum Genet 1985;37(1):1-31.

3. Welch GN, Loscalzo J. Homocysteine and atherothrombosis. NEngl JMed 1998;338(15):1042-50.

4. Selhub J, Jacques PF, Wilson PWF, Rush D, Rosenberg JH. Vitamin status and intake as primary determinants of homocysteinemia in an elderly population. JAMA 1993;270:2693-98.

5. Selhub J, Jacques PF, Bostom AG, D'Agostino RB, Wilson PW, Belanger AJ, et al. Relationship between plasma homocysteine, vitamin status and extracranial carotid-artery stenosis in the Framingham Study population. J Nutr 1996;126(4 Suppl):1258S-65S.

6. Boushey CJ, Beresford SAA, Omenn GS, Motulsky AG. A quantative assessment of plasma homocysteine as a risk factor for vascular disease. Probable benefits of increasing folic acid intakes. JAMA 1995;274:1049-57.

7. den Heijer M, Koster T, Blom HJ, Bos GM, Briet E, Reitsma PH, et al. Hyperhomocysteinemia as a risk factor for deep-vein thrombosis [see comments]. NEngl JMed 1996;334(12):759-62.

8. Petri M, Roubenoff R, Dallal GE, Nadeau MR, Selhub J, Rosenberg IH. Plasma homocysteine as a risk factor for atherothrombotic events in systemic lupus erythematosus. Lancet 1996;348(9035):1120-4.

168     *Ivan J Perry*

9. Bell IR, Edman JS, Selhub J, Morrow FD, Marby DW, Kayne HL, et al. Plasma homocysteine in vascular disease and in nonvascular dementia of depressed elderly people. Acta Psychiatr Scand 1992;86(5):386-90.

10. McCaddon A, Davies G, Hudson P, Tandy S, Cattell H. Total serum homocysteine in senile dementia of Alzheimer type [In Process Citation]. Int J Geriatr Psychiatry 1998; 13(4):235-9.

11. Dekker GA, de Vries JI, Doelitzsch PM, Huijgens PC, von Blomberg BM, Jakobs C, et al. Underlying disorders associated with severe early-onset preeclampsia. Am JObstet Gynecol 1995;173(4):1042-8.

12. Rajkovic A, Catalano PM, Malinow MR. Elevated homocyst(e)ine levels with preeclampsia. Obstet Gynecol 1997;90(2):168-71.

13. Stampfer MJ, Malinow MR. Can lowering homocysteine levels reduce cardiovascular disease risk? NEngl JMed 1995;332:328-29.

14. Brattstrom L, Lindgren A, Israelsson B, Andersson A, Hultberg B. Homocysteine and cysteine: determinants of plasma levels in middle-aged and elderly subjects. JIntern Med 1994;236(6):633-41.

15. Nygard O, Vollset SE, Refsum H, Stensvold I, Tverdal A, Nordrehaug JE, et al. Total plasma homocysteine and cardiovascular risk profile. The Hordaland Homocysteine Study. Jama 1995;274(19):1526-33.

16. Kang SS, Wong PW, Zhou JM, Cook HY. Total homocyst(e)ine in plasma and amniotic fluid of pregnant women. Metabolism 1986;35(10):889-91.

17. Malinow MR. Homocyst(e)ine and arterial occlusive diseases. JIntern Med 1994;236(6):603-17.

18. Subar AF, Harlan LC, Mattson ME. Food and nutrient intake differences between smokers and non-smokers in the US. Am JPublic Health 1990;80(11):1323-9.

19. Vermaak WJ, Ubbink JB, Barnard HC, Potgieter GM, van Jaarsveld H, Groenewald AJ. Vitamin B-6 nutrition status and cigarette smoking. Am J Clin Nutr 1990;51(6):1058-61.

20. Bates CJ, Mansoor MA, van der Pols J, Prentice A, Cole TJ, Finch S. Plasma total homocysteine in a representative sample of 972 British men and women aged 65 and over. Eur JClin Nutr 1997;51(10):691-7.

21. Dalery K, Lussier-Cacan S, Selhub J, Davignon J, Latour Y, Genest J, Jr. Homocysteine and coronary artery disease in French Canadian subjects: relation with vitamins $B_{12}$, $B_6$, pyridoxal phosphate, and folate. Am JCardiol 1995;75(16):1107-11.

22. Sutton-Tyrrell K, Bostom A, Selhub J, Zeigler-Johnson C. High homocysteine levels are independently related to isolated systolic hypertension inolderadults. Circulation 1997;96(6):1745-9.

23. Clarke R, Woodhouse P, Ulvik A, Frost C, Sherliker P, Refsum H, et al. Variability and determinants of total homocysteine concentrations in plasma in an elderly population. Clin Chem 1998;44(1):102-7.

24. Nakata Y, Katsuya T, Takami S, Sato N, Fu Y, Ishikawa K, et al. Methylenetetrahydrofolate reductase gene polymorphism: relation to blood pressure and cerebrovascular disease [In Process Citation]. Am JHypertens 1998;11(8 Pt 1):1019-23.

25. Frosst P BH, Milos R, Goyette P, Sheppard CA, Matthews RG, Boers GJH, Den Heijer M, Kluijtmans LAJ, van den Heuvel LP, Rosen R. A candidate genetic risk factor for vascular

disease: a common mutation in methylenetetrahydrofolate reductase. Nature Gen 1995; 10: 111-3.

26. Markus HS, Ali N, Swaminathan R, Sankaralingam A, Molloy J, Powell J. A common polymorphism in the methylenetetrahydrofolate reductase gene, homocysteine, and ischemic cerebrovascular disease [see comments]. Stroke 1997;28(9): 1739-43.

27. Brattstrom L. Common mutation in the methylenetetrahydrofolate reductase gene offers no support for mild hyperhomocysteinemia being a causal risk factor for cardiovascular disease [letter; comment]. Circulation 1997;96(10):3805-7.

28. Araki A, Sako Y, Ito H. Plasma homocysteine concentrations in Japanese patients with non- insulin-dependent diabetes mellitus: effect of parenteral methylcobalamin treatment. Atherosclerosis 1993;103(2):149-57.

29. Fiorina P, Lanfredini M, Montanari A, Peca MG, Veronelli A, Mello A, et al. Plasma homocysteine and folate are related to arterial blood pressure in type 2 diabetes mellitus [In Process Citation]. Am JHypertens 1998;11(9):1100-7.

30. Giltay EJ, Hoogeveen EK, Elbers JM, Gooren LJ, Asscheman H, Stehouwer CD. Insulin resistance is associated with elevated plasma total homocysteine levels in healthy, non-obese subjects [letter] [In Process Citation].Atherosclerosis 1998;139(1):197-8.

31. Phillips AN, Smith GD. How independent are "independent" effects? Relative risk estimation when correlated exposures are measured imprecisely. J Clin Epidemiol 1991 ;44(11): 1223-31.

32. Nygard O, Refsum H, Ueland PM, Vollset SE. Major lifestyle determinants of plasma total homocysteine distribution: the Hordaland Homocysteine Study [see comments]. Am J Clin Nutr 1998;67(2):263-70.

33. Boers GHJ. Hyperhomocysteinemia: a newly recognized risk factor for vascular disease. Neth JMed 1994;45:34-41.

34. Boers GH. Hyperhomocysteinemia as a risk factor for arterial and venous disease. A review of evidence and relevance [In Process Citation]. Thromb Haemost 1997;78(1):520-2.

35. Graham IM, Daly LE, Refsum HM, Robinson K, Brattstrom LE, Ueland PM, et al. Plasma homocysteine as a risk factor for vascular disease. The European Concerted Action Project. Jama 1997;277(22):1775-81.

36. Lindgren A, Brattstrom L, Norrving B, Hultberg B, Andersson A, Johansson BB. Plasma homocysteine in the acute and convalescent phases after stroke [see comments]. Stroke 1995;26(5):795-800.

37. Alfthan G, Pekkanen J, Jauhiainen M, Pitkaniemi J, Karvonen M, Tuomilehto J, et al. Relation of serum homocysteine and lipoprotein(a) concentrations to atherosclerotic disease in a prospective Finnish population based study. Atherosclerosis 1994;106(1):9-19.

38. Verhoef P, Hennekens CH, Malinow MR, Kok FJ, Willett WC, Stampfer MJ. A prospective study of plasma homocyst(e)ine and risk of ischemic stroke. Stroke 1994;25(10):1924-30.

39. Perry I, Refsum H, Morris R, Ebrahim S, Ueland P, Shaper A. Prospective study of serum total homocysteine concentration and risk of stroke in middle- aged British men. Lancet 1995;346:1395-8.

40. Perry IJ. Serum total homocysteine concentration and risk of stroke [letter]. Lancet 1996;348(9040):1526.

41. Bots ML, Witteman JCM, Hoes AW, Koudstaal PJ, Grobbee DE. Homocysteine and risk of cardiovascular disease in the elderly. The Rotterdam Study [Abstract]. Can JCardiol 1997;13 SupplB:150B.

42. Clarke R, Fitzgerald D, O'Brien C, O'Farrell C, Roche G, Parker RA, et al. Hyperhomocysteinemia: a risk factor for extracranial carotid artery atherosclerosis. Ir JMed Sci 1992;161(3):61-5.

43. Malinow MR, Nieto FJ, Szklo M, Chambless LE, Bond G. Carotid artery intimal-medial wall thickening and plasma homocyst(e)ine in asymptomatic adults. The Atherosclerosis Risk in Communities Study. Circulation 1993;87(4):1107-13.

44. Selhub J, Jacques PF, Bostom AG, D'Agostino RB, Wilson PW, Belanger AJ, et al. Association between plasma homocysteine concentrations and extracranial carotid-artery stenosis [see comments]. NEngl JMed 1995;332(5):286-91.

45. Tonstad S, Joakimsen O, Stensland-Bugge E, Leren TP, Ose L, Russell D, et al. Risk factors related to carotid intima-media thickness and plaque in children with familial hypercholesterolemia and control subjects. Arterioscler Thromb VascBiol 1996;16(8):984-91.

46. Aronow WS, Ahn C, Schoenfeld MR. Association between plasma homocysteine and extracranial carotid arterial disease in older persons. Am J Cardiol 1997;79(10):1432-3.

47. Ridker PM, Rifai N, Pfeffer MA, Sacks FM, Moye LA, Goldman S, et al. Inflammation, pravastatin, and the risk of coronary events after myocardial infarction in patients with average cholesterol levels. Cholesterol and Recurrent Events (CARE) Investigators. Circulation 1998;98(9):839-44.

48. Beck JD, Offenbacher S, Williams R, Gibbs P, Garcia R. Periodontitis: a risk factor for coronary heart disease? Ann Periodontol 1998;3(1): 127-41.

49. Kuller LH, Evans RW. Homocysteine, vitamins, and cardiovascular disease [editorial; comment]. Circulation 1998;98(3):196-9.

50. Giles WH, Kittner SJ, Anda RF, Croft JB, Casper ML. Serum folate and risk for ischemic stroke. First National Health and Nutrition Examination Survey epidemiologic follow-up study. Stroke 1995;26(7):1166-70.

51. Robinson K, Arheart K, Refsum H, Brattstrom L, Boers G, Ueland P, et al. Low circulating folate and vitamin $B_6$ concentrations: risk factors for stroke, peripheral vascular disease, and coronary artery disease. European COMAC Group [see comments] . Circulation 1998;97(5):437-43.

52. Folsom AR, Nieto FJ, McGovern PG, Tsai MY, Malinow MR, Eckfeldt JH, et al. Prospective study of coronary heart disease incidence in relation to fasting total homocysteine, related genetic polymorphisms, and B vitamins: the Atherosclerosis Risk in Communities (ARIC) study [see comments]. Circulation 1998;98(3):204-10.

53. Nilsson K, Gustafson L, Faldt R, Andersson A, Brattstrom L, Lindgren A, et al. Hyperhomocysteinemia--a common finding in a psychogeriatric population. Eur J Clin Invest 1996;26(10):853-9.

54. Joosten E, Lesaffre E, Riezler R, Ghekiere V, Dereymaeker L, Pelemans W, et al. Is metabolic evidence for vitamin B-12 and folate deficiency more frequent in elderly patients with Alzheimer's disease? J Gerontol A Biol Sci Med Sci 1997;52(2):M76-9.

55. Parnetti L, Bottiglieri T, Lowenthal D. Role of homocysteine in age- related vascular and non-vascular diseases. Aging (Milano) 1997;9(4):241-57.

56. Clarke R, Smith AD, Jobst KA, Refsum H, Sutton L, Ueland PM. Folate, vitamin $B_{12}$, and serum total homocysteine levels in confirmed Alzheimer disease [In Process Citation]. Arch Neurol 1998;55(11): 1449-55.

57. Goodwin JS, Goodwin JM, Garry PJ. Association between nutritional status and cognitive functioning in a healthy elderly population. Jama 1983;249(21):2917-21.

58. Riggs KM, Spiro A, 3rd, Tucker K, Rush D. Relations of vitamin $B_{12}$, vitamin $B_6$, folate, and homocysteine to cognitive performance in the Normative Aging Study. Am JClin Nutr 1996;63(3):306-14.

59. Stampfer MJ, Malinow MR, Willett WC, Newcomer LM, Upson B, Ullmann D, et al. A prospective study of plasma homocyst(e)ine and risk of myocardial infarction in US physicians. Jama 1992;268(7):877-81.

60. Wald NJ, Watt HC, Law MR, Weir DG, McPartlin J, Scott JM. Homocysteine and ischemic heart disease: results of a prospective study with implications regarding prevention. Arch Intern Med 1998;158(8):862-7.

61. Arnesen E, Refsum H, Bonaa KH, Ueland PM, Forde OH, Nordrehaug JE. Serum total homocysteine and coronary heart disease. Int JEpidemiol 1995 ;24(4):704-9.

62. Nygard O, Nordrehaug JE, Refsum H, Ueland PM, Farstad M, Vollset SE. Plasma homocysteine levels and mortality in patients with coronary artery disease. NEngl JMed 1997;337(4):230-6.

63. Hoogeveen EK, Kostense PJ, Beks PJ, Mackaay AJ, Jakobs C, Bouter LM, et al. Hyperhomocysteinemia is associated with an increased risk of cardiovascular disease, especially in non-insulin-dependent diabetes mellitus: a population-based study. Arterioscler Thromb Vasc Biol 1998; 18(1): 133-8.

64. Roberts JM. Endothelial dysfunction in preeclampsia. Semin Reprod Endocrinol 1998;16(1):5-15.

65. Hornberger J. A cost-benefit analysis of a cardiovascular disease prevention trial, using folate supplementation as an example. Am JPublic Health 1998;88(1):61-7.

66. Ness AR, Powles JW. Fruit and vegetables, and cardiovascular disease: a review. Int JEpidemiol 1997;26(1):1-13.

67. Hu FB, Stampfer MJ, Manson JE, Rimm EB, Colditz GA, Rosner BA, et al. Frequent nut consumption and risk of coronary heart disease in women: prospective cohort study [In Process Citation]. l~mj 1998;317(7169):1341-5.

68. Brattstrom LE, Hardebo JE, Hultberg BL. Moderate homocysteinemia--a possible risk factor for arteriosclerotic cerebrovascular disease. Stroke 1984;15(6):1012-6.

69. Boers GH, Smals AG, Trijbels FJ, Fowler B, Bakkeren JA, Schoonderwaldt HC, et al. Heterozygosity for homocystinuria in premature peripheral and cerebral occlusive arterial disease [see comments]. N Engl J Med 1985;313(12):709-15.

70. Araki A, Sako Y, Fukushima Y, Matsumoto M, Asada T, Kita T. Plasma sulfhydryl-containing amino acids in patients with cerebral infarction and in hypertensive subjects. Atherosclerosis 1989;79(2-3): 139-46.

71. Brattstrom L, Israelsson B, Norrving B, Bergqvist D, Thorne J, Hultberg B, et al. Impaired homocysteine metabolism in early-onset cerebral and peripheral occlusive arterial disease. Effects of pyridoxine and folic acid treatment. Atherosclerosis 1990;81 (1):51 -60.

72. Coull BM, Malinow MR, Beamer N, Sexton G, Nordt F, de Garmo P. Elevated plasma homocyst(e)ine concentration as a possible independent risk factor for stroke. Stroke 1990;21(4):572-6.

73. Clarke R, Daly L, Robinson K, Naughten E, Cahalane S, Fowler B, et al. Hyperhomocysteinemia: an independent risk factor for vascular disease [see comments]. NEngl JMed 1991 ;324(17): 1149-55.

74. Brattstrom L, Lindgren A, Israelsson B, Malinow MR, Norrving B, Upson B, et al. Hyperhomocysteinemia in stroke: prevalence, cause, and relationships to type of stroke and stroke risk factors. Eur J Clin Invest 1992;22(3):214-21.

75. Dudman NP, Wilcken DE, Wang J, Lynch JF, Macey D, Lundberg P. Disordered methionine/homocysteine metabolism in premature vascular disease. Its occurrence, cofactor therapy, and enzymology. Arterioscler Thromb 1993;13(9):1253-60.

76. Perry IJ. Homocysteine, hypertension and stroke. J Hum Hypertens 1999 (In press).

# 11. HOMOCYSTEINE AS A RISK FACTOR FOR CORONARY ARTERY DISEASE

P. BARTON DUELL AND M. RENÉ MALINOW

## SUMMARY

Hyperhomocysteinemia is an important addition to the growing list of potentially reversible risk factors for coronary heart disease (CHD). A compelling case can be made for performing screening measurements of plasma homocysteine concentrations in most if not all patients with myocardial infarction or a high risk of coronary artery disease. The genetic basis for regulation of plasma homocysteine levels suggests that approximately 50% of first-degree relatives of patients with hyperhomocysteinemia also may be hyperhomocysteinemic. Appropriate intervention includes correction of secondary causes of elevated homocysteine levels and treatment with folic acid, possibly in combination with vitamins $B_6$ and $B_{12}$. This intervention can effectively reduce plasma homocysteine concentrations in most patients and is predicted to prevent cardiovascular complications. Aggressive treatment of traditional CHD risk factors also is indicated, particularly among patients known to have atherosclerotic vascular disease. Verification of the clinical benefit and safety of homocysteine-lowering will require the completion during the next 5 to 10 years of 10 ongoing large scale prospective randomized clinical intervention trials involving more than 61,000 subjects.

*K. Robinson (ed.), Homocysteine and Vascular Disease, 173-202.*
© 2000 *Kluwer Academic Publishers. Printed in the Netherlands.*

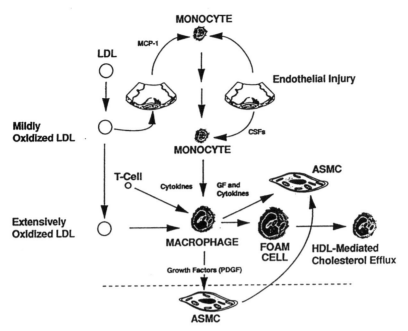

*Figure 1. Potential mechanisms of atherogenesis in the artery wall. Homocysteine may contribute to LDL oxidation, cell activation, and endothelial injury in this model (adapted from Bierman [3]).*

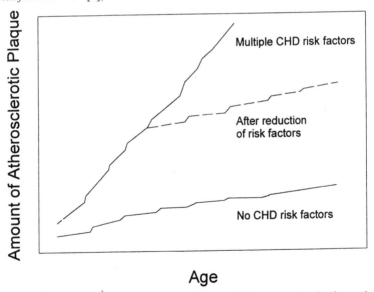

*Figure 2. The relationship between age and cumulative amount of atherosclerotic plaque. The gradual development of atherosclerotic plaques is believed to be characterized by episodes of accelerated atherogenesis. The slope of the line, which reflects the rate of accumulation of atherosclerotic plaque, is increased in individuals with multiple CHD risk factors. It is hypothesized that a reduction in risk factors reduces the slope of the line (dashed line), which may delay or prevent the development of CHD.*

## INTRODUCTION

Coronary atherosclerosis is a multifactorial disease that results from a complex series of events occurring over many decades. The initiating event is believed to be focal micro-injuries to the arterial endothelium and intima [1,2], a process that probably occurs in all individuals. In patients who are resistant to the development of atherosclerosis, it is likely that such injuries may be repaired by normal mechanisms without further sequelae. In contrast, among patients with a sufficiently atherogenic metabolic milieu, micro-injuries are believed to initiate a gradual, but inexorable, process of cellular proliferation, inflammatory responses, and lipid deposition that culminates in the formation of advanced atherosclerotic plaques (Figure 1)[3]. In some regards, atherosclerosis should not be thought of as a consequence of abnormal mechanisms, but rather as a consequence of normal repair processes gone awry under the influence of ongoing endothelial injury, inflammatory stimulation, or excessive activation of cellular responses to injury. A central step in atherogenesis appears to be the deposition of lipids in the arterial wall. As a consequence, individuals with low plasma concentrations of low density lipoprotein (LDL) cholesterol (<80–90 mg/dl) and triglyceride tend to be resistant to atherosclerosis, even in the presence of other risk factors. The gradual development of atherosclerosis is likely to be characterized by episodes of acceleration induced by transient periods of increased injury or enhanced cellular responses (Figure 2).

Traditional risk factors for coronary atherosclerosis include potentially reversible characteristics such as tobacco smoking, hypercholesterolemia, elevated plasma LDL cholesterol, low concentrations of plasma high density lipoprotein (HDL) cholesterol, hypertriglyceridemia, hypertension, diabetes mellitus, obesity (especially visceral adiposity), insulin resistance syndrome, and sedentary lifestyle (Table 1) [4]. Other traditional risk factors, which are not reversible, include age, menopause, family history of coronary heart disease (CHD) and male sex [4]. Although menopause is not reversible, estrogen replacement therapy may partially reverse the atherogenic effects of this condition. In addition to these risk factors, a rapidly growing list of nontraditional risk factors for coronary atherosclerosis has been accumulating (Table 2). A prominent, and well-documented, condition among these alternative risk factors is hyperhomocysteinemia [5,6], which will be the focus of this chapter. The list of other nontraditional risk factors includes multiple proven and theoretical conditions such as elevated plasma lipoprotein (a) [7], elevated plasma apoprotein B [8], small dense LDL [9,10], elevated plasma fibrinogen [11], increased oxidation of LDL (multiple mechanisms) [12,13], homozygosity for the deletion/deletion variant in the deletion/insertion angiotensin converting

*Table 1. Traditional risk factors for coronary atherosclerosis*

| Potentially Reversible | Irreversible |
|---|---|
| Tobacco smoking | Age |
| Hypercholesterolemia | Menopause |
| Elevated plasma LDL cholesterol | Family history of CHD |
| Low HDL cholesterol | Male sex |
| Hypertriglyceridemia | |
| Hypertension | |
| Diabetes mellitus | |
| Obesity | |
| Insulin Resistance Syndrome | |
| Sedentary lifestyle | |

*Table 2. Nontraditional risk factors for coronary atherosclerosis*

| | |
|---|---|
| Hyperhomocysteinemia | Deletion/Insertion ACE gene polymorphism |
| Elevated plasma lipoprotein (a) | Increased oxidation of LDL (multiple mechanisms) |
| Elevated plasma apoprotein B | Mutations affecting platelet activation |
| Small dense LDL | Paraoxonase deficiency |
| Elevated remnant lipoproteins | Infectious agents (e.g. CMV, C. pneumoniae, H. pylori) |
| Elevated plasma fibrinogen | Low plasma vitamin $B_6$ (independent from homocysteine) |
| Impaired glucose tolerance | |

enzyme (ACE) gene polymorphism (controversial) [14], mutations affecting platelet activation [15], reduced serum paraoxonase activity [16], and infectious agents such as cytomegalovirus (CMV), chlamydia pneumoniae (C. pneumoniae), and Helicobacter pylori (H. pylori) [17,18]. Additional new genetic risk factors for atherosclerosis are being frequently reported.

Elevated plasma concentrations of lipoprotein (a) (Lp(a)) appear to interact synergistically with elevated levels of LDL cholesterol, resulting in a 2 to 3-fold increase of risk of atherosclerosis [7]. Among individuals with familial hypercholesterolemia, a genetic disorder associated with severely elevated levels of LDL cholesterol and >85% lifetime risk of CHD, those with elevated Lp(a) have a 2-fold higher risk of early CHD compared to those with low levels of Lp(a) [19]. Lp(a) may contribute to atherosclerosis by accumulating at sites of endothelial injury, where it may cause lipid deposition, might inhibit plasminogen-mediated fibrinolysis, and undergo atherosclerosis-enhancing oxidative modification [7]. As with many other CHD risk factors, elevated levels of Lp(a) may be non-atherogenic when plasma LDL cholesterol concentrations are below 80 to 90 mg/dl [20]. The results of recent studies have suggested that homocysteine may interact synergistically with lipoprotein (a) to enhance the risk of atherosclerosis [21]. Elevated plasma levels of apoprotein B were recognized more than 15 years ago as a risk factor for CHD [8]. This association is due in part to the strong correlation between apoprotein B and LDL cholesterol concentrations, but increased apoprotein B also is a marker for atherogenic remnant lipoproteins and small dense LDL. Small dense LDL, sometimes referred to as "pattern B" LDL (in contrast to larger "pattern A" LDL), is a genetically related condition that is associated with a 2 to 3-fold increased risk of CHD [9,10]. It is unclear whether small dense LDL is directly atherogenic or is merely a marker for other atherogenic factors, but several lines of evidence suggest that small dense LDL is atherogenic. For example, small dense LDL is more readily oxidized than larger buoyant LDL and appears to enter more readily into the artery wall, where it may be undergo enhanced retention in the subendothelial space. Plasma concentrations of fibrinogen are also an independent predictor of risk of coronary atherosclerosis, as demonstrated in the PROCAM [11] and other studies. Among male patients with elevated plasma LDL cholesterol concentrations, the risk of CHD is 2-fold higher if the plasma fibrinogen concentration is in the highest versus lowest tertile [11]. The concept that oxidation of LDL contributes to atherogenesis has gained considerable support during the last decade [12,13]. Currently, a large body of evidence from in vitro tissue culture experiments, animal studies, and more limited human studies suggests that oxidative modification of LDL and other lipoproteins may play a central role in endothelial dysfunction and development of CHD. The results from some, but not all, studies suggest that increased plasma concentrations of homocysteine may stimulate oxidation of LDL [22,23]. This topic is extensively reviewed in chapter 19. The deletion/insertion ACE gene polymorphism was identified in 1992 [24] as an apparent CHD risk factor in patients who were deemed to be at low risk on the basis of other traditional risk factors. Individuals who are homozygous for the deletion/deletion polymorphism tend to have elevated plasma levels of angiotensin, a compound that has potent pro-atherosclerotic effects in the artery wall. Subsequent studies have both supported and contradicted the association between homozygosity for the deletion/deletion ACE gene polymorphism and CHD. One interpretation of the data is that this polymorphism may confer increased CHD risk in some [14], but not necessarily all, patient populations. A growing number of studies have suggested that mutations in various platelet genes, such as the glycoprotein IIb/IIIa receptor [15], may increase the risk of thrombosis and thereby enhance the risk of myocardial infarction in some patients. Paraoxonase is an enzyme that is carried primarily in HDL particles in blood and facilitates protection of LDL against oxidation [16]. The results of recent human and animal studies have suggested that individuals with reduced serum paraoxonase activity (due to polymorphisms in the paraoxonase gene) have increased risk of CHD [16]. The link between infectious agents such as CMV and C. pneumoniae remains controversial, but is based on the hypothesis that such factors may stimulate the inflammatory aspects of atherogenesis [17,18]. H. pylori may contribute to atherogenesis indirectly by causing vitamin $B_{12}$ deficiency and secondary hyperhomocysteinemia. Although plasma concentrations of homocysteine and vitamin $B_6$ are inversely related, the results of 2 recent studies have suggested that plasma levels of pyridoxine may predict risk of coronary artery disease independently from plasma levels of homocysteine [25,26]. Further studies are required to clarify the mechanism responsible for this association.

## PLASMA HOMOCYSTEINE

The concentration of total plasma homocysteine, referred to as homocysteine in this book, is the sum of the concentrations of the thiol amino acid homocysteine and the homocysteinyl moieties of the oxidized disulfides, homocystine and homocysteine-cysteine [27]. Moderate hyperhomocysteinemia, commonly defined as plasma concentrations of homocysteine between 15 and 30 μmol/L [28], has been detected in 10 to 20% of patients with coronary artery disease [29]. Optimal levels of homocysteine are still being defined, but are believed to be below 9 to 10 μmol/L, which approximates mean values in the United States. Plasma homocysteine levels are modulated by a variety of genetic (e.g. C677T polymorphisms in the gene for methylenetetrahydrofolate reductase), environmental (e.g. deficiencies of folate and vitamins $B_6$ and $B_{12}$, drug effects), various disease states (such as hypothyroidism), male sex, and aging-related factors (such as renal insufficiency and menopause). The biochemistry, determinants and metabolism of homocysteine have been extensively reviewed in chapters 3-6.

## HISTORY OF HOMOCYSTEINE AND CORONARY ARTERY DISEASE

The history of homocysteine and cardiovascular disease is extensively discussed in chapter 2. The association between homocystinuria and early atherothrombotic complications was first recognized about 35 years ago in patients with homocystinuria, a rare genetic disorder associated with cystathionine β-synthase deficiency, severe hyperhomocysteinemia, premature atherothrombotic disease, and early death [30]. Without treatment of severe hyperhomocysteinemia, it is estimated that 50% of such subjects will have a vascular event before age 30 years. Despite the intriguing link between severely elevated plasma homocysteine concentrations and atherosclerosis in this rare disorder, research in the field of homocysteine and atherosclerosis progressed slowly until the last decade. In 1975, McCully proposed [31], and Wilcken and Wilcken subsequently confirmed [32], that individuals with modestly elevated plasma concentrations of homocysteine also experienced increased risk of diffuse atherosclerotic vascular disease. Since that time the number of publications on the topic of homocysteine and coronary disease has grown exponentially (increased from 5.8 publications/year on blood homocysteine between 1966-1975 to 226 publications/year during 1995-1998). At the present time, despite the results of some studies showing no association between plasma homocysteine and CHD [33], the pooled data from more than 80 clinical studies involving more than 11,000 patients [34] indicate that moderate hyperhomocysteinemia is a common independent risk factor for myocardial infarction, stroke, peripheral vascular disease, and total mortality [29,32,35-112].

## HYPERHOMOCYSTEINEMIA AND MECHANISMS OF ATHEROGENESIS

A cause and effect relationship between hyperhomocysteinemia and atherogenesis remains unproven, but nonetheless, several lines of evidence suggest that homocysteine is atherogenic in addition to being a marker for increased risk of CHD. Several plausible mechanisms have been identified by which homocysteine may contribute to atherogenesis. These mechanisms include direct cytotoxic effects [109-116], generation of reactive oxygen species [109,112], diminished release of nitric oxide [109,117] [a primary mediator of endothelium-dependent vasodilation [118]], endothelial dysfunction [119-122], potentiation of LDL oxidation [22,23] and lipid peroxidation [165], stimulation of smooth muscle cell e cell proliferation [123], possible abnormalities in platelet function [114,115,124-128], and activation or repression of gene transcription [129]. Prothrombotic effects of homocysteine also may be related to abnormalities in antithrombin activity [130,131], factors V and VII [132,133], protein C [134], cell surface thrombomodulin cofactor activity [135], tissue-type plasminogen activator [136], prothrombin activation of Factor Xa [132], and antithrombin III and von

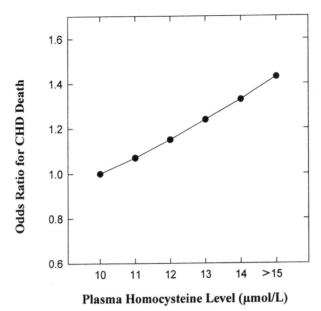

*Figure 3. The relationship between CHD death and plasma homocysteine for homocysteine concentrations within the upper half of the "normal" range (approximately 50th to 95th percentiles). Data from Boushey et al [36].*

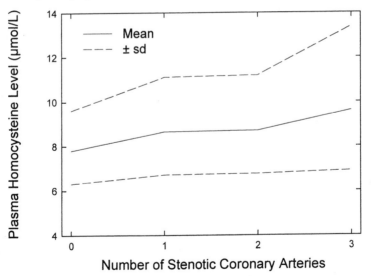

*Figure 4. The relationship between plasma homocysteine concentrations and severity of coronary artery disease in 156 controls (zero stenotic arteries) and 199 patients with coronary artery disease (1 to 3 stenotic arteries). Data from von Eckardstein et al [48].*

Willebrand factor [137,138]. The results of additional recent studies indicate that homocysteine also may interact synergistically with lipoprotein (a) to potentiate increased risk of atherosclerosis [21]. Thus, several plausible mechanisms for homocysteine-induced atherogenesis have been identified that are supported by extensive evidence from in vitro studies. These findings suggest that homocysteine probably plays a causative role in thrombosis and atherogenesis. This conclusion also lends support to the notion that lowering plasma homocysteine concentrations will reduce the risk of atherosclerosis. The pathology of homocysteine-mediated atherogenesis have been reviewed in greater detail in chapter 7.

## HOMOCYSTEINE AND RISK OF MYOCARDIAL INFARCTION

Elevated plasma concentrations of homocysteine are associated with a graded and continuous increased risk of myocardial infarction [29,36,93] which mirrors the curvilinear relationship between hypercholesterolemia and coronary heart disease. Even "normal" homocysteine levels in the range of 10 to 15 $\mu$mol/L (approximating the $50^{th}$ and $95^{th}$ percentiles) are associated with progressively higher risk of death from coronary heart disease (Figure 3). Moreover, the odds ratio in men for death from coronary heart disease attributable to hyperhomocysteinemia was 1.43 for homocysteine concentrations $\geq$ 15 $\mu$mol/L compared to 10 $\mu$mol/L [36]. In other studies, the severity of coronary artery disease, quantified as the number of stenotic coronary arteries identified by angiography, was proportional to the plasma homocysteine concentration in 156 controls and 199 patients with coronary artery disease (Figure 4). Preliminary data from Alfthan and colleagues showed that cardiovascular mortality in 11 countries was highly correlated with mean plasma homocysteine concentrations (r=0.71) [65], but these data must be interpreted with caution due to small numbers of subjects from each country (n=20 or 40).

In a meta-analysis by Boushey and colleagues of 14 case-control studies involving 1830 controls and 2927 cases, the odds ratio for coronary artery disease in individuals with elevated levels of homocysteine was 1.7 (95% confidence interval 1.5 to 1.9) (Figure 5) [36]. A recent nested case-control study showed that a 4 $\mu$mol/L increase in plasma homocysteine was associated with a relative risk of CAD of 1.32 (95% confidence interval 1.05 to 2.65) in men and women [55]. An additional recent study showed that the risk of death in 587 men and women with coronary artery disease was highly correlated with plasma levels of homocysteine [38] (Figure 6). In this study, the 4-year risk of

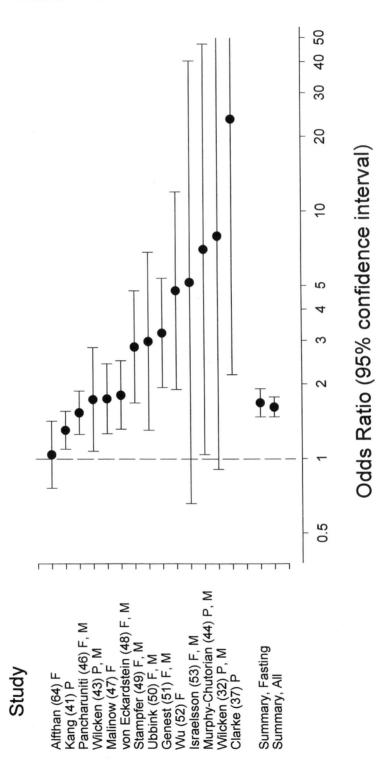

*Figure 5. Meta-analysis of the relationship between fasting (F) and post-methionine (P) plasma homocysteine concentrations and odds ratio for coronary artery disease. M=men only. Adapted from Boushey et al [36].*

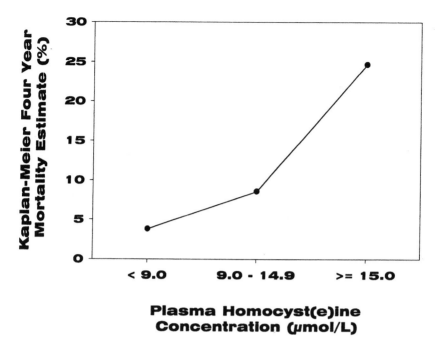

*Figure 6. The prospective relationship between four-year risk of total mortality and plasma homocysteine concentrations patients with coronary artery disease. Data from Nygard et al [38]. Figure from Duell and Malinow [6].*

death was 6 times higher in patients with plasma homocysteine concentrations ≥ 15.0 µmol/L compared to < 9.0 µmol/L [38].

Refsum and colleagues recently reviewed the results of 42 additional epidemiological and clinical studies of the association between plasma homocysteine and cardiovascular disease that have been published since the Boushey meta-analysis [34] (table 3). Seven of the 42 studies (17%) did not show an association between plasma homocysteine concentrations and risk of atherosclerosis and thrombosis, and two other studies showed mixed results (significant association only for fasting or post-methionine plasma homocysteine concentrations), but 23 of the studies (79%) showed a significant statistical relationship between plasma homocysteine and atherothrombotic complications [34]. Since the publication of the Refsum review, 11 additional studies have been published or were not previously cited [25,42,78,78B,97B,98,102-104,107,108] (Table 3). Nine of the 11 studies showed a positive association between CHD and plasma homocysteine, although one showed a positive relationship between CHD and fasting, but not post-methionine homocysteine concentrations [98] (table 3). One of the other 2 studies demonstrated a positive association in women, but not in men [25]. In contrast, the remaining nested

Table 3. Epidemiological and clinical studies of the association between homocysteine and cardiovascular disease published since the review by Boushey and colleagues in 1995. Modified and revised from Refsum and colleagues (34).

| Study Type and Endpoint | Sample Size | Cases/Events | Controls | Age (yrs) | Sex | tHcy | Result | Reference |
|---|---|---|---|---|---|---|---|---|
| **Epidemiological** | | | | | | | | |
| CVD mortality in 11 countries | 260 | | | 40-49 | M | B | Positive | 65 |
| **Cross-Sectional** | | | | | | | | |
| Atherosclerosis severity in PAD | 185 | | | <55 | M/F | B/M | Pos/Pos | 66 |
| Atherosclerosis in hyperlipidemia | 482 | | | mean 60 | M/F | B | Positive | 67 |
| Arterial occlusive disease in HD | 50 | 24 | | 26-84 | M/F | B | Positive | 68 |
| Intervention failure in PAD | 66 | | | mean 52 | M/F | B | Positive | 69 |
| Carotid wall thickness in FH/healthy subjects | 115 | | | 10-19 | M/F | B | Positive | 70 |
| Atherosclerotic complications in HD | 176 | 85 | | mean 56 | M/F | B | Positive | 71 |
| Extend of CAD in pt with suspected CAD | 367 | | | mean 73 | M/F | B | Negative | 72 |
| CHD death in male relatives of children | 756 | 42 | | 8-12 | M/F | B | Positive | 73 |
| CHD in male relatives of FH children | 165 | 39 | | 7-17 | M/F | B | Positive | 74 |
| Macrovascular disease in diabetes | 28 | 17 | | <60 | M/F | B/M | Neg/Pos | 75 |
| Venous thromboembolic events | 208 | | | 19-91 | M/F | B | Positive | 76 |
| CHD, PAD, CVD in the general population | 630 | | | ≥ 55 | M/F | B | Positive | 77 |
| Extent of CAD (1, 2, or 3 vessel) | 297 | | | mean 58 | M/F | B | Positive | 78 |
| Extent of aortic atherosclerotic plaque | 156 | 60 | | 30-89 | M/F | B | Positive | 78B |
| **Case-Control** | | | | | | | | |
| Recurrent venous thromboembolic events | 185 | | 220 | 23-88 | M/F | B,M | Pos/Pos | 79 |
| Acute MI - population control | 68 | | 80 | 28-81 | M/F | B | Negative | 80 |
| Acute stroke - population control | 162 | | 60 | 51-98 | M/F | B | Negative | 61 |
| CAD - healthy workers | 150 | | 584 | <60 | M/F | B | Positive | 81 |
| CHD - mixed control source | 162 | | 155 | 38-68 | M/F | B | Positive | 82 |
| Venous/arterial occlusions-mixed control | 157 | | 60 | mean 33 | M/F | B/M | Pos/Pos | 83 |

| | | | | | | | |
|---|---|---|---|---|---|---|---|
| Venous thromboembolic events-blood donors | 35 | 39 | 20-56 | M/F | B/M | Neg/Neg | 84 |
| CAD - healthy executives | 304 | 231 | mean 62 | M/F | B | Positive | 85 |
| PAD - population control | 65 | 65 | 36-62 | M/F | B/M | Pos/Pos | 86 |
| PAD - mixed control source | 50 | 45 | mean 46 | M | B | Negative | 87 |
| Venous thromboembolic events-neighbor | 269 | 269 | <70 | M/F | B | Positive | 88 |
| First MI - population control | 130 | 118 | <76 | M/F | B | Positive | 40 |
| CAD - population control | 70 | 45 | 28-79 | M/F | B | Positive | 89 |
| CAD - mixed control source | 45 | 23 | mean 48 | M/F | B/M | Pos/Pos | 90 |
| CHD - mixed control source | 111 | 105 | <55 | M/F | B/M | Pos/Neg | 91 |
| Thromboangiitis obliterans-healthy subjects | 12 | 30 | mean 33 | M/F | B | Positive | 92 |
| MI in N. Ireland - general practice control | 191 | 171 | 25-64 | M | B | Negative | 93 |
| MI in France - population control | 229 | 315 | 25-64 | M | B | Positive | 93 |
| CHD,PAD,CVD - general practice control | 58 | 111 | 13-68 | M/F | B/M | Pos/Pos | 94 |
| CHD,PAD,CVD - mixed control source | 750 | 800 | <60 | M/F | B | Positive | 95 |
| CAD - healthy workers | 152 | 121 | <60 | M/F | B | Positive | 96 |
| CAD - mixed control source | 131 | 189 | 25-65 | M/F | B | Positive | 97 |
| CAD - healthy control patients | 140 | 102 | 45-85 | M/F | B | Positive | 42 |
| MI - population control | 79 | 386 | <45 | F | B | Positive | 97B |
| CHD (UK Asian Indians and Caucasians) | 173 | 395 | mean 52 | ----- | B/M | Pos/Neg | 98 |

Nested Case-Control

| | | | | | | | |
|---|---|---|---|---|---|---|---|
| Stroke - 12.8 yr follow-up | 107 | 118 | 40-59 | M/F | B | Positive | 99 |
| CHD - 4 yr follow-up | 122 | 478 | 12-61 | M/F | B | Positive | 55 |
| Venous thromboembolic events-10 yr follow-up | 145 | 646 | 25-68 | M | B | Positive | 100 |
| CAD without prior MI - 9 yr follow-up | 149 | 149 | 25-68 | M | B | Negative | 101 |
| Nonfatal MI, CHD death - 6 yr follow-up | 240 | 472 | 35-57 | M | B | Negative | 102 |
| Ischemic heart disease death | 229 | 1126 | 35-64 | M | B | Positive | 103 |
| MI,stroke,CABG,PTCA,CHD death - 3 yr follow-up | 122 | 244 | ----- | F | B | Positive | 104 |

Cohort

| Cohort | | | | | | | |
|---|---|---|---|---|---|---|---|
| Venous thromboembolic events in SLE (4.8 yr) | 337 | 94 | mean 35 | M/F | B | Positive | 105 |
| CHD events in hemodialysis patients (1.4 yr) | 73 | 16 | mean 56 | M/F | B | Positive | 106 |
| Mortality in CAD patients (4.6 yr) | 587 | 64 | 32-80 | M/F | B | Positive | 38 |
| CHD incidence (3.3 yr) | 759 | 232 | 45-64 | M/F | B | Pos-F/Neg-M | 25 |
| CHD events and death in renal failure (1.5 yr) | 167 | 86 | mean 56 | M/F | B | Positive | 107 |
| Mortality after MI or unstable angina (3.5 yr) | 444 | 68 | ------ | ---- | B | Positive | 108 |

B=basal or fasting plasma homocysteine concentration, CAD=angiographically documented coronary artery disease, CABG=coronary artery bypass graft surgery, CHD=coronary heart disease, CVD=cerebrovascular disease, FH=familial hypercholesterolemia, HD=hemodialysis, M=post-methionine plasma homocysteine concentration, MI=myocardial infarction, PAD=peripheral arterial disease, PTCA=percutaneous coronary angioplasty, SLE=systemic lupus erythematosis, tHcy=total homocysteine measurement (fasting/basal (B) or post-methionine (M))

case-control study found no association between homocysteine and nonfatal MI or CHD death in 712 men participating in the Multiple Risk Factor Intervention trial [102]. The study by Al-Obaidi et al demonstrated that elevated plasma homocysteine concentrations are associated with increased risk of death in patients admitted with acute myocardial infarction or unstable angina [108]. During 3.5 years of follow-up, the number of subjects who died were 4.8%, 5.9%, 5.8%, 18.52%, and 18.07%, respectively, among quintiles for plasma homocysteine concentrations (mean values for homocysteine quintiles: 8.4, 10.1, 12.2, 15.7, and 127.9 $\mu$mol/L). The 3.5 year risk of nonfatal myocardial infarction also was proportional to homocysteine quintiles, associated with a 9.6% versus 30.1% incidence of myocardial infarction in the bottom and top quintiles of plasma homocysteine.

In summary, the results of more than 80 studies involving more than 11,000 patients suggest that elevated plasma homocysteine is a common and independent risk factor for atherosclerosis. Although the results of some well-designed studies did not show a relationship between plasma homocysteine and CHD, such studies are overshadowed by a wealth of additional studies (78% of studies of homocysteine and CHD published during the last 4 years) showing a strong relationship between homocysteine and CHD risk.


## REDUCTION OF CHD RISK BY HOMOCYSTEINE-LOWERING

At the present time, no studies have been completed that test the hypothesis that treatment to reduce plasma homocysteine concentrations will reduce the risk of atherothrombotic complications. However, provocative results were recently published from a small uncontrolled study of progression of carotid atherosclerosis in 38 patients with plasma homocysteine > 14 $\mu$mol/L who were evaluated before and after a mean of 4.4 $\pm$ years of treatment with folic acid 2.5 to 5.0 mg daily, plus vitamin $B_6$ 25 mg daily, and vitamin $B_{12}$ 250$\mu$g daily [139] (figure 7). The rate of increase in the area of carotid atherosclerosis was about 0.3 $cm^2$ per year before treatment and decreased to about -0.05 $cm^2$ per year after treatment. Although this difference was statistically significant (P=0.002), the results of this study need to be interpreted with caution due to the lack of a placebo control group and small numbers of subjects. Recently, long-term survival of a patient with homocystinuria to 50 years of age was reported [140]. The unusually prolonged event-free survival of this patient was attributed to normalization of his plasma homocysteine concentration with B-vitamin therapy since the age of 18 years. Although this anecdotal report is consistent with a reduction in CHD risk by homocysteine lowering, the influence of confounding variables on the results cannot be accurately asses-

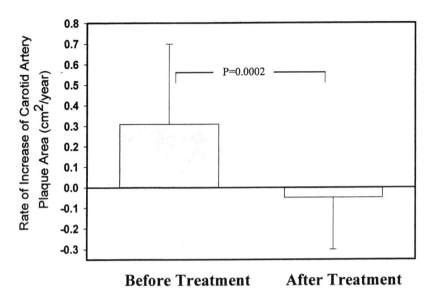

*Figure 7. The relationship between rate of increase of carotid artery plaque area (cm²/year) measured by ultrasound and treatment with multivitamins in 38 men and women with atherosclerosis. Serial measurements of carotid artery plaque area were made before and after treatment with folic acid 2.5-5.0 mg daily, vitamin B₆ - 25 mg daily, and vitamin B₁₂ - 250 μg daily with mean follow-up of 4.4 ± 1.5 years. Data from Peterson et al [139].*

sed. Ten major intervention trials involving more than 61,000 subjects are currently in progress (or will begin soon) that were designed to assess the effects of homocysteine lowering on prevention of cardiovascular endpoints. The primary endpoint for 6 of the trials is coronary artery disease (BERGEN=Bergen vitamin study, CHAOS-2=Cambridge heart antioxidant study, NORVIT=Norwegian study of homocysteine lowering with B-vitamins in myocardial infarction, PACIFIC=Prevention with a combined inhibitor and folate in coronary heart disease, SEARCH=Study of the effectiveness of additional reductions in cholesterol and homocysteine, WACS=Women's antioxidant and cardiovascular disease study). The primary endpoint for the 4 other trials is stroke (HOPE-2=Health outcome and prevention evaluation number 2, IST-2=International strokes trial number 2, VISP=Vitamin intervention for stroke prevention, VITATOPS=Vitamins to prevent strokes). The results of these trials will be anxiously awaited during the next few years.

## SCREENING FOR HYPERHOMOCYSTEINEMIA

Debate continues regarding whether screening for hyperhomocysteinemia is cost-effective or even clinically indicated [141]. Despite the lack of proof that homocysteine-lowering will reduce the risk of cardiovascular disease, there are several compelling reasons to measure plasma homocysteine levels in patients at high risk of cardiovascular disease, such as those with atherosclerotic vascular disease, a history of unexplained thrombosis, or a significant family history of vascular disease. First, hyperhomocysteinemia (plasma homocysteine $> 90^{th}$ or $95^{th}$ percentile) is common in such individuals, occurring in 10 to 40 percent (10-20% of CAD patients, about 30% of stroke patients, and 30-50% of patients with peripheral vascular disease) [28]. Second, if a desirable level for plasma homocysteine is < 9 or 10 μmol/L, approximately half of the general population and a larger proportion of CHD patients will have plasma homocysteine concentrations that are higher than desirable. Third, although the benefit of reducing plasma homocysteine levels on clinical outcome remains untested, hyperhomocysteinemia is a strong predictor of mortality in patients with coronary artery disease (four year estimated mortality 3.8% and 24.7% for plasma homocysteine concentrations < 9.0 μmol/L vs ≥ 15.0 μmol/L, respectively) [38]. Thus, the identification of individuals with hyperhomocysteinemia and coronary artery disease provides an opportunity to administer relatively nontoxic and potentially efficacious therapy to patients who have a strikingly increased risk of death [38,108]. Fourth, since the occurrence of hyperhomocysteinemia often follows an autosomal dominant pattern of inheritance [64], testing of first degree relatives allows the identification of additional individuals who may also have increased risk of atherosclerosis due to hyperhomocysteinemia. Fifth, if post-treatment measurements of homocysteine are not done, the clinician cannot be certain that the patient's plasma homocysteine concentration has decreased to an acceptable level. However, empiric therapy with folic acid and other B-vitamins is likely to normalize plasma homocysteinemia in many, but not all patients, especially those with occult cobalamin deficiency or defects in cystathionine β-synthase. In view of these considerations and the relatively low cost of homocysteine measurements (< $45-60 in many laboratories), routine screening of high risk patients for hyperhomocysteinemia appears to be a justifiable and valuable tool in the endeavor to prevent morbidity and mortality from CHD. The most prudent approach is to quantify pretreatment plasma homocysteine concentrations in high risk individuals and to re-check the levels after therapy to ensure that homocysteine concentrations have been adequately reduced.

*Table 4. Suggestions for Treatment of Hyperhomocysteinemia (adapted from reference 6)*

Initial Therapy
Increase dietary folate, pyridoxine, and vitamin $B_{12}$ (legumes are a good source of folate)
Folic Acid 1-2 mg/d (as little as 200-400 µg/d may be sufficient in some patients)
Addition of a multivitamin containing cobalamin may help prevent masking of B12 deficiency

Supplemental Therapy
Pyridoxine (vitamin $B_6$) 10 to 25 mg/d (higher doses may be required in patients with heterozygous cystathione ß-synthase deficiency)

Vitamin $B_{12}$ 400 µg orally/d in deficient patients or 1000 µg IM monthly in those with intrinsic factor deficiency or achlorhydria (2 mg/d given orally may be sufficient to partially overcome intrinsic factor deficiency in some patients [157])

Additional Therapy for Resistant Hyperhomocysteinemia
Betaine 6 g/d [161]

Choline (dose undefined) [162-164]

Although fasting plasma samples are preferable, nonfasting samples often yield similar values [142]. However, the results of recent studies suggested that homocysteine levels may significantly increase (+12%) or decrease (-8%) after some types of meals [143]. The methionine loading test has been valuable as a research tool to identify individuals who have normal fasting plasma concentrations of homocysteine and latent abnormalities in homocysteine metabolism [144,145], but the increased expense and inconvenience rules against routine use of such testing in most clinical settings. Thus, from a practical standpoint, fasting measurements of plasma homocysteine are sufficient for most clinical applications, but non-fasting measurements also can be used when fasting samples are unavailable. Proper handling of blood samples is important to prevent spurious elevations of plasma homocysteine [166,167]. Chilling of blood on ice after phlebotamy [166] and separation of plasma from cells as son as possible will help prevent a 50 to 300% increase in plasma homocysteine concentrations caused primarily by release of homocysteine from red blood cells [167].

## TREATMENT FOR HYPERHOMOCYSTEINEMIA IN PATIENTS WITH CORONARY ARTERY DISEASE

The first line of therapy needs to be directed toward proven strategies for management of traditional risk factors, such as hypercholesterolemia [4,146]. In this endeavor, it should be noted that niacin (nicotinic acid) and probably bile acid sequestrants, can dramatically increase plasma homocysteine concentrations [147,148]. Although treatment with niacin alone or in combination with a bile acid sequestrant reduces the risk of MI and decreases progression of atherosclerosis, the significance of niacin-induced hyperhomocysteinemia is unclear, since an increase in the plasma homocysteine concentration could potentially counteract or decrease the benefits of cholesterol reduction.

Elevated levels of homocysteine can be significantly reduced or normalized with vitamin therapy in most individuals [149,150], with the exception of patients with homocystinuria, renal failure, or niacin-induced hyperhomocysteinemia. Appropriate therapy also needs to include correction of secondary causes of hyperhomocysteinemia [151]. The optimal doses and combinations of therapeutic vitamins have not been defined, but the several suggestions for treatment have been outlined in table 4. After appropriate dietary modification, folic acid in doses of 1 to 2 mg daily is the primary mode of therapy, although doses as low as 200 µg daily may be adequate in many patients [152,153]. Many multivitamin supplements contain 400 µg or more of folic acid and therefore may be sufficient for treatment of hyperhomocysteinemia in many patients. Other investigators have used 5 to 10 mg of folic acid daily, but doses in this range have not been shown to be more efficacious than 0.5 mg daily [154]. Breakfast cereals fortified with $\geq$ 400 µg folic acid per serving also can significantly reduce plasma homocysteine concentrations in patients with coronary artery disease [155]. Administration of pyridoxine at a dose of 10 to 25 mg daily may be useful as adjunctive therapy in patients who do not achieve adequate lowering of plasma homocysteine levels with folic acid therapy. Patients with heterozygous deficiency of cystathionine $\beta$-synthase deficiency may be more likely to require adjunctive therapy with pyridoxine. Dosages of 250 mg or more have been used in some studies [156], but may be unnecessary in most patients [157] and could increase the risk of neuropathy. Vitamin $B_{12}$ therapy alone has little effect on plasma homocysteine concentrations [154] except in the setting of vitamin $B_{12}$ deficiency [158], which can be associated with plasma homocysteine concentrations > 100 µmol/L [159]. However, in patients treated with folic acid and vitamin $B_6$, the addition of vitamin $B_{12}$ therapy may decrease the plasma homocysteine concentration by an additional 5-7% [152]. To prevent masking of vitamin $B_{12}$ deficiency with possible neurologic complications, it is imperative to correct vitamin $B_{12}$ deficiency prior to beginning treatment with folic acid. It has been suggested that this potential complication can be averted by providing 400 to 1000 μg of oral vitamin $B_{12}$ daily in conjunction with folic acid supplementation. Moreover, in patients with documented vitamin $B_{12}$ deficiency, daily oral administration of cyanocobalamin 2 mg may be a satisfactory alternative to parenteral therapy [160]. Patients who do not respond adequately to therapy with folic acid and vitamins $B_6$ and $B_{12}$ also may be treated with betaine [161] or choline (a betaine precursor) [162-164], both of which are believed to act by increasing activity of betaine-homocysteine methyltransferase [163].

*Acknowledgements. This work was supported in part by the Oregon Health Sciences Foundation, the National Institutes of Health (RR00163-34), and the American Heart Association.*

## REFERENCES

1. Ross R: Atherosclerosis - and inflammatory disease. N Engl J Med 1999;340:115-126.
2. Ross R: Cell biology of atherosclerosis. Ann Rev Physiol 1995;57:791-804.
3. Bierman EL: Atherogenesis in diabetes. Arterioscler Thromb 1992;12:647-656.
4. Summary of the second report of the National Cholesterol Education Program (NCEP) expert panel on detection, evaluation, and treatment of high blood cholesterol in   adults. JAMA 1993;269:3015-3023.
5. Welch GN, Loscalzo J: Homocysteine and atherothrombosis N Engl J Med 1998;338:1042-1050.
6. Duell PB, Malinow MR: Homocyst(e)inemia and risk of atherosclerosis: a clinical approach to evaluation and management. The Endocrinologist 1998;8:170-177.
7. Scanu AM, Lawn RM, Berg K: Lipoprotein (a) and atherosclerosis. Ann Int Med 1991;115:209-218.
8. Sniderman AD, Wolfson C, Teng B, Franklin FA, Bachorik PS, Kwiterovich PO Jr: Association of hyperapobetalipoproteinemia with endogenous hypertriglyceridemia and atherosclerosis. Ann Int Med 1982;97:833-839.
9. Austin MA: Triacylglycerol and coronary heart disease. Proc Nutr Soc 1997;56:667-670.
10. Krauss RM: Triglycerides and atherogenic lipoproteins: rationale for lipid management. Am J Med 1998;105:58S-62S.
11. Heinrich J, Balleisen L, Schulte H, Assmann G, van de Loo J: Fibrinogen and factor VII in the prediction of coronary risk. Results from the PROCAM study in healthy men. Arterioscler Thromb 1994;14:54-59.
12. Steinberg D: Oxidative modification of LDL and atherogenesis. Circulation 1997;95:1062-1071.

13. Steinberg D: Low density lipoprotein oxidation and its pathobiological significance. J Biol Chem 1997;272:20963-20966.

14. O'Malley JP, Maslen CL, Illingworth DR: Angiotensin-converting enzyme DD genotype and cardiovascular disease in heterozygous familial hypercholesterolemia. Circulation 1998;97:1780-1783.

15. Clemetson KJ, Clemetson JM: Integrins and cardiovascular disease. Cell Mol Life Sci 1998;54:502-513.

16. Mackness MI, Mackness B, Durrington PN, Fogelman AM, Berliner J, et al: Paraoxonase and coronary heart disease. Curr Opin Lipidology 1998;9:319-324.

17. Gibbs RG, Carey N, Davies AH: Chlamydia pneumoniae and vascular disease. British J Surg 1998; 85:1191-1197.

18. Cook PJ, Lip GY: Infectious agents and atherosclerotic vascular disease. QJM 1996;89:727-735.

19. Seed M, Hoppichler F, Reaveley D, McCarthy S, Thompson GR, et al: Relation of serum lipoprotein (a) phenotype to coronary heart disease in patients with familial hypercholesterolemia. N Engl J Med 1990;322:1494-1499.

20. Maher VM, Brown BG, Marcovina SM, Hillger LA, Zhao XQ, Albers JJ: Effects of lowering elevated LDL cholesterol on the cardiovascular risk of lipoprotein(a). JAMA 1995;274:1771-1774.

21. Foody JM, Robinson K, Jacobsen DW, Milberg JA, Sprecher DL: Homocysteine and lipoprotein (a) interaction: enhanced prediction of CAD in women. Circulation 1998;98:I-602 (abstract).

22. Hirano K, Ogihara T, Miki M, et al: Homocysteine induces iron-catalyzed lipid peroxidation of low-density lipoprotein that is prevented by $\alpha$-tocopherol. Free Rad Res 1994;21:267-276.

23. Blom HJ, Kleinveld HA, Boers GH, et al: Lipid peroxidation and susceptibility of low density lipoprotein to in vitro oxidation in hyperhomocysteinemia. Eur J Clin Invest 1995;25:149-154.

24. Cambien F, Poirier O, Lecerf L, Evans A, Cambou JP, Arveiler D, Luc G, Bard JM, Bara L, Ricard S, et al: Deletion polymorphism in the gene for angiotensin-converting enzyme is a potent risk factor for myocardial infarction. Nature 1992;359:641-644.

25. Folsom AR, Nieto FJ, McGovern PG, Tsai MY, Malinow MR, Eckfeldt JH, Hess DL, Davis CE: Prospective study of coronary heart disease incidence in relation to fasting total homocysteine, related genetic polymorphisms, and B vitamins: the Atherosclerosis Risk in Communities (ARIC) study. Circulation 1998;98:204-210.

26. Robinson K, Arheart K, Refsum H, Brattstrom L, Boers G, Ueland P, Rubba P, Palma-Reis R, Meleady R, Daly L, Witteman J, Graham I: Low circulating folate and vitamin $B_6$ concentrations: risk factors for stroke, peripheral vascular disease, and coronary artery disease. European COMAC Group. Circulation 1998;97:437-443.

27. Malinow MR: Plasma homocyst(e)ine and arterial occlusive diseases: a mini-review. Clin Chem 1995;41:173-176.

28. Kang SS, Wong PWK, Malinow MR: Hyperhomocyst(e)inemia as a risk factor for occlusive vascular disease. Ann Rev Nutr 1992;12:279-298.

29. Malinow MR: Plasma homocyst(e)ine : a risk factor for arterial occlusive diseases. J Nutr 1996;126:1238S-1243S.

30. Mudd SH, Levy HL, Skovby F: Disorders in transsulfuration. In: The Metabolic and Molecular Basis of Metabolic Disease, Scriver CR, Beaudet AL, Sly WS, Valle D, eds. McGraw Hill: New York, 1995:1279-1327.

31. McCully KS and Wilson RB: Homocysteine theory of arteriosclerosis. Atherosclerosis 1975;22:215-227.

32. Wilcken DEL, Wilcken B: The pathogenesis of coronary artery disease. A possible role for methionine metabolism. J Clin Invest 1976;57:1079-1082.

33. Refsum H, Ueland PM: Recent data are not in conflict with homocysteine as a cardiovascular risk factor. Curr Opin Lipidology 1998;9:533-539.

34. Refsum H, Ueland PM, Nygard O, Vollset SE: Homocysteine and cardiovascular disease. Ann Rev Med 1998;49:31-61.

35. Malinow MR. Homocyst(e)ine and arterial occlusive diseases. J Intern Med 1994;236:603-617.

36. Boushey CJ, Beresford SA, Omen GS, Motulsky AG: A quantitative assessment of plasma homocysteine as a risk factor for vascular disease. JAMA 1995;274:1049-1057.

37. Clarke R, Daly L, Robinson K, Naughten E, Cahalane S, Fowler B, Graham I: Hyperhomocysteinemia: an independent risk factor for vascular disease. N Engl J Med 1991;324:1149-1155.

38. Nygard O, Nordrehaug JE, Refsum H, Ueland PM, Farstad M, Vollset SE: Plasma homocysteine levels and mortality in patients with coronary artery disease. N Engl J Med 1997;337:230-236.

39. Mayer EL, Jacobsen DW, Robinson KR: Homocysteine and coronary atherosclerosis. J Am Coll Cardiol 1996;27:517-527.

40. Verhoef P, Stampfer MJ, Buring JE, Gaziano JM, Allen RH, Stabler SP, Reynolds RD, Kok FJ, Hennekens CH, Willett WC: Homocysteine metabolism and risk of myocardial infarction: relation with vitamins $B_6$, $B_{12}$, and folate. Am J Epidemiol 1996;143:845-859.

41. Kang SS, Wong PWK, Cook HY, Norusis M, Messer JV: Protein-bound homocyst(e)ine. A possible risk factor for coronary artery disease. J Clin Invest 1986;77:1482-1486.

42. Malinow MR, Nieto FJ, Kruger WD, Duell PB, Hess DL, Gluckman RA, Block PC, Holzgang CR, Anderson PH, Seltzer D, Upson B, Lin QR: The effects of folic acid supplementation on plasma total homocysteine are modulated by multivitamin use and the methylenetetrahydrofolate reductase genotype. Arteriosclerosis and Thrombosis 1997;17:1157-1162.

43. Wilcken DEL, Reddy SG, Gupta VJ: Homocysteinemia, ischemic heart disease, and the carrier state for homocystinuria. Metabolism 1983;32:363-370.

44. Murphy-Chutorian DR, Wexman MP, Grieco AJ, Heininger JA, Glassman E, Gaull GE, Ng SK, Feit F, Wexman K, Fox AC: Methionine intolerance: a possible risk factor for coronary artery disease. J Am Coll Cardiol 1985;6:725-730.

45. Dudman NPB, Wilcken DEL, Wang J, Lynch JF, Macey D, Lundberg P: Disordered methionine/homocysteine metabolism in premature vascular disease. Arterioscler Thromb 1993;13:1253-1260.

46. Pancharuniti N, Lewis CA, Sauberlich HE, Perkins LL, Go RC, Alvarez JO, Macaluso M, Acton RT, Copeland RB, Cousins AL, et al: Plasma homocysteine, folate, and vitamin $B_{12}$ concentrations and risk for early-onset coronary artery disease. Am J Clin Nutr 1994;59:940-948.

47. Malinow MR, Sexton G, Averbuch M, Grossman M, Wilson D, Upson B: Homocyst(e)inemia in daily practice. Coron Artery Dis 1990;1:215-220.

48. von Eckardstein A, Malinow MR, Upson B, Heinrich J, Schulte H, Schonfeld R, Kohler E, Assmann G: Effects of age, lipoproteins, and hemostatic parameters on the role of homocyst(e)inemia as a cardiovascular risk factor in men. Atheroscler Thromb 1994;14:460-464.

49. Stampfer MJ, Malinow MR, Willett WC, Newcomer LM, Upson B, Ullmann D, Tishler PV, Hennekens CH: A prospective study of plasma homocyst(e)ine and risk of myocardial infarction in US physicians. JAMA 1992;268:877-881.

50. Ubbink JB, Vermaak WJH, Bennett JM, Becker PJ, van Staden DA, Bissbort S: The prevalence of homocysteinemia and hypercholesterolemia in angiographically defined coronary artery disease. Klin Wochenscr 1991;69:527-534.

51. Genest JJ, McNamara JR, Salem DN, Wilson PWF, Schaefer EJ, Malinow MR: Plasma homocyst(e)ine levels in men with premature coronary artery disease. J Am Coll Cardiol 1990;16:1114-1119.

52. Wu LL, Wu J, Hunt SC, James BC, Vincent GM, Williams RR, Hopkins PN: Plasma homocysteine as a risk factor for early familial coronary artery disease. Clin Chem 1994;40:552-561.

53. Israelsson B, Brattström LE, Hultberg BL: Homocysteine and myocardial infarction. Atherosclerosis 1988;71:227-233.

54. Graham I: Interactions between homocysteinemia and conventional risk factors in vascular disease. Eur Heart J 1994;15(suppl):530 (abstract).

55. Arnesen E, Refsum H, Bonaa KH, Ueland PM, Forde OH, Nordrehaung JE: Serum total homocysteine and coronary heart disease. Int J Epidemiol 1995;24:704-709.

56. Brattström LE, Harbebo JE, Hultberg BL: Moderate homocysteinemia. Stroke 1984;15:1012-1016.

57. Araki A, Sako Y, Fukushima Y, Matsumoto Asada T, Kita T: Plasma sulfhydryl-containing amino acids in patients with cerebral infarction and in hypertensive subjects. Atherosclerosis 1989;79:139-146.

58. Coull B, Malinow MR, Beamer N, Sexton G, Nordt F, deGarmo P: Elevated plasma homocyst(e)ine concentration as a possible independent risk factor for stroke. Stroke 1990;21:572-576.

59. Brattström LE, Israelsson B, Norrving B, Bergqvist D, Thorne J, Hultberg B, Hamfelt A: Impaired homocysteine metabolism in early-onset cerebral and peripheral occlusive arterial disease. Atherosclerosis 1990;81:51-60.

60. Brattström LE, Lindgren A, Israelsson B, Malinow MR, Norrving B, Upson B, Hamfelt A: Hyperhomocysteinemia in stroke. Eur J Clin Invest 1992;22:214-221.

61. Lindgren A, Brattstrom L, Norrving B, Hultberg B, Andersson A, Johansson BB: Plasma homocysteine in the acute and convalescent phases after stroke. Stroke 1995;26:795-800

62. Bergmark C, Mansoor MA, Swedenborg J, deFaire U, Svardal AM, Ueland PM: Hyperhomocysteinemia in patients operated for lower extremity ischemia below the age of 50: effect of smoking and extent of disease. Eur J Vasc Surg 1993;7:391-396.

63. Molgaard J, Malinow MR, Lassvik C, Holm A-C, Upson B, Olsson AG: Hyperhomocyst(e)inemia: an independent risk factor for intermittent claudication: J Intern Med 1992;231:273-279.

64.  Alfthan G, Pekkanen J, Jauhiainen M, et al: Relation of serum homocysteine and lipoprotein(a) concentrations to atherosclerotic disease in a prospective Finnish population based study. Atherosclerosis 1994;106:9-19.

64B. Genest JJ, McNamara JR, Upson B, Salem DN, Ordovaas JM, Schaefer EJ, Malinow MR: Prevalence of familial hyperhomocyst(e)inemia in men with premature coronary artery disease. Arterioscler Thromb 1991;11:1129-1136.

64C. Verhoef P, Hennekens CH, Malinow MR, Kok FJ, Willett WC, Stampfer MJ: A prospective study of plasma homocyst(e)ine and risk of ischemic stroke. Stroke 1994;25:1924-1930.

65.  Alfthan G, Aro A, Gey F: Plasma homocysteine and cardiovascular disease mortality. Lancet 1997;349:397 (letter).

66.  van den Berg M, Stehouwer CDA, Bierdrager E, et al.. Plasma homocysteine and severity of atherosclerosis in young patients with lower-limb atherosclerotic disease. Arterioscler Thromb Vasc Biol 1996;16:165-71

67.  Glueck CJ, Shaw P, Lang JE, et al.. Evidence that homocysteine is an independent risk factor for atherosclerosis in hyperlipidemic patients. Am. J. Cardiol. 1995;75:132-36

68.  Bachmann J, Tepel M, Raidt H, et al.. Hyperhomocysteinernia and the risk for vascular disease in hemodialysis patients. J Am. Soc. Nephrol. 1995;6:121-25

69.  Currie IC, Wilson YG, Scott J, et al: Homocysteine: an independent risk factor for the failure of vascular intervention. Br J Surg 1996;83:1238-1241.

70.  Tonstad S, Joakimsen 0, Stenslandbugge E, et al.. Risk factors related to carotid intima-media thickness and plaque in children with familial hypercholesterolemia and control subjects. Arterioscler Thromb Vasc Biol 1996;16:984-91

71.  Robinson K, Gupta A, Dennis V, et al: Hyperhomocysteinemia confers an independent increased risk of atherosclerosis in end-stage renal disease and is closely linked to plasma folate and pyridoxine concentrations. Circulation 1996;94: 2743-48

72.  Herzlich BC, Lichstein E, Schulhoff N, et al: Relationship among homocysteine, vitamin B-12 and cardiac disease in the elderly: association between vitamin B-12 deficiency and decreased left ventricular ejection fraction. J Nutr 1996;126:S1249-53

73.  Tonstad S, Refsum H, Siversten M, et al: Relation of total homocysteine and lipid levels in children to premature cardiovascular death in male relatives. Pediatr Res 1996;40:47-52.

74.  Tonstad S, Refsum H, Ueland PM: Association between total homocysteine and parental history of cardiovascular disease in children with familial hypercholesterolemia. Circulation 1997;96

75.  Munshi MN, Stone A, Fink L, Fonseca V: Hyperhomocysteinernia following a methionine load in patients with noninsulin-dependent diabetes mellitus and macrovascular disease. Metabolism 1996;45:133-135.

76.  Simioni P, Prandoni P, Burlina A, et al: Hyperhomocysteinemia and deep vein thrombosis - a case-control study. Thromb. Haemost. 1996;76:883-886

77.  Bots ML, Laurier LJ, Lindemans J, et al. Homocysteine, atherosclerosis and prevalent cardiovascular disease in the elderly: The Rotterdam study. J Intern Med 1997.

78.  Title LM, Dunn J, Cummings P, Zayed E, Dempsey GI, O'Neill BJ, Johnstone DE, Bata IR, Nassar BA: Relation between homocysteine, a mutation in methylenetetrahydrofolate reductase and extent of coronary artery disease. Circulation 1998;98:I-439-440 (abstract).

78B. Konecky N, Malinow MR, Tunick PA, Freedberg RS, Rosenzweig BP, Katz ES, Hess DL, Upson B, Leung B, Perez J, Kronzon I: Correlation between plasma homocyst(e)ine and aortic atherosclerosis. Am Heart J 1997;133:534-540.

79.  den Heijer M, Blom HJ, Gerrits WBJ, et al: Is hyperhomocysteinemia a risk factor for recurrent venous thrombosis? Lancet 1995;345:882-85

80.  Landgren F, Israelsson B, Lindgren A, et al: Plasma homocysteine in acute myocardial infarction: homocysteine lowering effect of folic acid. J Intern. Med 1995;237:381-388

81.  Dalery K, Lussier-Cacan S, Selhub J, et al.. Homocysteine and coronary artery disease in French Canadian subjects: relation with vitamins B 12, B₆, pyridoxal phosphate, and olate. Am. J Cardiol. 1995;75:1107-11

82.  Hopkins PN, Wu LL, Wit J, et al.. Higher plasma homocyst(e)ine and increased susceptibility to adverse effects of low folate in early familial coronary artery disease. Arterioscler Thromb Vasc Biol 1995;15:1314-20

83.  Fermo 1, Arcelloni C, Devecchi E, et al.. High-performance liquid chromatographic method with fluorescence detection for the determination of total homocysteine in plasma. J Chromatography 1992;593:171-76

84.  Amundsen T, Ueland PM, Waage A: Plasma homocysteine levels in patients with deep venous thrombosis. Arterioscler. Thromb. Vasc. Biol. 1995;15:1321-23.

85.  Robinson K, Mayer EL, Miller DP, et al.. Hyperhomocysteinemia and low pyridoxal phosphate: common and independent reversible risk factors for coronary artery disease. Circulation 1995;92:2825-30

86.  Mansoor MA, Bergmark C, Svardal AM, et al: Redox status and protein binding of plasma homocysteine and other aminothiols in patients with early-onset peripheral vascular disease. Arterioscler Thromb Vasc Biol 1995;15:232-240.

87.  Valentine RJ, Kaplan H S, Green R, et al.. Lipoprotein (a), homocysteine, and hypercoagulable states in young men with premature peripheral atherosclerosis: a prospective, controlled analysis, J. Vasc. Surg. 1996;23:53-63

88.  den Heijer M, Koster T, Blom HJ, et al: Hyperhomocysteinemia as a risk factor for deep-vein thrombosis. N Engl J Med 1996;334:759-62

89.  Loehrer FMT, Angst CP, Haefuli WE, et al: Low whole-blood s-adenosylmethionine and correlation between 5-methyltetrahydrofolate and homocysteine in coronary artery disease. Arterioscler Thromb Vasc Biol 1996;16:727-33

90.  Lolin YI, Sanderson JE. Cheng SK, et al.. Hyperhomocysteinemia and premature coronary artery disease in the Chinese. Heart 1996;76:117-22

91.  Gallagher PM, Meleady R, Shields DC, et al.. Homocysteine and risk of premature coronary heart disease. Evidence for a common gene mutation. Circulation 1996;94:2154-2158.

92.  Stammler F, Diehm C, Hsu E, et al.. Prevalence of hyperhomocysteinaernia in thrombangiitis obliterans (Buerger's disease): does homocysteine play a pathogenetic role? Dtsch. Med Wochenschr. 1996;121:1417-1423.

93.  Malinow MR, Ducimetiere P, Luc G, Evans AE, Arveiler D, Cambien F, Upson BM: Plasma homocyst(e)ine levels and graded risk for myocardial infarction: findings in two populations at contrasting risk for coronary heart disease. Atherosclerosis 1996;126:27-34.

94. Kluijtmans LA, van den Heuvel LP, Boers GH, Frosst P, Stevens EM, van Oost BA, den Heijer M, Trijbels FJ, Rozen R, Blom HJ: Molecular genetic analysis in mild hyperhomocysteinemia: a common mutation in the methylenetetrahydrofolate reductase gene is a genetic risk factor for cardiovascular disease. Am J Hum Genet 1996;58:35-41.

95. Graham IM, Daley LE, Refsum HM, et al: Plasma homocysteine as a risk factor for vascular disease: the European concerted action project. JAMA 1997;277:1775-1781.

96. Christensen B, Frosst P, Lussier-Cacan S, et al: Correlation of a common mutation in the methylenetetrahydrofolate reductase gene with plasma homocysteine in patients with premature coronary artery disease. Arterioscler Thromb Vasc Biol 1997;17:569-73.

97. Verhoef P, Kok FJ, Kruyssen DACM, et al.. Plasma total homocysteine, B vitamins and risk of coronary atherosclerosis. Arterioscler Thromb Vasc Biol 1997;17: 989-995.

97B. Schwartz SM, Siscovick DS, Malinow MR, Rosendaal FR, Beverly RK, Hess DL, Psaty BM, Longstreth WT Jr, Koepsell TD, Raghunathan TE, Reitsma PH: Myocardial infarction in young women in relation to plasma total homocysteine, folate, and a common variant in the methylenetetrahydrofolate reductase gene. Circulation 1997;96:412-417.

98. Chambers JC, Obeid O, Hooper J, Kemp M, Reilly P, Powell-Tuck J, Kooner JS: Hyperhomocysteinamia may account for the excess coronary heart disease risk in UK Indian Asians compared to European whites. Circulation 1998;98:I-169 (abstract).

99. Perry IJ, Refsum H, Morris RW, et al: Prospective study of serum total homocysteine concentration and risk of stroke in middle-aged British men. Lancet 1995;346:1395-1398.

100. Ridker PM, Hennekens CH, Selhub J, et al.. Interrelation of hyperhomocyst(e)inemia, factor V Leiden, and risk of future venous thromboembolism. Circulation 1997;95:1777-1782.

101. Verhoef P, Hennekens CH, Allen RH, et al: Plasma total homocysteine and risk of angina pectoris with subsequent coronary artery bypass surgery. Am. J Cardiol. 1997;79:799-801.

102. Evans RW, Shaten BJ, Hempel JD, Cutler JA, Kuller LH: Homocysteine and risk of cardiovascular disease in the Multiple Risk Factor Intervention Trial. Arteriosclerosis, Thrombosis & Vascular Biology 1997;17:1947-1953.

103. Wald NJ, Watt HC, Law MR, Weir DG, McPartlin J, Scott JM: Homocysteine and ischemic heart disease: results of a prospective study with implications regarding prevention. Arch Int Med 1998;158:862-867.

104. Ridker PM, Buring JE, Manson JE: A Prospective Study of Total Plasma Homocysteine and the Risk of Future Cardiovascular Events Among Apparently Healthy Women. Circulation 1998;98:I-810 (abstract).

105. Petri M, Roubenoff R, Dallal GE, et al: Plasma homocysteine as a risk factor for atherothrombotic events in systemic lupus erythematosus. Lancet 1996;348: 1120-1124.

106. Bostom AG, Shemin D, Verhoef P, Nadeau MR, Jacques PF, Selhub J, Dworkin L, Rosenberg IH: Elevated fasting total plasma homocysteine levels and cardiovascular disease outcomes in maintenance dialysis patients. A prospective study. Arterioscler Thromb Vasc Biol 1997;17:2554-2558.

107. Moustapha A, Naso A, Nahlawi M, Gupta A, Arheart KL, Jacobsen DW, Robinson K, Dennis VW: Prospective study of hyperhomocysteinemia as an adverse cardiovascular risk factor in end-stage renal disease. Circulation 1998;97:138-141.

108. Al-Obaidi MK, Stubbs PJ., Amersey R, Conroy R, Graham IM, Noble MI: Admission Plasma Homocysteine Predicts Long Term Mortality In Patients Presenting With Acute Coronary Syndromes. Circulation 1998;98:I-555 (abstract).

109. Stamler JS, Osborne JA, Jaraki O, et al: Adverse vascular effects of homocysteine are modulated by endothelium-derived relaxing factor and related oxides of nitrogen. J Clin Invest 1993;91:308-318.

110. Van Den Berg M, Boers GH, Franken DG, Blom HJ, Van Kamp GJ, Jakobs C, Rauwerda JA, Kluft C, Stehouwert CD: Hyperhomocysteinemia and endothelial dysfunction in young patients with peripheral arterial occlusive disease. Eur J Clin Invest 1995;25:176-181.

111. Dudman NPB, Hicks C, Lynch JF, Wilcken DEL, Wang J: Homocysteine thiolactone disposal by human arterial endothelial cells and serum in vitro. Arterioscler Thromb 1991;11:663-670.

112. Starkebaum G, Harlan JM: Endothelial cell injury due to copper-catalyzed hydrogen peroxide generation from homocysteine. J Clin Invest 1986;77:1370-1376.

113. Wall RT, Harlan JM, Harker LA, Striker GE: Homocysteine-induced endothelial cell injury in vitro: a model for the study of vascular injury. Thromb Res 1980;18:113-121.

114. Harker LA, Slichter SJ, Scott CR, Ross R: Homocystinemia. Vascular injury and arterial thrombosis. N Engl J Med 1974;291:537-543.

115. Harker LA, Ross R, Slichter SJ, Scott CR: Homocystine-induced arteriosclerosis. The role of endothelial cell injury and platelet response in its genesis. J Clin Invest 1976;58:731-741.

116. Harker LA, Harlan JM, Ross R: Effects of sulfinpyrazone on homocysteine-induced endothelial injury and atherosclerosis in baboons. Circ Res 1983;53:731-739.

117. Radomski MW, Salas E: Nitric oxide - biological mediator, modulator and factor of injury: its role in the pathogenesis of atherosclerosis. Atherosclerosis 1995;118:S69-S80.

118. Levine GN, Keaney JF, Jr, Vita JA: Medical progress: cholesterol reduction in cardiovascular disease - clinical benefits and possible mechanisms. N Engl J Med 1995;332:512-521.

119. Celermajer DS, Sorensen K, Ryalls M, et al: Impaired endothelial function occurs in the systemic arteries of children with homozygous homocystinuria but not their heterozygous parents. J Am Coll Cardiol 1993;22:854-858.

120. Lentz SR, Sobey CG, Piegors DJ, Bhopatkar MY, Faraci FM, Malinow MR, Heistad DD: Vascular dysfunction in monkeys with diet-induced hyperhomocyst(e)inemia. J Clin Invest 1996;98:24-29.

121. Tawakol A, Omland T, Gerhard M, Wu JT, Creager MA: Hyperhomocysteinemia is associated with impaired endothelium-dependent dysfunction in humans. Circulation 1997;95:1119-1121.

122. Duell PB, Malinow MR: Hyperhomocyst(e)inemia is associated with impaired flow-mediated arterial vasodilation. J Invest Med 1997;45:220A (abstract).

123. Tsai JC, Perella MA, Yoshizumi M, Hsieh CM, Haber E, Schlegel R, Lee ME: Promotion of vascular smooth muscle cell growth by homocysteine: a link to atherosclerosis. Proc Nat Acad Sci USA 1994;91:6369-6373.

124. McDonald L, Bray C, Field C, Love F, Davies B: Homocystinuria, thrombosis and the blood-platelets. Lancet 1964;1:745-746.

125. DiMinno G, Davi G, Margaglione M, Cirillo F, Grandone E, Ciabattoni G, Catalano I, Strisciuglio P, Andria G, Patrono C, et al: Abnormally high thromboxane biosynthesis in homozygous homocystinuria. Evidence for platelet involvement and probucol-sensitive mechanism. J Clin Invest 1993;92:1400-1406.

126. Uhlemann ER, TenPas JH, Lucky AW, Schulman JD, Mudd SH, Shulman NR: Platelet survival and morphology in homocystinuria due to cystathione synthase deficiency. N Engl J Med 1976;295:1283-1286.

127. Hill-Zobel RL, Pyeritz RE, Scheffel U, Malpica O, Engin S, Camargo EE, Abbott M, Guilarte TR, Hill J, McIntyre PA, Murphy EA, Tsan MF: Kinetics and distribution of [111]indium-labeled platelets in patients with homocystinuria. N Engl J Med 1982;307:781-786.

128. Graeber JE, Slott JH, Ulane RE, Schulman JD, Stuart M: Effect of homocysteine and homocystine on platelet and vascular arachidonic acid metabolism. Pediatr Res 1982;16:490-493.

129. Kokame K, Kato H, Miyata T: Homocysteine-respondent genes in vascular endothelial cells identified by differential display analysis. J Biol Chem 1996;271:29659-29665.

130. Giannini MJ, Coleman M, Innerfield I. Antithrombin activity in homocystinuria. Lancet 1975;1:1094 (letter).

131. Palareti G, Coccheri S: Lowered antithrombin III activity and other clotting changes in homocystinuria: effects of a pyridoxine-folate regimen. Haemostasis 1989;19 Suppl:24-28.

132. Hilden M, Brandt NJ, Nilsson IM, Schonheyder F: Investigation of coagulation and fibrinolysis in homocystinuria. Acta Med Scand 1974;195:533-535.

133. Rodgers GM, Kane WH: Activation of endogenous factor V by a homocysteine-induced vascular endothelial cell activator. J Clin Invest 1986;77:1909-1916.

134. Rogers GM, Conn MT: Homocysteine, an atherogenic stimulus, reduces protein C activation by arterial and venous endothelial cells. Blood 1990;75:895-901.

135. Hayashi T, Honda G, Suzuki K: An atherogenic stimulus homocysteine inhibits cofactor activity of thrombomodulin and enhances thrombomodulin expression in human umbilical vein endothelial cells. Blood 1992;79:2930-2936.

136. Hajjar KA: Homocysteine-induced modulation of tissue plasminogen activator binding to its endothelial cell membrane receptor. J Clin Invest 1993;91:2873-2879.

137. Nishinaga M Ozawa T, Shimada K: Homocysteine, a thrombogenic agent, suppresses anticoagulant heparin sulfate expression in cultured porcine aortic endothelial cells. J Clin Invest 1993;92:1381-1386.

138. Lentz SR, Sadler JE: Homocysteine inhibits von Willebrand factor processing and secretion by preventing transport from the endoplasmic reticulum. Blood 1993;81:683-689.

139. Peterson JC and Spence JD: Vitamins and progression of atherosclerosis in hyperhomocysteinemia. Lancet 1998;351:263 (letter).

140. Nugent A, Hadden DR, Carson NAJ: Long-term survival of homocystinuria: the first case. Lancet 1998;352:624-625.

141. Malinow MR, Bostom AG, Krauss RM. AHA Science Advisory: Homocyst(e)ine, Diet, and Cardiovascular Diseases. A Statement for Healthcare Professionals From the Nutrition Committee, American Heart Association. Circulation 1999;99:178-182.

142. Malinow MR, Kang, SS, Taylor LM, Wong PW, Coull B, Inahara T, Mukerjee D, Sexton G, Upson B: Prevalence of hyperhomocyst(e)inemia in patients with peripheral arterial occlusive disease. Circulation 1989;79:1180-1188.

143. Duell PB, Malinow MR, Gregory JF, Connor WE: Reduction of fasting and postprandial plasma homocysteine concentrations by a semi-vegetarian very low-fat diet. Circulation 1998;98:I192 (abstract).

144. Andersson A, Brattström L, Israelsson B, Isaksson A, Hamfelt A, Hultberg B: Plasma homocysteine before and after methionine loading with regard to age, gender, and menopausal status. Eur J Clin Invest 1992;22:79-87.

145. Bostom AG, Roubenoff R, Dellaripa P, et al: Validation of abbreviated oral methionine-loading test. Clin Chem 1995;41:948-949.

146. The 4S Investigators: Randomized trial of cholesterol lowering in 4444 patients with coronary heart disease: the Scandinavian Simvastatin Survival Study (4S). Lancet 1994;344:1383-1389.

147. Garg R, Malinow MR, Pettinger M, Hunninghake D: Treatment with niacin increases plasma homocyst(e)ine levels. Circulation 1996;94:I-457 (abstract).

148. Blankenhorn DH, Malinow MR, Mack WJ: Colestipol plus niacin therapy elevates plasma homocyst(e)ine levels. Coronary Artery Disease 1991;2:357-360.

149. Landgren F, Israelsson B, Lindgren A, et al: Plasma homocysteine in acute myocardial infarction: homocysteine-lowering effect of folic acid. J Intern Med 1995;237:381-388.

150. Malinow MR: Hyperhomocyst(e)inemia: a common and easily reversible risk factor for occlusive atherosclerosis. Circulation 1990;81:2004-2006.

151. Selhub J, Jacques PF, Wilson PWF, Rush D, Rosenberg IH: Vitamin status and intake as primary determinants of homocysteinemia in an elderly population. JAMA 1993;270:2693-2698.

152. Guttormsen AB, Ueland PM, Nesthus I, Nygard O, Schneede J, Vollset SE, Refsum H: Determinants and vitamin responsiveness of intermediate hyperhomocysteinemia (> or = 40 micromol/liter): the Hordaland homocysteine Study. J Clin Invest 1996;98:2174-83.

153. Kang SS, Wong PWK, Norusis M: Homocysteinemia due to folate deficiency. Metabolism 1987;36:458-462.

154. Lowering blood homocysteine with folic acid based supplements: meta-analysis of randomized trials. Homocysteine trialists' collaboration. BMJ 1998;316:894-898.

155. Malinow MR, Duell PB, Hess DL, Anderson PH, Kruger WD, Phillipson BE, Gluckman RA, Block PC, Upson BM: Reduction of plasma homocyst(e)ine levels by breakfast cereal fortified with folic acid in patients with coronary heart disease. N Engl J Med 1998;338:1009-1015.

156. Bostom AG, Shemin D, Lapane KL, et al: High dose B-vitamin treatment of hyperhomocysteinemia in dialysis patients. Kidney Int 1996;49:147-152.

157. Ubbink JB, Vermaak WJH, van der Merwe A, Becker PJ, Delport R, Potgieter HC: Vitamin requirements for the treatment of hyperhomocysteinemia in humans. J Nutr 1994;124:1927-1933.

158. Brattström L, Israelsson B, Lindgarde F, Hultberg B: Higher total plasma homocysteine in vitamin $B_{12}$ deficiency than in heterozygosity for homocystinuria due to cystathione ß-synthase deficiency. Metabolism 1988;37:175-178.

159. Lindenbaum J, Healton EB, Savage DG, Brust JC, Garrett TJ, Podell ER, Marcell PD, Stabler SP, Allen RH: Neuropsychiatric disorders caused by cobalamin deficiency in the absence of anemia or macrocytosis. N Engl J Med 1988;318:1720-1728.

160. Kuzminski AM, Del Giacco EJ, Allen RH, Stabler SP, Lindenbaum J: Effective treatment of cobalamin deficiency with oral cobalamin. Blood 1998;92:1191-1198.

161. Wilcken DE, Wilcken B, Dudman NP, Tyrell PA: Homocystinuria: the effects of betaine in the treatment of patients not responsive to pyridoxine. N Engl J Med 1983;309:448-453.

162. Malinow MR, Ryan M: unpublished data.

163. Emmert JL, Garrow TA, Baker DH: Hepatic betaine-homocysteine methyltransferase activity in the chicken is influenced by dietaary intake of sulfur amino acids, choline and betaine. J Nutrition 1996; 126:2050-2058.

164. Lobley GE, Connell A, Revell D: The importance of transmethylation reactions to methionine metabolism in sheep; effects of supplementation with creatine and choline. Brit J Nutr 1996;75:47-56.

165. Voutilainen S, morrow JD, Roberts LJ, Alfthan G, Alho H, Nyyssönen K, Salonen Jt: Enhanced in vivo lipid peroxidation at elevated plasma total homocysteine leveld. Arterioscler Thromb Basc Biol 1999;19:1263-1266.

166. Kittner SJ, Malnow MR, Seipp MJ, Upson B, Hebel Jr: Stability of blood homocysteine under epidemiological field conditions. J Clin Lab Anal 1995;9:75-76.

167. Manilow MR, Axthelm MK, Meredith MJ, MacDonald NA, Upson BM: Synthesis and transsulfuration of homocysteine in blood. J Lab Clin med 1994;123:421-9.

# 12. HOMOCYSTEINE AND FAMILY HISTORY OF CORONARY ARTERY DISEASE

JACQUES GENEST JR.

## SUMMARY

The risk of developing coronary artery disease (CAD) or atherosclerosis in other vascular beds can be estimated by determining the presence of conventional risk factors (age, gender, family history, plasma lipids and lipoproteins, diabetes, hypertension and cigarette smoking). Homocysteine is an emerging cardiovascular risk factor. As seen in previous chapters, plasma levels of homocysteine are determined by environmental factors (nutritional, gender, age, vitamin status, renal function) and by genetics. Homocysteine might thus represent a partly heritable cardiovascular risk factor and, in selected individuals, a more complete study of the family may allow the identification of asymptomatic patients at risk. Mutations at genes encoding for enzymes that metabolize homocysteine, such as the methylenetetrahydrofolate reductase (MTHFR) mutation at residue 677 may represent a disease susceptibility gene for the development of CAD.

## INTRODUCTION

The search for genetic factors associated with CAD stems from the observations made over many decades of the occurrence of CAD within families. Indeed, a family history of early-onset CAD is considered as a risk

*K. Robinson (ed.), Homocysteine and Vascular Disease, 203-216.*
© 2000 *Kluwer Academic Publishers. Printed in the Netherlands.*

factor for the development of CAD. Arbitrarily, a family history is considered positive if a first-degree relative is affected before age 55 years for a man and 65 years for a woman [1]. Barrett-Connor *et al.*[2,3] identified a positive family history of CAD as an independent determinant of disease in individual subjects. It should be noted that first-degree relatives will share half the chromosomes as the proband. In the case of monogenic disorders associated with premature CAD, the association with genetic factors is easy to make and relatively unequivocal. One of the best example of monogenic dominant autosomal disorders (i.e. not related to the sex chromosome) is familial hypercholesterolemia. In familial hypercholesterolemia, the gene coding for the low density lipoprotein receptor (LDL-R) is defective and affected individuals have a roughly twofold elevation in LDL-cholesterol levels. Based on the prevalence of familial hypercholesterolemia in a normal population (approximately 1:500) and in premature CAD (2-4:100), familial hypercholesterolemia represents an approximately 10-fold increase in cardiovascular risk. Affected individuals often develop CAD in the third to sixth decades of life [4,5]. In the very rare subjects homozygous for the disorder, who have two altered copies of the LDL-R gene, CAD is often present in the teenage years and, until recently, survival past age 30 years was unusual. As mentioned in the first chapter dealing with the historical aspects of homocysteine and vascular disease and in chapter 7 patients with homocystinuria present at a young age with thromboembolic disorders which prove debilitating and often fatal in youth [6-10].

There are, however, few gene disorders with such a dramatic presentation. Many familial traits associated with CAD, such as familial combined hyperlipidemia [5,11] and mild to moderate hyperhomocysteinemia are thought to be polygenic or oligogenic with strong environmental influences [12-15]. Other complex traits that are associated with CAD, such as high blood pressure and diabetes have so far eluded a simple genetic characterization in part because age of expression, incomplete penetrance and gender effects play a role in the phenotypic expression.

In the past 20 years, rapid advances in genetics have allowed the cloning and sequencing of thousands of genes. Many gene products are involved in proteins associated with conventional risk factors. The finding of polymorphisms within these genes (more often than not these polymorphisms are either intronic or do not alter the function of the mature protein) has allowed the study of associations between allele frequencies of these polymorphisms in a normal population and plasma levels of specific variables (for instance, polymorphisms of the apolipoprotein genes and plasma lipoprotein cholesterol levels) or between allele frequencies in CAD cases compared with controls. Not surprisingly, few such polymorphisms have been useful from a clinical standpoint. Coronary artery disease is a chronic disease and its etiology is multifactorial [16]. Multiple genes contribute to the phenotypic manifestation of a single risk factor and multiple risk factors are associated with CAD in a given individual. Thus, the lack of association between single gene polymorphisms does not exonerate the role of a particular gene with CAD. The biological inference between a single gene and a complex disease such as CAD is simply too large a biological step.

We have to consider intermediate steps in the events leading to CAD. The term "middle distance reality" has been used to describe this approach. In the case of homocysteine, the association between elevated plasma homocysteine levels and vascular disease has been shown in the previous chapter. In the present chapter, I shall review the genetics of CAD, the prevalence of elevated homocysteine in subjects with CAD and the familial occurrence of hyperhomocysteinemia and discuss the genetic aspects of elevated plasma homocysteine. Because some genes may influence plasma homocysteine levels, especially under nutritional or environmental condition, the concept of "disease susceptibility genes" is brought forth. Simply stated, subjects with a genetic background that predispose to elevated homocysteine levels under certain conditions (for example a relative nutritional folate deficiency) may have a higher risk of developing CAD than subjects without this disposition. Nonetheless, proper lifestyle changes, including vitamin supplementation can compensate for a genetic predisposition.

## GENETICS OF CAD

In the search for familial metabolic disorders associated with CAD, much attention has been given to the lipoprotein field. The seminal work of Goldstein, in a now classic paper in 1973 [5] defined familial lipoprotein disorders in coronary artery disease. The authors studied subjects who survived a myocardial infarction and their families. They identified syndromes of lipoprotein disorders in CAD and characterized a novel disorder, familial combined hyperlipidemia. Since then, the characterization of complex biochemical traits that were partly inherited opened the field of cardiovascular genetics. The first genetic disorders associated with coronary artery disease that were examined were dyslipoproteinemias, with familial hypercholesterolemia representing the best characterized monogenic disorder associated with premature CAD. The importance of genetics in the epidemiology of CAD was shown by Barrett-Connor over 15 years ago and in studies of men with premature CAD. In a study of 4014 adult men and women from the Rancho Bernardo study, a family history of myocardial infarction was associated with a marked increase in risk of developing CAD [2,3].

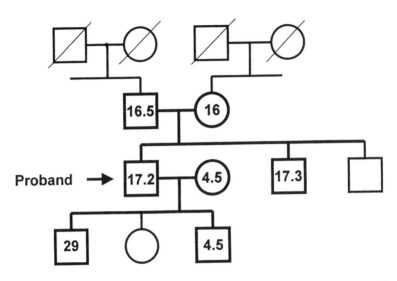

*Figure 1. Pedigree of a kindred with familial hyperhomocysteinemia. Plasma homocysteine level is indicated within the symbol (μmol/L).*

Interestingly, two studies suggested that although conventional risk factors for CAD are considered to be heritable, children of parents with premature myocardial infarction do not have marked abnormalities in cholesterol or glucose metabolism of high blood pressure. Several reasons for this observation might be considered: first, expression of a polygenic disorder might not occur until adult age, second, affected children may be "diluted" with normal children and third, factors other than conventional risk factors may play a role in the familial occurrence of CAD [17,18].

Tonstad *et al.* [19] examined 756 school children aged 8 to 12 years. A mild elevation of homocysteine levels was associated with early onset cardiovascular disease in male relatives. In this group of children, the distribution of plasma homocysteine was shifted towards higher values and serum folate levels were a strong determinant of homocysteine levels. In a subsequent study of 155 children with a parental history of cardiovascular disease, these children had higher mean homocysteine levels than children who did not have a parental history of cardiovascular disease [20]. There was a trend towards an increase in the prevalence of the homozygous state for the $MTHFR_{C677T}$ mutation in children whose parents had cardiovascular disease. Homocysteine, therefore,

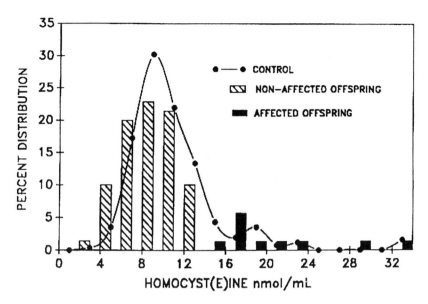

*Figure 2. Frequency distribution of homocysteine levels in the offspring of probands with elevated levels. From reference 12.*

may be one of the non-conventional cardiovascular risk factors that is heritable.

## PREVALENCE OF ELEVATED HOMOCYSTEINE IN SUBJECTS WITH CAD

Elevated plasma homocysteine has been recognized as a risk factor in early familial CAD, defined as the presence of two or more first-degree relatives with onset of CAD by age 55 years in men and 65 in women [1]. As discussed in Chapter 10, the prevalence of hyperhomocysteinemia in subjects with CAD is higher than in control subjects. The prevalence of hyperhomocysteinemia is dependent on cut-points and the population examined. In our populations, the $90^{th}$ percentile corresponds to approximately 15 μmol/L for men and approximately 14 μmol/L for women. Based on this definition, 20-40% of subjects with premature CAD have elevated plasma concentrations [12,21].

We studied 71 probands and their nuclear families to determine the prevalence of familial hyperhomocysteinemia in premature CAD [12]. Of these probands, all men, 20 (28%) had hyperhomocysteinemia, defined as a total plasma homocysteine level >15 μmol/L. There were 60 spouses and 239 first-degree relatives (an average of 5.2 subjects per kindred). Segregation of hyperhomocysteinemia, defined as the proband and at least one first-degree relative having a plasma homocysteine level >90th percentile was found in 10/20 families or 14% of 71 kindred. The prevalence of familial hyperhomocysteinemia was thus estimated to be 14% in our premature CAD population. An example of familial hyperhomocysteinemia is shown in Figure 1.

Wu *et al.* [22] examined 266 CAD patients from 170 such families and found a significant increase in plasma homocysteine levels compared with controls. Hyperhomocysteinemia (defined as >95th percentile) was seen in 17.6% of the probands. Concordant elevated homocysteine levels were seen in 10/85 families (12%) with two or more affected siblings. The trait "hyperhomocysteinemia" is not transmitted as a simple Mendelian trait because the effects of genetic predisposition are modulated by environmental variables, especially vitamin status. Thus, the number of affected offspring from a proband with elevated homocysteine do not follow a simple 1:2 ratio as would be expected from a co-dominant trait. The frequency distribution of homocysteine levels in offspring of parents with hyperhomocysteinemia is shown in figure 2. Only 25% of these offspring had homocysteine levels > 15 μmol/L [12].

## FAMILIAL OCCURRENCE OF HYPERHOMOCYSTEINEMIA

The prevalence of familial hyperhomocysteinemia depends on the population studied (normal subjects, subjects with elevated homocysteine levels, patients with atherosclerosis), cut-points used to define abnormal levels (e.g. the 90th or 95th percentiles of a normal distribution) and the method used for measurement (fasting or post methionine load homocysteine levels). In a study of 21 subjects with vascular disease (cerebral occlusive disease (10), peripheral vascular disease (3), CAD (3), anterior spinal syndrome (2), and venous thrombosis (3)) in whom elevated post methionine load homocysteine levels were documented, Franken et al. [14] examined 96 family members for the presence of elevated homocysteine levels. An elevated post methionine load homocysteine level was seen in at least 15 family members of the 21 screened families (71%). This is in contrast to the 50% we observed in probands with premature CAD (10 out of 20 families of male probands) [12]. In a study of 107 patients with venous thromboembolism and arterial occlusive disease occurring at a young age (mean age 32 and 31 years, respectively), moderate hyperhomocysteinemia was identified in 13% of patients with venous thromboembolism and in 19% of patients with arterial disease [23]. The prevalence of hyperhomocysteinemia

Table 1. Parent-Offspring correlations for homocysteine [reference 12]

| Groups compared pairwise | r | p |
|---|---|---|
| Mean Parent - mean Offspring | 0.356 | 0.002 |
| Proband-Spouse | 0.264 | 0.041 |
| Proband-Mean offspring | 0.248 | 0.037 |
| Spouse-Mean offspring | 0.224 | 0.084 |

was nearly twice as high when post methionine load (8 hours) homocysteine levels were used. Out of 12 families with hyperhomocysteinemia studied, 8 (66%) had familial hyperhomocysteinemia.

## GENETIC ASPECTS OF ELEVATED PLASMA HOMOCYSTEINE

The major factors modulating plasma homocysteine levels have been reviewed in Chapter 5; these include: the male gender, increasing age, renal function, diet (including vitamin status), drugs and genetics [24-29]. Plasma homocysteine levels are considered to be in part genetically determined [12,25,30-32]. Several lines of evidence support this concept. First, the study of families reveals that plasma homocysteine levels correlate between parents and offspring. As shown in Table 1, the mean plasma homocysteine levels between parents (taken as the mean between a proband and the spouse) and the mid-value of their offspring have a high degree of correlation, indicating a possible genetic influence in the determination of homocysteine levels. There is also a statistically significant correlation between proband and spouse, suggesting that shared household (diet, socioeconomic status, smoking) also plays an important role in determining homocysteine levels within kindred.

The study of monozygotic twins has shed light on the genetics of homocysteine. Reed *et al.* [31] studied plasma homocysteine levels in 82 pairs of twins. The intraclass correlation coefficient for log-transformed homocysteine levels was r=0.55 in 43 pairs of monozygotic twins and r=0.19 in 39 pairs of dizygotic twins. The difference between correlation coefficients for homocysteine between mono- and dizygotic twins was statistically significant (p<0.05). On the basis of these observations, plasma homocysteine levels have a strong genetic determinant. Several genes involved in the metabolism of homocysteine have been identified and mutations causing human diseases have been identified. The genes for cystathionine β-synthase (CBS) [33,34], MTHFR [35] and for methionine synthase [36] have recently been cloned and sequenced.

*CBS.* The chromosomal localization for the CBS gene is 21q22.3. Several mutations have been identified in the CBS gene that lead to a defective enzyme with reduced affinity for any of its substrates (serine, homocysteine or the vitamin $B_6$ derivative, pyridoxal 5'-phosphate) [34,37-42,49-52]. Homocystinuria is predominantly caused by mutations at the CBS gene in the homozygous or compound heterozygous state. The prevalence of homocystinuria due to CBS mutations is approximately 1:335 000 worldwide but varies between 1:65 000 in Ireland to 1:900 000 in Japan [32]. Heterozygotes for CBS deficiency have enzymatic activity that may be as low as 50% of normal but values frequently overlap with those of normal individuals. Thus the diagnosis of heterozygous CBS deficiency may not be accurate based solely on enzyme activity [43]. Over 60 mutations of the CBS gene have been reported causing a defective enzyme [34,37-39,40-44]. The most frequent mutations include CBS G307S ($CBS_{G919A}$) seen in 31% of cases and I278T ($CBS_{T833C}$), or C341T, with the first two being the most prevalent (in a cohort of Irish descent) [44]. Thought initially to be frequent in subjects with CAD, CBS mutations appear uncommon in CAD subjects [37,41] . A 68 bp insertion in exon 8 of the CBS gene ($CBS_{844ins68}$) has been associated with CAD in one study, despite the fact that this mutation appears not to impart functional significance. A more recent study questions this association [41]. Thus, CBS mutations are infrequent and lead to homocystinuria in the homozygous state. In subjects with CAD, such mutations are seen infrequently.

*MTHFR* (located on 1p36.3) [35]. Mutations of the MTHFR gene have been identified in patients with severe elevations of homocysteine. Since the description of the gene, over 20 mutations have been identified in patients with markedly elevated plasma homocysteine levels. These mutations are a cause of severe hyperhomocysteinemia in children [35,45]. In the past 15 years, Kang described a frequent isoform of MTHFR that has no residual activity after heating at 46°C [46]. This thermolabile variant was seen in greater frequency in premature CAD patients and was considered a novel genetic risk factor for the disease. The molecular basis of this thermolability is caused by the $MTHFR_{C677T}$ mutation resulting in a alanine for valine substitution [13]. Thermolability of MTHFR is seen in increased frequency in subjects with elevated homocysteine levels [46]. In 625 subjects, the prevalence of homozygous $MTHFR_{C677T}$ was seen in 48.4%, 35.5% and 23.5% of those in the top 5, 10 and 20% of the distribution of homocysteine level, compared with a frequency of 11.5% in the study population [48]. Similarly, in 121 subjects with premature CAD, there was a significant increase in the prevalence of at least one allele of the $MTHFR_{C677T}$ mutation in subjects separated by the median of homocysteine levels (30/120 alleles versus 50/122 alleles in the elevated homocysteine group) ($\chi^2$=5.8, p=0.016) [Genest, unpublished observations]. In subjects homozygous for the $MTHFR_{C677T}$ mutation, plasma homocysteine levels are increased only in subjects with decreased plasma levels of folate; when folate levels are normal, plasma homocysteine levels are similar in subjects homozygous, heterozygous or not carrying the $MTHFR_{C677T}$ variant [13]. This is an example of gene-environment interaction where a genetic predisposition can be modulated in a favorable environment and, conversely, the effects of an altered environment can be synergistic with a genetic predisposition to produce a markedly altered phenotype.

Several studies have shown an increased allele frequency of the $MTHFR_{C677T}$ mutation in patients with CAD [reviewed in 13,2,47,53,63] but others have not. The association between allele frequency of the $MTHFR_{C677T}$ mutation and coronary artery disease may thus be modulated by environmental influences, especially plasma folate levels.

*Methionine synthase (MS)* (1q42.3) [36,54]. Methionine synthase catabolizes the remethylation of homocysteine to methionine, a step that involves methyltetrahydrofolate and methyl cobalamin. The gene maps to chromosome 1q42.3 [36,54] and several mutations have been identified that lead to the molecular basis of the cblG complementation group of folate/cobalamin disorders. A frequent polymorphism D919G ($MS_{A2756G}$) has been reported and may modulate homocysteine levels in the presence of abnormal vitamin $B_{12}$ levels.

*Methionine synthase reductase (MSR)* (5p15.2) [55]. The recent cloning of the MS gene [55] has allowed the identification of mutations in the cblE complementation group of disorders of folate/cobalamin metabolism. Several mutations have been identified to date in patients with the cblE phenotype, confirming the molecular basis of the cblE mutation.


GENE-ENVIRONMENT INTERACTIONS

The study of the genes associated with homocysteine metabolism has allowed the characterization of mutations leading to severe elevations in plasma homocysteine levels. Common polymorphisms of the MTHFR gene have revealed a strong gene-environment interaction in the modulation of homocysteine levels. In patients with CAD in whom at least one first-degree relative also had CAD, plasma homocysteine levels were strongly modulated by plasma folate levels such that patients with low folate levels had marked increases in homocysteine levels; this relationship between folate and homocysteine was more marked than in healthy controls [57]. The interaction between the homozygous state for $MTHFR_{C677T}$ and folate in the modulation of homocysteine levels has already been described. The response to folic acid used for therapeutic purposes has been examined in subjects with large variations in plasma homocysteine levels. All patients then received supplemental folate and the effects were examined according to plasma folate levels and the presence of the $MTHRF_{C677T}$ mutation. Interestingly, patients with normal folate levels had relatively little benefit from supplemental folate whereas those with plasma folate levels less than the median benefited to a greater extent. The best response to exogenous folate occurred in subjects with low plasma folate levels and the homozygous state for the $MTHFR_{C677T}$ mutation [56]. This strongly supports the concept that the effects of disease susceptibility genes may be compensated by appropriate lifestyle changes.

## CONCLUSIONS

A family history of early onset coronary artery disease has been established as an independent risk factor for CAD. The pathogenesis of CAD is very complex and the role of a single biochemical variable in modulation the development and expression of CAD depends on the absolute level of this variable (e.g. extreme cholesterol elevation in familial hypercholesterolemia) and the interactions of the variable with other risk factors [58]. It has long been suspected that genetic factors such as hyperhomocysteinemia play a role in vascular diseases [59]. Indeed, the pioneering work of McCully [61] is being recognized after being largely ignored by a large segment of the scientific community. Only recently have public health measures been applied to the population at large by fortifying grains with folic acid. Intended to increase dietary folate to decrease the incidence of neural tube defect in the developing fetus, these measures may have little impact on preventive cardiovascular health. Malinow recently studied the impact of vitamins fortified with folate according to the Food and Drug administration guidelines in the US. This increase in dietary folate may not be sufficient to decrease plasma homocysteine levels to produce clinically significant results [60]. In patients surviving an acute myocardial infarction, an elevated plasma homocysteine level is a strong, graded and independent risk factor for mortality [62]. There is, to date, no evidence that vitamin supplementation with folic acid reduces mortality in the secondary prevention of cardiovascular disease. Physician judgement must thus be exercized as to when and in whom should be measured and in whom should it be treated.

## REFERENCES

1.  The Expert Panel. Summary of the Second report of the National Cholesterol Education Program (NCEP) expert panel on detection, evaluation, and treatment of high blood cholesterol in adults (Adult Treatment Panel II). J Am Med Ass 1993;269:3015-3023
2.  Barrett-Connor E. Khaw K. Family history of heart attack as an independent predictor of death due to cardiovascular disease. Circulation. 1984;69:1065-9
3.  Khaw KT. Barrett-Connor E. Family history of heart attack: a modifiable risk factor. Circulation. 1986;74:239-244

4. Dammerman M, Breslow JL. Genetic basis of lipoprotein disorders. *Circulation* 1995;91:505-511

5. Goldstein JL, Schrott HG, Hazzard WR, Bierman EL, Motulsky AG. Hyperlipidemia in coronary heart disease. II. Genetic analysis of lipid levels in 176 families and delineation of a new inherited disorder, combined hyperlipidemia. J Clin Invest 1973;52:1544-1568

6. Harker LA, Slichter SJ, Scott CR, Ross R. Homocystinemia. Vascular injury and arterial thrombosis. N Engl J Med. 1974;291:537-543

7. Kang SS, Wong PWK, Norusis M. Homocysteinemia secondary to folate deficiency. Metabolism 1987;36:458-462

8. McCully KS. Vascular pathology of homocysteinemia: implications for the pathogenesis of arteriosclerosis. Am J Pathol 1969;56:111-128

9. Mudd SH, Levy HL, Skovby F. Disorders of transsulfuration, in: Scriver CR, Beaudet AL, Sly WS, Valle D. (eds):The Metabolic Basis of Inherited Disease 6th ed. McGraw-Hill Book Co., New York 1989:693-734

10. Schimke RN, McKusick VA, Huang T, Pollack AD. Homocystinuria. JAMA 1965;193:711-719

11. Genest J Jr, Martin-Munley SS, McNamara JR, Ordovas JM, Jenner JL, Meyers RH, Silberman SR, Wilson PWF, Salem DN, Schaefer EJ. Familial Lipoprotein Disorders in Patients With Premature Coronary Artery Disease. Circulation 1992;85:2025-2033

12. Genest J Jr, McNamara JR, Upson B, Salem DN, Ordovas JM, Schaefer EJ, Malinow MR. Prevalence of familial hyperhomocyst(e)inemia in men with premature coronary artery disease. Arterioscler Thromb 1991;11:1129-1136

13. Christensen B, Frosst P, Lussier-Cacan S, Selhub J, Goyette P, Rosenblatt DS, Genest J Jr, Rozen R. Correlation of a common mutation in methylenetetrahydrofolate reductase gene with plasma homocysteine in patients with premature coronary artery disease. Arterioscler Thromb Vasc Biol 1997;17:569-573

14. Franken DG, Boers GHJ, Blom HJ, Cruysberg JR, Trijbels FJM, Hamel BC. Prevalence of familial mild hyperhomocysteinemia. Atheroscler 1996;125:71-80

15. Williams RR, Malinow MR, Hunt SC et al. Hyperhomocyst(e)inemia in Utah siblings with early coronary artery disease. Coronary Art Dis 1990;1:681-5

16. Ross R. The pathogenesis of atherosclerosis – an update. N Engl J Med 1986;314:488-500

17. Thelle DS, Forde OH. The cardiovascular study in Finnmark county: coronary risk factors and the occurrence of myocardial infarction in first degree relatives and in subjects of different ethnic origin. Am J Epidemiol 1979;110:708-15

18. Levine RS, Hennekens CH, Rosner B, Gourley J, Gelband H, Jesse MJ. Cardiovascular risk factors among children of men with premature myocardial infarction. Public Health Reports 1981;96:58-60

19. Tonstad S, Refsum H, Sivertsen M, Christophersen B, Ose L, Ueland PM. Relation of total homocysteine and lipid levels in children to premature cardiovascular deaths in male relatives. Pediatric Res. 1996;40:47-52

20. Tonstad S, Refsum H, Ueland PM. Association between plasma total homocysteine and parental history of cardiovascular disease in children with familial hypercholesterolemia. Circ 1997;96:1803-1808

21. Dalery K, Lussier-Cacan S, Selhub J, Davignon J, Latour Y, Genest J Jr. Homocysteine and coronary artery disease in French Canadian subjects: relation with vitamins $B_{12}$, $B_6$, pyridoxal phosphate, and folate. Am J Cardiol 1995;75:1107-1111

22. Wu LL, Wu J, Hunt SC, James BC, Vincent GM, Williams RR, Hopkins PN. Plasma homocyst(e)ine as a risk factor for early familial coronary artery disease. Clin Chem 1994;40:552-561

23. Fermo I, Vigano' D'Angelo S, Paroni R, Mazzola G, Calori G, D'Angelo A. Prevalence of moderate hyperhomocysteinemia in patients with early-onset venous and arterial occlusive disease. Ann Intern Med 1995;123:747-753

24. Selhub J, Jacques PF, Wilson PWF, Rush D, Rosenberg IH. Vitamin status and intake as primary determinants of homocysteinemia in an elderly population. JAMA 1993;270:2693-2698

25. Berg K, Malinow MR, Kierulf P, Upson B. Population variation and genetics of plasma homocyst(e)ine levels. Clin Genet 1992;41:315-321

26. Lussier-Cacan S, Davignon J, Selhub J, Genest J Jr. Plasma homocyst(e)ine levels in a population selected for health: relationship with vitamins $B_{12}$, $B_6$, pyridoxal phosphate and folate and cardiovascular risk factors. Circulation 1993;88:1563

27. Mayer EL, Jacobsen DW, Robinson K. Homocysteine and coronary atherosclerosis. J Am Coll Cardiol 1996;27:517-527

28. Refsum H, Ueland PM, Nygard O, Vollset SE. Homocysteine and cardiovascular disease. Annu Rev Med 1998;49:31-62

29. Ubbink JB, Vermaak WJ, van der Merwe A, Becker PJ. Vitamin B-12, vitamin B-6, and folate nutritional status in men with hyperhomocysteinemia. Am J Clin Nutr 1993;57:47-53

30. Kang SS, Wong PWK, Susmano A, Sora J, Norusis M, Ruggie N. Thermolabile methylenetetrahydrofolate reductase: an inherited risk factor for coronary artery disease. Am J Hum Genet 1991;48:536-545

31. Reed T, Malinow MR, Christian JC, Upson B. Estimates of heritability of plasma homocyst(e)ine levels in aging adult male twins. Clin Genet 1991;39:425-428

32. Naughten ER. Yap S. Mayne PD. Newborn screening for homocystinuria: Irish and world experience. European Journal of Pediatrics. 1998;157 Suppl 2:S84-7

33. Kraus JP, Williamson CL, Firgaira FA, Yang-Feng IL, Munke M, Francke U, Rosenbert LE. Cloning and screening with nanogram amounts of immunopurified mRNAs: cDNA cloning and chromosomal mapping of cystathionine beta-synthase and the beta subunit of propionyl-CoA carboxylase. Proc Natl Acad Sci USA 1986;83:2047-2051.

34. Tsai MY, Gard U, Key NS, Hanson NQ, Suh A, Schwichtenberg K. Molecular and biochemical approaches in the identification of heterozygotes for homocystinuria. Atheroscler 1996;122:69-77

35. Frosst P, Blom HJ, Milos R, Goyette P, Sheppard CA, Matthews RG, Boers GJH, den Heijer M, Kluijtmans LAJ, van den Heuvel LP, Rozen R. A candidate genetic risk factor for vascular disease: a common mutation in methylenetetrahydrofolate reductase. Nature Genetics 1995;10:111-113

36. Chen LH, Liu ML, Hwang HY, Chen LS, Korenberg J, Shane B. Human methionine synthase. cDNA cloning, gene localization, and expression. J Biol Chem 1997;272:3628-34

37. Tsai MY, Bignell M, Schwichtenberg K, Hanson NQ. High prevalence of a mutation in the cystathionine beta-synthase gene. Amer J Human Gen 1996;59:1262-1267

38. Tsai MY, Hanson NQ, Bignell MK, Schwichtenberg KA. Simultaneous detection and screening of T833C and G919A mutations of the cystathionine beta-synthase gene by single-strand conformational polymorphism. Clin Biochem 1996;29:473-477

39. Tsai MY, Wong PW, Gard U, Hanson NQ, Schwichtenberg K. Identification of a splice site mutation in the cystathionine beta-synthase gene resulting in variable and novel splicing defects of pre-mRNA. Biochem & Molec Med 1997;61:9-15

40. Kluijtmans LA, Blom HJ, Boers GH, van Oost BA, Trijbels FJ, van den Heuvel LP. Two novel missense mutations in the cystathionine beta-synthase gene in homocystinuric patients. Human Genetics 1995;96:249-250

41. Kluijtmans LA, Boers GH, Trijbels FJ, van Lith-Zanders HM, van den Heuvel LP, Blom HJ. A common 844INS68 insertion variant in the cystathionine beta-synthase gene. Biochemical & Molecular Medicine. 1997;62:23-25

42. Kluijtmans LA, Boers GH, Verbruggen B, Trijbels FJ, Novakova IR, Blom HJ. Homozygous cystathionine beta-synthase deficiency, combined with factor V Leiden or thermolabile methylenetetrahydrofolate reductase in the risk of venous thrombosis. Blood. 1998;91:2015-2018

43. McGill JJ, Mettler G, Rosenblatt DS, Scriver CR. Detection of heterozygotes for recessive alleles. Homocysteinemia: paradigm of pitfalls in phenotypes. Am J Med Genet 1990;36:45-52

44. Kraus JP. Biochemistry and molecular genetics of cystathionine beta-synthase deficiency. European Journal of Pediatrics. 1998;157:S50-3

45. Goyette P, Sumner JS, Milos R, Duncan AMV, Rosenblatt DS, Matthews RG, Rozen R. Human methylenetetrahydrofolate reductase: isolation of cDNA, mapping and mutation identification. Nature Genet 1994;7:195-200

46. Kang SS, Passen EL, Ruggie N, Wong PWK, Sora H. Thermolabile defect of methylenetetrahydrofolate reductase in coronary artery disease. Circulation 1993;88:1463-1469

47. Kluijtmans LAJ, van den Heuvel LPWJ, Boers GHJ, Frosst P, Stevens EM, van Oost BA, den Heijer M, Trijbels FJ, Rozen R, Blom HJ. Molecular genetic analysis in mild hyperhomocysteinemia: a common mutation in the methylenetetrahydrofolate reductase gene is a genetic risk factor for cardiovascular disease. Am J Hum Genet 1996;58:35-41

48. Harmon DL, Woodside JV, Yarnell JW, McMaster D, Young IS, McCrum EE, Whitehead AS, Evans AE. The common 'thermolabile' variant of methylenetetrahydrofolate reductase is a major determinant of mild hyperhomocysteinemia. Quarterly J Med 1996;89:571-577

49. Dawson PA, Cochran DA, Emmerson BT, Kraus JP, Dudman NP, Gordon RB. Variable hyperhomocysteinemia phenotype in heterozygotes for the Gly307Ser mutation in cystathionine beta-synthase. Australian & New Zealand Journal of Medicine. 1996;26:180-5

50. Dawson PA, Cox AJ, Emmerson BT, Dudman NP, Kraus JP, Gordon RB. Characterisation of five missense mutations in the cystathionine beta-synthase gene from three patients with $B_6$-nonresponsive homocystinuria. Eur J Human Gen 1997;5:15-21

51. Sebastio G, Sperandeo MP, Panico M, de Franchis R, Kraus JP, Andria G. The molecular basis of homocystinuria due to cystathionine beta-synthase deficiency in Italian families, and report of four novel mutations. American J Human Gen 1995;56:1324-1333

52. Sperandeo MP, Candito M, Sebastio G, Rolland MO, Turc-Carel C, Giudicelli H, Dellamonica P, Andria G. Homocysteine response to methionine challenge in four obligate heterozygotes for homocystinuria and relationship with cystathionine beta-synthase mutations. J Inher Metab Dis 1996;19:351-35

53. Wilcken DE, Wang XL, Sim AS, McCredie RM. Distribution in healthy and coronary populations of the methylene tetrahydrofolate reductase (MTHFR) $C_{677}T$ mutation. Atheroscler Thromb Vasc Biol 1996;16:878-882

54. Leclerc D, Campeau E, Goyette P, Adjalla CE, Christensen B, Ross M, Eydoux P, Rosenblatt DS, Rozen R, Gravel RA. Human methionine synthase: cDNA cloning and identification of mutations in patients of the cblG complementation group of folate/cobalamin disorders. Hum Mol Genet 1996;5:1867-1874

55. Leclerc D, Wilson A, Dumas R, Gafuik C, Song D, Watkins D, Heng HH, Rommens JM, Scherer SW, Rosenblatt DS, Gravel RA. Cloning and mapping of a cDNA for methionine synthase reductase, a flavoprotein defective in patients with homocystinuria. PNAS 1998;95:3059-3064

56. Malinow MR, Nieto FJ, Kruger WD, Duell PB, Hess DL, Gluckman RA, Block PC, Holzgang CR, Anderson PH, Seltzer D, Upson B, Lin QR. The effects of folic acid supplementation on plasma total homocysteine are modulated by multivitamin use and methylenetetrahydrofolate reductase genotypes. Arterioscler, Thromb Vasc Biol. 1997;17:1157-1162

57. Hopkins PN, Wu LL, Wu J, Hunt SC, James BC, Vincent GM, Williams RR. Higher plasma homocyst(e)ine and increased susceptibility to adverse effects of low folate in early familial coronary artery disease. Arterioscler Thromb Vasc Biol 1995;15:1314-1320

58. Fuster V, Badimon L, Badimon JJ, Chesebro JH. The pathogenesis of coronary artery disease and the acute

59. Boers GHJ, Smals AGH, Trijbels FJM, Fowler B, Bakkeren JAJM, Schoonderwaldt HC, Kleijer WJ, Kloppenborg PWC. Heterozygosity for homocystinuria in premature peripheral and cerebral occlusive arterial disease. N Engl J Med 1985;313:709-715

60. Malinow MR, Duell PB, Hess DL, Anderson PH, Kruger WD, Phillipson BE, Gluckman RA, Block PC, Upson BM. Reduction of plasma homocyst(e)ine levels by breakfast cereal fortified with folic acid in patients with coronary heart disease. N Engl J Med 1998;338:1009-1015

61. McCully KS. Homocysteine and vascular disease. Nature Med. 1996;2:386-389

62. Nygard O, Vollset SE, Refsum H, Stensvold I, Tverdal A, Nordrehaug JE, Ueland PM, Kvale G. Total plasma homocysteine and cardiovascular risk profile. The Hordaland homocysteine study. JAMA 1995;274:1526-1533

63. Schwartz SM, Siscovick DS, Malinow MR, Rosendaal FR, Beverly RK, Hess DL, Psaty BM, Longstreth WT Jr., Koepsell TD, Raghunathan TE, Reitsma PH. Myocardial infarction in young women in relation to plasma total homocysteine, folate, and a common variant in the methylenetetrahydrofolate reductase gene. Circulation 1997;96:412-417

# 13. HOMOCYSTEINE AS A RISK FACTOR FOR CARDIOVASCULAR DISEASE IN WOMEN

PETRA VERHOEF

SUMMARY

Elevated plasma levels of total homocysteine are considered a risk factor for cardiovascular disease (CVD). Levels are generally lower in women than men, and in premenopausal than postmenopausal women. Differences in circulating estrogens may be partly responsible for these observations.

The present chapter reviews studies that have investigated associations of homocysteine with risk of CVD by gender or by menopausal status. Furthermore, the evidence for a homocysteine-lowering effect of estrogen replacement therapy in postmenopausal women is discussed.

Six out of 10 of the epidemiologic studies that included both men and women found elevated homocysteine to be a stronger risk factor in women than in men. Several of these studies estimated that the risk was about twice as high in women as in men. Three studies observed no effect modification, and one a weaker effect in women. Two studies that consisted (almost) entirely of women observed a direct association of elevated homocysteine with CVD risk as well, comparable to effects in male populations.

The stronger effect among women in some studies may be explained by aspects of the study design, such as young age at inclusion, or aspects of the data-analysis, such as use of an overall instead of a gender-specific cutoff-point. Also, one cannot exclude the possibility that women are somehow more susceptible to detrimental effects of homocysteine than men, although there is

K. Robinson (ed.), Homocysteine and Vascular Disease, 217-238.
© 2000 Kluwer Academic Publishers. Printed in the Netherlands.

clear evidence from other studies that estrogens have a "protective" effect on the vascular wall and favorable effect on hemostasis.

Elevation of homocysteine is found to be a risk factor in populations of both young and elderly women, but only few studies have compared the relation between homocysteine and risk of CVD among premenopausal and postmenopausal women. Generally, it appears that women are not protected against CVD before the menopause. Several, mostly uncontrolled, intervention studies have indicated that estrogen replacement therapy, either alone, sequentially or continuously combined with progestogen, lowers homocysteine by about 11-13% during postmenopausal years.

In conclusion, we should consider elevated homocysteine as an equally strong, potential risk factor for CVD in both men and women, before and after the menopause. Results from randomized trials of B-vitamins, that are currently being conducted among large populations of men and women, will tell us whether homocysteine-lowering gives a CVD benefit.


INTRODUCTION

Retrospective case-control studies and cross-sectional studies have very consistently shown that moderately elevated plasma levels of homocysteine (in most studies measured as total homocysteine) are more prevalent among patients of CVD than among control subjects [1,2]. Several prospective studies – in which homocysteine was measured before onset of CVD – have confirmed this finding [3,4], but others observed weaker or no associations [3,5,6]. Results from ongoing randomized prevention trials will reveal whether homocysteine-reduction through B-vitamin supplementation will indeed reduce CVD incidence.

Circulating levels of homocysteine are generally lower in women than in men [7-12]. Most [13-17] but not all [12] studies have indicated that the menopause may lead to a rise in plasma homocysteine concentrations. Some investigators have suggested that this could in part account for the markedly increased risk of CVD which is observed in women after the menopause [18]. Circulating estrogens may largely explain the lower homocysteine concentrations in women compared to men, and in premenopausal women compared to postmenopausal women.

The present chapter reviews studies that have compared associations of homocysteine with risk of CVD for women and men, or for premenopausal and postmenopausal women. Some findings on B-vitamins and risk of CVD are included as well. Furthermore, results from intervention studies that tested effects of estrogen replacement therapy on homocysteine levels in postmenopausal women are discussed.


CONCENTRATIONS OF HOMOCYSTEINE IN WOMEN: COMPARISON
WITH MEN AND EFFECT OF THE MENOPAUSE

Concentrations of homocysteine are generally lower in women than in men [7-12]. This applies to fasting levels as well as those after an oral load with L-methionine (referred to as post-methionine loading homocysteine), although one study observed no difference between men and women in post-load concentrations [12].

Plasma concentrations of homocysteine increase with age in both men and women [2]. This is most likely due to declining renal function associated with ageing [9]. Except for one study [12], studies have shown that plasma concentrations are higher in postmenopausal than premenopausal women [13-17]. Some studies indicated that this rise cannot totally be accounted for by the generally observed age-related increase in plasma homocysteine levels. In the Hordaland study [10], a population-based study conducted in Norway among 7591 men and 8585 women, the male-to-female ratio in geometric mean levels was 1.19 in subjects 40-42 years old, and 1.12 in subjects 65-67 years old. Furthermore, the age-related increase appeared to be steeper in women than in men, suggesting that the menopause influences homocysteine levels. Kang *et al.* [13] observed an abrupt increase of protein-bound homocysteine concentrations in females after 50 years of age. In the age group of 60-69 years, mean protein-bound homocysteine concentrations were higher in women than in men. In a European multi-center case-control study, using data for controls only, homocysteine concentrations were plotted against age. In the postmenopausal age range, levels post-load, but not fasting, of women surpassed levels of men [19]. Similarly, Andersson *et al.* [12] observed that post-load levels among postmenopausal women were similar to levels in men of the same age, whereas fasting levels were lower compared to those in men of similar age. Wouters *et al.* observed higher mean plasma levels, fasting and post-methionine loading, in postmenopausal women than premenopausal women [17]. The contrast was stronger for post-methionine loading than fasting homocysteine. However, the investigators did not compare levels of pre- and postmenopausal women to levels of men of comparable age.

In summary, men have higher levels than women, but it appears that the menopause induces an additional increase in homocysteine concentration above the generally observed age-related increase. Possibly, this effect of the menopause is more evident for post-methionine loading than for fasting levels.

## BIOLOGIC MECHANISMS

Likely explanations for differences between men and women are differences in muscle mass, vitamin status, and hormonal differences. The higher levels of men are believed to be related to their larger muscle mass, since about 75% of homocysteine is formed in conjunction with creatine-creatinine synthesis [20]. This is reflected by the fact that men usually have higher creatinine concentrations than women. This relationship between creatinine and homocysteine was nicely illustrated in a cross-sectional study by Brattström *et al.*, in which sex differences disappeared within strata of serum creatinine concentrations [9]. A large cross-sectional study of elderly participants in the Framingham study [7] found that the difference in basal (nonfasting) homocysteine between the sexes was largely attributable to differences in vitamin status. However, the Hordaland study [10] observed that gender-differences remained virtually unchanged after multivariate adjustment for intake of vitamin supplements, fruits and vegetables.

Besides muscle mass and vitamin status, hormonal differences may be responsible for differences between the sexes. Also, the menopause-related increase in homocysteine concentrations, as observed in some studies, is very likely to be due to hormonal changes, as no corresponding age-related changes are seen in men. The hypothesized homocysteine-lowering effect of estrogens is derived from the observation that concentrations are lower in pregnant than in nonpregnant women [21,22]. Also, the level was observed to be lower during the peak hormonal (i.e. high estrogen) phase than in the low hormonal phase, in women using oral contraceptives [23]. However, this was not confirmed by others [24,25]. Furthermore, Wouters *et al.* [17] observed an inverse association between post-methionine loading, but not fasting, plasma homocysteine and serum estradiol levels in premenopausal women. Strong evidence for effects of hormones on plasma levels is derived from a study [26] in which male-to-female (M→F) transsexuals were treated with ethinyl estradiol and an anti-androgen, and female-to-male (F→M) transsexuals were treated with testosterone esters, all for 4 months. M→F transsexuals showed a decreased geometric mean homocysteine, and F→M transsexuals an increase. Effects were partly explained by changes in creatinine. Therefore, it is likely that part of the effect of hormones is explained through effects on muscle mass.

## EPIDEMIOLOGIC STUDIES OF CVD RISK: ASSOCIATIONS AMONG MEN AND WOMEN

Previously, researchers have suggested that the lower homocysteine concentrations among premenopausal women compared to men may protect them against CVD [14,16]. Is that true and does the possible protective effect disappear after the menopause? Unfortunately, in most epidemiologic studies, women formed only a small part of the study population or were not included at all. Therefore, in most studies, estimates of CVD risk associated with elevated homocysteine are given for the sexes combined, usually multivariately adjusted for sex and other CVD risk factors. A recent meta-analysis [1] indicated that the effect of homocysteine elevation on coronary heart disease [CHD] risk is stronger in women than in men: the odds ratio (OR) for CHD of a 5 $\mu$mol/L increment (about 1 SD) was 1.6 (95% confidence interval [CI], 1.4 - 1.7) in men and 1.8 (95% CI, 1.3 to 1.9) in women.

Table 1 lists 10 recent epidemiologic studies which showed separate estimates of CVD risk for men and (a reasonable sample of) women [5,27-33,35,37]. Furthermore, the table includes one study that consisted of women only [34] and one [36] that consisted for 93% of women. With the exception of the study by Graham *et al.* [33] – the European multi-center case-control study – and the Finnish prospective study by Alfthan *et al.* [35], none of the studies were included in the meta-analysis of Boushey *et al.* [1]. Only the European study [33] measured both fasting and post-methionine loading homocysteine concentrations. Some of the studies showed gender-specific associations of circulating vitamin levels with risk of CVD [5,29,33,34], which will be discussed later in this chapter.

Inevitably, the studies vary with respect to definition of case status or endpoint, the age of the population, the cutoff-points used to define elevation of homocysteine (some studies looked at the relationship continuously or per quantiles), adjustment for confounding factors, et cetera. However, the main aim is to compare the strength of associations among the sexes.

## HOMOCYSTEINE AND CVD RISK

Of the 10 studies [5, 27-33,35,37] that included both men and women, 6 studies observed stronger associations of homocysteine with CVD risk among women than men [5, 27,30,32,33,37]. The other 4 studies observed a weaker effect among women than men [28] or no difference between the sexes [29,31,35]. Below, some key findings will be described in more detail.

With data of the Atherosclerosis Risk in Communities (ARIC) Study, Malinow et al. [27] observed a graded, positive association between homocysteine

**Table 1** Epidemiologic studies on total homocysteine and risk of cardiovascular disease that studied possible effect modification by gender or included women only

| Study | Study design | Case status or endpoint | # of Cases/controls or events (by gender)[1] | Age (year) | Risk Factor(s)[2] | Results for tHcy-CVD association |
|---|---|---|---|---|---|---|
| Malinow[27] | Cross-sectional; sample from ARIC study | Increased[3] IMT of carotid wall | 287 case-control pairs (164 M, 123 F); matched on age | 45-64 | B-tHcy | Positive association; stronger among F than M |
| Selhub[28] | Cross-sectional; Framingham Heart Study | Maximal degree of ECAS ≥ 25% | 392 cases (180 M, 212 F) / 649 controls (238 M, 411 F) | 67-96 | B-tHcy | Positive association; weaker among F than M |
| Aronow[29] | Cross-sectional | CHD | 219 cases (69 M, 150 F) / 281 controls (84 M, 197 F) | 60 to 99 | B-tHcy Vitamin B₁₂ Folate | Positive association; similar associations for M and F |
| Robinson[30] | Case-control | CHD | 304 cases (201 M, 103 F) / 231 controls (187 M, 44 F) | 62 ± 11 / 51 ± 10 | B-tHcy | Positive association; slightly stronger among F than M |
| Hopkins[31] | Case-control | Early familial CHD | 162 cases (120 M, 42 F) / 155 controls (85 M, 70 F) | 38 to 68 | B-tHcy | Positive association among M and F; data suggest that there is a continuous effect in F, and a threshold effect in M |
| Den Heijer[22] | Case-control | First episode of DVT | 269 case-control pairs (117 M, 152 F); matched on age | 16-70 (mean 44) | B-tHcy | Positive association; much stronger among F than M |

| Study | Study design | Case status or endpoint | # of Cases/controls or events (by gender)[1] | Age (year) | Risk Factor(s)[2] | Results for tHcy-CVD association |
|---|---|---|---|---|---|---|
| Graham[33] | Case-control; European COMAC Study | Vascular disease (cardiac, cerebral, peripheral) | 750 cases (544 M, 206 F)<br>800 controls (570 M, 230 F) | mean 47<br>mean 44<br>all < 60 | B-tHcy<br>PML-tHcy<br>Folate<br>PLP<br>Vitamin $B_{12}$ | Positive association for both fasting and PML tHcy among both sexes; stronger association for PML tHcy in F than in M |
| Schwartz[34] | Case-control | MI | 79 cases, 386 controls (all F) | <45 | B- tHcy<br>Folate<br>Vitamin $B_{12}$ | Positive association |
| Alfthan[35] | Prospective study among 7424 subjects; nested case-control design; follow-up of 9 years | MI or stroke | 265 case-control pairs (134 M, 131 F); matched on age | 40-64 | B-tHcy | No association; no difference between the sexes |
| Petri[36] | Prospective cohort study among 337 patients with SLE (313 women); mean follow-up of 4.8 years | Stroke and thrombotic events | 29 events of stroke<br>31 events of ATD<br>33 events of VTD | $35 \pm 12$ | B-tHcy | Positive association for stroke and ATD but not for VTD |
| Nygard[37] | Prospective cohort study among 587 patients (109 F) with CAD; median follow-up 4.6 years | Mortality | 64 deaths (53 M, 11 F) | median: 62 | B-Hcy | Postive association for both sexes |

| Study | Study design | Case status or endpoint | # of Cases/controls or events (by gender)[1] | Age (year) | Risk Factor(s)[2] | Results for tHcy-CVD association |
|---|---|---|---|---|---|---|
| Folsom[5] | Prospective study in ARIC study (n=15792); case-cohort design; median follow-up 3.3 years | CHD | 232 events (75% M)<br>537 controls (75% M) | 45-64 | B-tHcy<br>Folate<br>PLP<br>Vitamin B$_{12}$ | Positive association for tHcy in F, and no association in M |

ARIC=Atherosclerosis Risk in Communities; ATD=arterial thrombotic disease; B-tHcy = baseline or fasting total homocysteine; CHD = coronary heart disease; DVT=deep-vein thrombosis; ECAS=extracranial carotid artery stenosis; F=females; IMT=intimal-medial thickness; M=males; MI=myocardial infarction; NHANES=National Health and Nutrition Examination Survey; PLP=pyridoxal phosphate; PML=post-methionine loading total homocysteine; SLE=systemic lupus erythematosus; VTD=venous thrombotic disease

[1] Not all studies provide complete information on numbers of males and females
[2] Listed are the factors for which the authors show gender-specific results; the table discusses tHcy-effects only (see text for vitamin-effects)
[3] See original paper for definition of increased IMT

and thickening of the carotid artery intima-media complex [27], a measure for atherosclerosis. For men, the association was not statistically significant, and it was weaker than in women. Adjusting for age, study center, race, and examination period, the OR for subjects in the highest quintile (> 10.5 μmol/L) compared to subjects in the lowest quintile (< 5.9 μmol/L) was 2.3 (n.s.) among men and 4.8 (p < 0.01) among women. When additionally adjusting for other risk factors for CVD, these ORs were 1.4 and 2.5, respectively (n.s.). In a case-control study, Robinson *et al.* [30] also observed a slightly stronger association among women than men. As a cutoff-point for hyperhomocysteinemia they used levels of homocysteine above the sex-adjusted 80th percentile for control subjects (13.5 μmol/L in men and 11.8 μmol/L in women). These levels conferred a multivariately-adjusted OR of 2.9 (95% CI, 1.7 - 4.7) in men and of 3.5 (95% CI, 1.4 - 8.5) in women. Furthermore, Den Heijer *et al.* [32], observed that homocysteine concentrations above 18.5 μmol/L (the 95th percentile for control subjects) conferred an age-adjusted OR of 1.4 (95% CI, 0.6 - 3.4) in men and of 7.0 (95% CI, 1.6 - 30.8) in women. When using gender-specific cutoff-points, the ORs were 1.8 (95% CI, 0.6 - 5.4) and 3.8 (95% CI, 1.4 - 10.2) among men and women, respectively. In the European multi-center case-control study [33], the positive association between post-methionine loading homocysteine and CVD was stronger for women than men. Taking those with levels below the 80th percentile among controls as the reference and adjusting for age, center, and conventional risk factors, the ORs for those with post-load homocysteine at or above the 80th percentile (38 μmol/L) were 1.7 (1.2 - 2.3) in men and 2.4 (1.4 - 4.2) in women. ORs for elevated fasting homocysteine were similar among the sexes. Folsom *et al.* [5] studied the association between homocysteine and risk of CHD, using a prospective case-cohort design nested within the ARIC study. Only in women there was a statistically significant positive trend for the association of homocysteine with CHD. The ORs for the highest (≥ 11.5 μmol/L) *versus* the lowest quintile (< 6.3 μmol/L) were 0.9 (95% CI, 0.3 - 2.6) among men and 2.5 (95% CI, 0.9 - 7.5) among women, respectively. These were adjusted for age, race and center. In the prospective study among CHD patients as published by Nygård *et al.* [37], it was observed that the positive association between homocysteine concentration and mortality was apparent for both men and women. In a recent review from the same group [2], they show data that suggest a stronger association for women than for men: during the follow-up period the Kaplan-Meier survival plots of patients with homocysteine below and above 15 μmol/L diverged more for women than for men.

Studies that found no difference between the sexes or a weaker effect in women are described below. There was a weaker association between basal homocysteine and stenosis of the extracranial carotid arteries among elderly

**Table 2** Epidemiologic studies on folate and risk of cardiovascular disease that studied possible effect modification by gender or included women only

| Study | Study design | Case status or endpoint | # of Cases/controls or events (by gender) | | Age (year) | Risk Factor(s) | Results |
|---|---|---|---|---|---|---|---|
| Giles[38] | Propsective cohort study in NHANES 1; n=2006; follow-up 13 years | Ischemic stroke | 98 events 1908 no event | (58 M, 40 F) (851 M, 1057 F) | mean: 62 mean: 52 | Serum folate | Inverse association; similar for the sexes |
| Morrison[39] | Retrospective cohort study; Nutrition Canada Survey; n= 5056; follow-up 15 years | CHD | 165 events | (112 M, 53 F) | 35–79 | Serum folate | Inverse association for both sexes; stronger association in F |
| Rimm[40] | Prospective cohort study; Nurses' Health Study; n= 80082; follow-up 14 years | Fatal and nonfatal CHD | 658 nonfatal 281 fatal | | 30–55 | Intake of folate and vitamin $B_6$ | Inverse associations for both vitamins |

CHD=coronary heart disease; F=females; M=males; NHANES=National Health and Nutrition Examination Survey

female than male subjects of the Framingham Heart Study [28]. Among men, the prevalence of stenosis $\geq 25\%$ was 58% (95% CI, 49% - 67%) among those with homocysteine in the highest quartile ($\geq 14.4$ µmol/L) and 27% (95% CI, 17% - 38%) among those with levels in the lowest quartile ($\leq 9.0$ µmol/L). For women, these prevalences were 39% (95% CI, 31% - 47%) and 31% (95% CI, 24% - 38%), respectively. However, a test of interaction between sex and homocysteine was not statistically significant. In another cross-sectional study among elderly subjects [29], there was no difference between men and women: elevated homocysteine levels ($> 17$ µmol/L) were associated with a four-fold increased risk of CHD among both sexes. In a case-control study, Hopkins et al. [31] observed similar ORs for early familial CHD among men and women. The ORs for those with homocysteine levels of 19 µmol/L and above, compared to those with levels of 9 µmol/L or less, were 13.8 (95% CI, 3.5 - 55) in men and 12.8 (95% CI, 2.0 - 82) in women. Alfthan *et al.* [35], in a prospective study, observed no association between homocysteine and risk of stroke or myocardial infarction, for neither of the sexes.

Finally, there was one study that included women only [34] and one that included 93% women [36]. In a case-control study, Schwartz *et al.* [34] observed a statistically significant positive trend for the association of homocysteine with risk of myocardial infarction. The OR was 2.3 (95% 0.9 - 5.6) for women in the upper quartile ($\geq 15.6$ µmol/L) of fasting concentrations, compared to women in the lowest quartile ($< 10.0$ µmol/L). Petri *et al.* [36], in a population of patients of systemic lupus erythematosus, found that elevated homocysteine ($> 14.1$ µmol/L) conferred an OR for stroke of 2.2 (95% CI, 1.2 - 4.1) and an OR for arterial thrombotic events of 3.7 (95% CI, 2.0-7.1). There was no association with venous thrombotic disease.

Summarizing, 6 out of 10 of the epidemiologic studies that included both men and women found elevated homocysteine to be a stronger risk factor in women than in men. Three observed no effect modification, and one a weaker effect in women. Two studies that consisted (almost) entirely of women observed a strong positive association of elevated homocysteine with CVD risk as well, comparable to effects in male populations.

## FOLATE, VITAMINS B$_6$ AND B$_{12}$ AND CVD RISK

Table 2 lists two prospective studies on the association between serum folate and risk of ischemic stroke [38] and myocardial infarction [39], respectively, and a prospective study on dietary intake of folate and vitamin B$_6$ and risk of CHD [40]. These studies did not measure plasma homocysteine concentrations. The latter study consists of women only. Furthermore, several of the studies of

**Table 3** Epidemiologic studies on total homocysteine and risk of cardiovascular disease that studied possible effect modification by menopause

| Study | Study design | Case status or endpoint | # of Cases/controls | (by gender and menopause)[1] | Age (year) | Risk Factor(s) | Result |
|---|---|---|---|---|---|---|---|
| Kang[13] | Cross-sectional; sample size of 443 subjects | ≥ 70% obstruction of one or more major coronary arteries | 241 cases 202 controls | (173 M, 68 F[2]) (93 M, 109 F[2]) | < 69 | Protein-bound Hcy | Similar effect in young and older women |
| Dudman[41] | Case-control | Vascular disease (cardiac, cerebral, peripheral) | 131 cases 56 controls | (84 M, 38 PREF, 9 POSTF) (20 M, 24 PREF, 11 POSTF) | wide age-range | Free PML-Hcy | The data suggested a slightly stronger effect in POSTF than PREF |
| Verhoef, unpublished | Case-control; subset of population of European COMAC Study | Vascular disease (cardiac, cerebral, peripheral) | 206 cases 230 controls | (107 PREF, 64 POSTF) (155 PREF, 52 POSTF) | mean 45 mean 41 all < 60 | B- and PML-tHcy | Stronger positive association for PML tHcy in POSTF than PREF; opposite observation for fasting tHcy |

B-tHcy = baseline or fasting total homocysteine; F = females; Hcy = homocysteine; PML = post-methionine loading total homocysteine; POSTF = postmenopausal females; PREF = premenopausal females

[1] For the European COMAC Study only the numbers for women are shown
[2] This study categorized subjects by 10-year age intervals; women aged 50 and over were considered postmenopausal (52 cases, 68 controls)

Table 1 showed gender-specific associations of circulating vitamin levels with risk of CVD [35,29,33,34].

Aronow *et al.* [29] observed that low circulating levels of folate and vitamin $B_{12}$ were associated with increased risk of CHD in a similar way among the sexes. In the European multi-center study, blood concentrations of pyridoxal phosphate (PLP, the metabolically active form of vitamin $B_6$) below the 20th percentile conferred a slightly stronger increased risk in women (especially premenopausal) than in men (unpublished findings, Verhoef *et al.*). Folsom *et al.* [5], however, observed a similar inverse association of plasma PLP with risk of CHD in both men and women. However, an inverse association of plasma folate with risk of CHD was observed in women only. Similarly, Morrison *et al.* [39] when calculating relative risks (RRs) for those in the lowest quartile of serum folate compared to the highest, observed a higher RR among women (2.8;95% CI, 1.3 - 6.2) than among men (1.4;95% CI, 0.8 - 2.3). Another prospective study (Giles *et al.*[38]), observed a nonsignificant inverse association between serum folate and risk of ischemic stroke. The authors stated that the association was not modified by sex, as the test for folate-sex interaction was not statistically significant. However, the data suggested a stronger association among women: the RR for those with serum folate $\leq$ 9.2 nmol/L, relative to those with higher levels was 1.6 (95% CI, 0.8 - 3.6) among women and 1.2 (95% CI, 0.6 - 2.4) among men.

There were two studies that looked at the association between vitamins and CVD in women only [34,40]. In a case-control study, Schwartz *et al.* [34] observed an inverse association between plasma folate and risk of CHD. The OR for women in the highest quartile of folate was 0.5 (95% CI, 0.2 - 1.3) compared to those in the lowest quartile. There was no association for vitamin $B_{12}$. In the Nurses' Health Study, Rimm *et al.* [40] found a 30% decreased risk of CHD among women in the highest quintile of folate intake (median intake of 696 $\mu$g/d), compared to those in the lowest quintile (median intake 157 $\mu$g/d). A similar inverse association was observed for vitamin $B_6$.

In summary, the studies on vitamins and CVD risk seem to indicate that low circulating levels of folate and PLP are slightly more strongly inversely associated with risk of CVD in women than in men.


EPIDEMIOLOGIC STUDIES OF CVD RISK: ASSOCIATIONS BY MENOPAUSAL STATUS

Table 3 lists 3 studies that have compared the association between some measure of homocysteine and risk of CVD among subgroups of pre- and postmenopausal women. Kang *et al.* [13] compared mean plasma protein-bound homocysteine concentrations of patients and controls within 10-year age groups, for men and women separately. Overall, mean plasma protein-bound concentrations were 29% higher in patients than controls. The difference was about 50% larger in women than in men, but there was no difference between women of premenopausal and postmenopausal age. In the study by Kang et al. [13], free homocysteine levels 4 hours after methionine loading were studied. Although there were only few postmenopausal women, the data suggested that the case-control contrast in free homocysteine levels was stronger in postmenopausal than premenopausal women. In the European multi-center case-control study, elevated post-methionine loading homocysteine showed a slightly stronger association in postmenopausal women than premenopausal women (unpublished findings, Verhoef *et al.*). Adjusting for age, center, and conventional risk factors, elevated post-methionine loading homocysteine conferred an OR of 2.1 (95% CI, 0.9 - 4.5) in premenopausal women and 2.6 (95% CI, 0.8 - 8.9) in postmenopausal women. For elevated fasting homocysteine, the opposite was observed: ORs were 1.5 (95% 0.6 - 3.6) in premenopausal women and 0.5 (95% CI, 0.1 - 2.1) in postmenopausal women. As all 95% CIs overlapped, it is difficult to infer an effect modification by menopause.

Thus, based on these few studies that have specifically studied effects of menopausal status there is no reason to presume that elevated homocysteine is not a risk factor in premenopausal women. In the study by Kang *et al.* [13] and the unpublished findings of the European study, there was a slight suggestion of post-methionine loading homocysteine being a stronger risk factor after the menopause than before.

## EFFECTS OF ESTROGEN REPLACEMENT THERAPY ON HOMOCYSTEINE CONCENTRATIONS

The observed inverse relationship between estrogen concentrations and homocysteine concentrations in premenopausal women and the apparent rise (especially post-methionine-loading) after the menopause have prompted investigation of possible homocysteine-lowering effects of estrogen replacement therapy [42-45]. Unfortunately, all studies tested effects on fasting and not post-methionine-load levels.

In a randomized, double-blind, placebo-controlled study among 27 postmenopausal women (14 in the treatment group, 13 in the control group), Mijatovic *et al.* [42] observed a significant 13% reduction in fasting homocysteine after 15 months of daily treatment with 17ß-estradiol in combination with dydrogesterone. During the first 12 months, the dose of 17ß-estradiol was 1 mg/d, followed by 2 mg/d for 3 months (months 13-15). The data suggested that there was an extra drop in homocysteine during months 13-15, compared to month 12, i.e. a dose-related effect. Effects were independent of (dose of) dydroges-terone, which was confirmed in another study of the same group [43]. Fur-thermore, it confirms findings of a previous, uncontrolled study [44] among 21 healthy postmenopausal women, who took 2 mg of micronized 17 ß-estradiol (in combination with 10 mg cyclic dydrogesterone for the first half of each 28 day cycle), daily for two years. After 6 months there was a statistically signifi-cant reduction of homocysteine concentration of 10.9%, after which no further statistical significant changes were observed. In another uncontrolled study, Anker *et al.* [45] observed a 11.3% reduction in fasting homocysteine concen-tration after 3 to 4 months of tamoxifen treatment in postmenopausal women with breast cancer (n=22). After 9-12 months, levels had dropped by 30%, and after 13-18 months by 25%, compared to baseline. However, since tamoxifen is both an estrogen agonist and antagonist, results are difficult to interpret.

In a randomized, double-blind, placebo-controlled, crossover trial, in 19 postmenopausal women from the Boston area, no effect of estrogen treatment on fasting homocysteine levels was observed (unpublished findings, Verhoef *et al.*). Dosages of 1 mg and 2 mg estradiol were tested against placebo for a pe-riod of 9 weeks each. To determine whether any effect of estradiol was medi-ated through effects on cofactors involved in homocysteine metabolism, chan-ges in plasma levels of folate and pyridoxal 5'-phosphate were measured as well. Compared to placebo, plasma concentrations of homocysteine were not statistically significantly different during treatment with 1 mg estradiol (-1%, $P=0.73$) or 2 mg estradiol (-9%, $P=0.21$). Mean concentrations of plasma pyri-doxal 5'-phosphate were markedly lower during treatment with 1 mg (-32%, $P=0.007$) and 2 mg estradiol (-45%, $P < 0.001$). Thus, pyridoxal 5'-phosphate reduction may be an unwanted side-effect of hormone replacement therapy. Mean plasma folate concentrations were nonsignificantly higher during treat-ment with estradiol.

## MEN AND WOMEN SHARE ELEVATED HOMOCYSTEINE AS A RISK FACTOR FOR CVD

The majority of epidemiologic studies reviewed in this chapter have observed that associations between homocysteine and risk of CVD are as strong, or even stronger, in women than in men. Several studies found the risk to be about twice as high in women as in men. Based on the available data there is no reason to assume that elevated homocysteine is not a risk factor in premenopausal women, although only few studies have specifically compared associations among subgroups of premenopausal and postmenopausal women.

However, elevation of homocysteine is a risk factor in studies that included young women [34,36] as well as in studies that included elderly women [28]. The studies on vitamins and CVD risk are few; they seem to indicate that low circulating levels of folate and pyridoxal 5'-phosphate are slightly more strongly inversely associated with risk of CVD in women than in men.

What explains the suggested stronger association between homocysteine and CVD risk among women compared to men ? Is it caused by differences between sexes with respect to susceptibility to adverse effects of homocysteine elevation ? Before discussing possible biologic differences between men and women, several methodologic issues will be discussed.

## METHODOLOGIC CONSIDERATIONS

*Interaction-effect* First of all, it should be noted that, with exception of one study [32], none of the studies observed a statistically significant sex-homocysteine interaction. Some studies did a formal interaction-analysis [5,28,38], whereas for others we can infer lack of interaction by the fact that the 95 %CIs of the risk estimates for men and women overlapped. The interaction-effect in the study by Den Heijer *et al.* [32] was statistically significant when using an overall cutoff-point for hyperhomocysteinemia, but 95% CI overlapped when using sex-specific cutoff-points. Limited sample size may often be the reason for the interactions not to be statistically significant. However, one can hardly ignore the suggestion of effect modification by sex. The Homocysteine Studies Collaboration, a currently ongoing project in which individual data of many epidemiologic studies are pooled, will most likely be able to study effect modification by gender with sufficient statistical power.

*Age at event* The CVD incidence in women before menopause is much lower than in men of similar age. After the menopause, the incidence gradually increases to rates that come close to those observed in men [18]. Hence, when studying premature CVD (usually defined as CVD before age 55 or 60 years) the effect of a risk factor may be stronger in women than in men. For example, studies of premature CVD may have included female patients that were somehow more susceptible to adverse effects of CVD risk factors, such as hypertension, smoking, hypercholesterolemia and maybe elevated homocysteine. With respect to susceptibility, one could think of genetic background or environmental factors. In fact, the European multi-center case-control study, which studied CVD before age 60, indicated that not only elevated homocysteine, but also hypertension and smoking (and to a lesser extent hypercholesterolemia) were stronger risk factors in women than in men. In the present review, the studies that included both men and women of postmenopausal age [28,29] showed similar associations in men and women [29] or even a weaker association in women than in men [28]. This may indeed indicate that studies of premature CVD tend to "overestimate" effects in women.

*Gender-specific cutoff-points* The distribution of homocysteine in women generally lies more to the left than in men. Consequently, when using an overall cutoff-point for hyperhomocysteinemia, less women than will than men will be categorized as hyperhomocysteinemic. In general, this should not be a problem, as the same cutoff points are applied to cases and controls, leaving estimates unaffected. A problem could arise when very few women are in the hyperhomocysteinemic category and estimates are based on very small numbers. There is less of a problem for estimates per quantiles, as male and female distributions overlap to a great extent, but the estimate for the upper quantile may be based on small numbers also. Nevertheless, there is no reason to assume that this should lead to bias towards a stronger effect in women. Only the studies by Robinson *et al.* [30] and Den Heijer *et al.* [32] used gender-specific cutoff-points. The first study [30] showed a slightly stronger effect in women compared to men, but this difference was not statistically significant. The second study [32] demonstrated that use of gender-specific cutoff-points attenuated the contrast in estimated risks between men and women, but the effect was still about twice as strong in women as in men.

## IS POST-METHIONINE LOADING HOMOCYSTEINE A SPECIAL CASE IN WOMEN ?

Some of the reviewed studies seemed to indicate that the possible menopause-induced increase in homocysteine concentration was more evident for post-methionine loading than fasting levels [17,19]. Furthermore, in the European multi-center case-control study [33], the positive association between post-methionine loading homocysteine and CVD was stronger for women than men. This raises the possibility that post-methionine loading homocysteine is somehow a special case in women. However, the explanation may partly lie in the current protocol for the methionine-loading test [46], i.e. the fact that the methionine dose is based on body weight and not on the amount of lean body mass (the metabolically active tissue). Therefore, it is very likely that women receive an overdose of methionine per kg of lean body mass compared to men. Moreover, postmenopausal women, who usually have more body fat than premenopausal women, may receive an overdose as well. This may explain the observed increase of post-methionine loading homocysteine after the menopause. The effect of body composition is illustrated by findings from the European multi-center study (unpublished findings, Verhoef *et al.*). In that study, after adjustment for age and center, women had 9% lower plasma concentrations of post-methionine loading homocysteine than men, but expressed per unit of body mass index males and females had similar levels post-load. As previously suggested by other investigators [47], it may be advisable in future research to standardize the methionine dose to body mass index rather than to bodyweight, especially when looking at differences between the sexes or between pre- and postmenopausal women.

The stronger association of post-load homocysteine with risk of CVD in women compared to men is in concordance with the described stronger effect of low circulating levels of pyridoxal 5'-phosphate among women than men, as pyridoxal 5'-phosphate is a cofactor for two key-enzymes in the transsulfuration pathway, the main route for homocysteine catabolism [2]. This pathway is generally accepted as the one which determines rise in homocysteine after methionine loading. The larger effect of post-methionine loading homocysteine in women is unlikely to be explained by the higher dose of methionine per kg metabolically active tissue, as there is no reason to assume that the overdose was higher in female cases than female controls. Therefore, the findings seem to indicate that low efficiency of homocysteine catabolism is a more significant risk factor for CVD in women than in men.

## ARE THERE BIOLOGIC EXPLANATIONS FOR EFFECT MODIFICATION BY GENDER ?

What biologic mechanism could explain the stronger association in women compared to men ? Is the vascular endothelium of women more vulnerable to detrimental effects of elevated homocysteine than that of men ? Is hemostasis easier disturbed in women than in men ? One would expect the opposite, as — at least before menopause — women's vascular endothelium is believed to receive "protection" from estrogens through all kinds of mechanisms. For example, there are indications that estrogens can interact with the endothelium-dependent arterial wall functions and vascular smooth muscle cells, thereby favoring vasodilatation. Also, estrogens may slow down progression of atherosclerosis through effect on vascular connective tissue [18]. Furthermore, studies of postmenopausal hormone replacement therapy indicate that estrogens may lead to a increased fibrinolytic capacity [18], which suggests that the presence of estrogens will enable women to cope better with thrombus formation than men. Therefore, at first sight it seems unlikely that a hormonal difference explains differences in effect of elevated homocysteine between men and women. Of course, one cannot exclude other differences between men and women.

## CONCLUSION

Men and women share elevated homocysteine as a risk factor for CVD. More research is needed to investigate whether a possible stronger association between homocysteine and CVD in women has a biologic background or whether it is explained by aspects of study design, such as age at inclusion, or methods of analysis, such as choice of the cutoff-point. Although levels are lower before than after the menopause, elevated homocysteine is associated with CVD risk in premenopausal as well as postmenopausal women. Several – mostly uncontrolled – clinical trials have indicated that estrogen replacement therapy may be useful in lowering homocysteine during postmenopausal years. However, a recently completed randomized, placebo-controlled secondary prevention trial of estrogen plus progestin did not find a reduced overall rate of CHD in postmenopausal women with established CHD [48]. Therefore, it seems advisable to test B-vitamin therapy rather than hormone replacement when it comes to reduction of CVD rate in postmenopausal women. Of course, we will have to wait for results from randomized clinical trials of B-vitamins and CVD, that are currently being conducted.

## REFERENCES

1. Boushey CJ, Beresford SAA, Omenn GS, Motulsky AG. A quantitative assessment of plasma homocysteine as a risk factor for vascular disease. Probable benefits of increasing folic acid intakes. JAMA 1995;274:1049-57.
2. Refsum H, Ueland PM, Nygård O, Vollset MD. Homocysteine and cardiovascular disease. Annu Rev Medicine 1998;49:31-62.
3. Stampfer MJ, Verhoef P. Prospective studies of homocysteine and cardiovascular disease. In: Graham I, Refsum H, Rosenberg IH, Ueland PM, Shuman JM, eds. Homocysteine Metabolism: From Basic Science to Clinical Medicine. Kluwer Academic Publishers, Boston, USA 1997, p. 239-44.
4. Wald NJ, Watt HC, Law MR, Weir DG, McPartlin J, Scott JM. Homocysteine and ischemic heart disease: results of a prospective study with implications regarding prevention. Arch Intern Med 1998;158:862-7.
5. Folsom AR, Nieto FJ, McGovern PG *et al.* Prospective study of coronary heart disease incidence in relation to fasting total homocysteine, related genetic polymorphisms, and B vitamins. The Atherosclerosis Risk in Communities (ARIC) Study. Circulation 1998;98:204-10.
6. Evans RW, Shaten BJ, Hempel JD, Cutler JA, Kuller LH. Homocyst(e)ine and risk of cardiovascular disease in the Multiple Risk Factor Intervention Trial. Arterioscler Thromb Vasc Biol 1997;17:1947-53.

7.  Selhub J, Jacques PF, Wilson PWF, Rush D, Rosenberg IH. Vitamin status and intake as primary determinants of homocysteinemia in an elderly population. JAMA 1993;270:2693-8.
8.  Jacobsen DW, Gatautis VJ, Green R *et al.* Rapid HPLC determination of total homocysteine and other thiols in serum and plasma: sex differences and correlation with cobalamin and folate concentrations in healthy subjects. Clin Chem 1994;40:873-81.
9.  Brattström L, Lindgren A, Israelsson B, Andersson A, Hultberg B. Homocysteine and cysteine: determinants of plasma levels in middle-aged and elderly subjects. J Intern Med 1994;236:633-41.
10. Nygård O, Vollset SE, Refsum H *et al.* Total plasma homocysteine and cardiovascular risk profile: The Hordaland homocysteine study. JAMA 1995;274:1526-33.
11. Lussier-Cacan S, Xhignesse M, Piolot A, Selhub J, Davignon J, Genest J Jr. Plasma total homocysteine in healthy subjects: sex specific relation with biological traits. Am J Clin Nutr 1996;64:587-3.
12. Andersson A, Brattström L, Israelsson B, Isaksson A, Hamfelt A, Hultberg B. Plasma homocysteine before and after methionine loading with regard to age, gender and menopausal status. Eur J Clin Invest 1992;22:79-87.
13. Kang SS, Wong PW, Cook HY, Norusis M, Messer JV. Protein-bound homocyst(e)ine. A possible risk factor for coronary artery disease. J Clin Invest 1986;77:1482-6.
14. Boers GH, Smals AG, Trijbels FJ, Leermakers AI, Kloppenborg PW. Unique efficiency of methionine metabolism in premenopausal women may protect against vascular disease in the reproductive years. J Clin Invest 1983;72:1971-6.
15. Brattström LE, Hultberg BL, Hardebo JE. Folic acid responsive post-menopausal homocysteinemia. Metabolism 1985;34:1073-7.
16. Blom HJ, Boers GH, Van den Elzen JP, Van Roessel JJ, Trijbels JM, Tangerman A. Differences between premenopausal women and young men in the transamination pathway of methionine catabolism, and the protection against vascular disease. Eur J Clin Invest 1988;18:633-8.
17. Wouters MGAJ, Moorrees MThEC, Van der Mooren MJ, et al. Plasma homocysteine and menopausal status. Eur J Clin Invest 1995;25:801-5.
18. Gensini GF, Micheli S, Prisco D, Abbate R. Menopause and risk of cardiovascular disease. Thromb Res 1996;84:1-19.
19. Verhoef P. Homocysteine, B-vitamins and cardiovascular disease: epidemiologic evidence. Dissertation, Agricultural University, Wageningen, The Netherlands, 1996.
20. Mudd SH, Pool JR. Labile methyl balance for normal humans on various dietary regimens. Metabolism 1975;24:721-3.
21. Kang SS, Wong PWK, Zhou J, Cook HY. Total homocyst(e)ine in plasma and amniotic fluid of pregnant women. Metabolism 1986;35:889-91.
22. Andersson A, Hultberg B, Brattström L, Isaksson A. Decreased serum homocysteine in pregnancy. Eur J Clin Chem Clin Biochem 1992;30:377-9.
23. Steegers-Theunissen RPM, Boers GHJ, Steegers EAP, Trijbels FJM, Thomas CMG, Eskes TKAB. Effects of sub-50 oral contraceptives on homocysteine metabolism: a preliminary study. Contraception 1992;45:129-39.

24. Beaumont V, Malinow MR, Sexton G, Wilson D, Lemort N, Upson B, Beaumont JL. Hyperhomocyst(e)inemia, anti-estrogen antibodies and other risk factors for thrombosis in women on oral contraceptives. Atherosclerosis 1992;94:147-52.

25. Brattström L, Israelsson B, Olsson A, Andersson A, Hultberg B. Plasma homocysteine in women on oral oestrogen-containing contraceptives and in men with oestrogen-treated prostatic carcinoma. Scand J Clin Lab Invest 1992;52:283-7.

26. Giltay EJ, Hoogeveen EK, Elbers JMH, Gooren LJG, Asscheman H, Stehouwer CDA. Effects of sex steroids on plasma total homocysteine levels: a study in transsexual males and females. J Clin Endocrinol Metab 1998;83:550-3.

27. Malinow MR, Nieto JN, Szklo M, Chambless LE, Bond G. Carotid artery intimal-medial wall thickening and plasma homocyst(e)ine in asymptomatic adults. The Atherosclerosis Risk in Communities Study. Circulation 1993;87:1107-13.

28. Selhub J, Jacques PF, Bostom AG et al. Association between plasma homocysteine concentrations and extracranial carotid-artery stenosis. N Engl J Med 1995;332:286-91.

29. Aronow WS, Ahn C. Assocation between plasma homocysteine and coronary artery disease in older persons. Am J Cardiol 1997;80;1216-18.

30. Robinson K, Mayer EL, Miller DP et al. Hyperhomocysteinemia and low pyridoxal phosphate. Common and independent reversible risk factors for coronary artery disease. Circulation 1995;92:2825-30.

31. Hopkins PN, Wu LL, Wu J et al. Higher plasma homocyst(e)ine and increased susceptibility to adverse effects of low folate in early familial coronary artery disease. Arterioscler Thromb Vasc Biol 1995;15:1314-20.

32. Den Heijer M, Koster T, Blom HJ et al. Hyperhomocysteinemia as a risk factor for deep-vein thrombosis. N Engl J Med 1996;334:759-62.

33. Graham IH, Daly LE, Refsum HM et al. Plasma homocysteine as a risk factor for vascular disease: The European Concerted Action Project. JAMA 1997;277:1775-81.

34. Schwartz SM, Siscovich DS, Malinow MR et al. Myocardial infarction in young women in relation to plasma total homocysteine, folate, and a common variant in the methylenetetrahydrofolate reductase gene. Circulation 1997;96:412-7.

35. Alfthan G, Pekkanen J, Jauhiainen M et al. Relation of serum homocysteine and lipoprotein(a) concentrations to atherosclerotic disease in a prospective Finnish population based study. Atherosclerosis 1994;106:9-19.

36. Petri M, Roubenoff R, Dallal GE, Nadeau MR, Selhub J, Rosenberg H. Plasma homocysteine as a risk factor for atherothrombotic events in systemic lupus erythematosus. Lancet 1996;348:1120-4.

37. Nygård O, Nordrehaug JE, Refsum H, Ueland PM, Farstad M, Vollset SE. Plasma homocysteine levels and mortality in patients with coronary artery disease. N Engl J Med 1997;337:230-6.

38. Giles WH, Kittner SJ, Anda RA, Croft JB, Casper ML. Serum folate and risk for ischemic stroke. First National Health and Nutrition Examination Survey Epidemiologic Follow-up Study. Stroke 1995;26:1166-70.

39. Morrison HI, Schaubel D, Desmeules M, Wigle DT. Serum folate and risk of fatal coronary heart disease. JAMA 1996;275:1893-6.

40. Rimm EB, Willett WC, Hu FB et al. Folate and vitamin B-6 from diet and supplements in relation to risk of coronary heart disease among women. JAMA 1998;279;359-64.

41. Dudman NPB, Wilcken DEL, Wang J, Lynch JF, Macey D, Lundberg P. Disordered methionine/homocysteine metabolism in premature vascular disease. Its occurrence, cofactor therapy, and enzymology. Arterioscler Thromb 1993;13:1253-60.

42. Mijatovic V, Kenemans P, Jakobs C, Van Baal WM, Peters-Muller ER, Van der Mooren MJ. A randomized controlled study of the effects of 17beta-estradiol-dydrogesterone on plasma homocysteine in postmenopausal women. Obstet Gynecol 1998;91:432-6.

43. Mijatovic V, Kenemans P, Netelenbos C et al. Postmenopausal oral 17ß-estradiol continuously combined with dyhydrogesterone reduces fasting serum homocysteine levels. Fertil Steril 1998;69:876-82.

44. Van der Mooren MJ, Wouters MGAJ, Blom HJ, Schellekens LA, Eskes TKAB, Rolland R. Hormone replacement therapy may reduce high serum homocysteine in post-menopausal women. Eur J Clin Invest 1994;24:733-6.

45. Anker G, Lonning PE, Ueland PM, Refsum H, Lien EA. Plasma levels of the atherogenic amino acid homocysteine in post-menopausal women with breast cancer treated with tamoxifen. Int J Cancer 1995;60:365-8.

46. Boers G. Refinement of the methionine loading test. In: Robinson K ed. Homocysteinemia and vascular disease. Proceedings of an EC COMAC-Epidemiology Expert Group Workshop. Luxembourg: Commission of the European Communities, 1990:61-6.

47. Silberberg J, Crooks R, Fryer J et al. Gender differences and other determinants of the rise in plasma homocysteine after L-methionine loading. Atherosclerosis 1997;133:105-10.

48. Hulley S, Grady D, Bush T et al. Randomized trial of estrogen plus progestin for secondary prevention of coronary heart disease in postmenopausal women. JAMA 1998;280:605-13.

# 14.  HOMOCYSTEINE AND VENOUS THROMBOSIS

MARTIN DEN HEIJER

## SUMMARY

Classical homocystinuria is associated with arterial vascular diseases and venous thrombosis. Although the relation between mild hyperhomocysteinemia
and arterial vascular disease was established in many studies since the late
seventies the relation with venous thrombosis remained controversial. In the
last decade several studies were published indicating that hyperhomocysteinemia was a risk factor also for venous thrombosis.

Mutated MTHFR (C677T) is an important cause of mild hyperhomocysteinemia, explaining about 25 %. Despite this strong influence on homocysteine
levels this polymorphism does not seem to be a risk factor for venous thrombosis.

Although there is epidemiological evidence for the relationship between
hyperhomocysteinemia and venous thrombosis, little is known about its pathophysiology. Several of the possible mechanisms proposed with respect to vascular disease, may be applied to venous thrombosis as well. However, up to
now there is no satisfying model which might explain a thrombophilic state at
concentrations in the range of mild hyperhomocysteinemia

The clinical relevance of the finding that hyperhomocysteinemia is a risk
factor for venous thrombosis depends mainly on its treatability by vitamin
supplementation. Clinical intervention studies have been started, but results are
not awaited before 2002.

*K. Robinson (ed.), Homocysteine and Vascular Disease, 239-252.*

## INTRODUCTION

In the early sixties several researchers reported a high incidence of thrombotic complications in patients with strongly elevated homocysteine levels (measured as homocystine in urine). Although the reported complications were both arterial and venous most attention was drawn to the arterial vascular complications.[1]

In 1969 McCully launched his 'homocysteine theory of arteriosclerosis'.[2] This marked the beginning of large number of studies on the relation between moderate hyperhomocysteinemia and vascular disease. Remarkably, the relation with venous thrombosis remained in the background. However, in the last decade this area advanced, by the appearance of several studies on the relation between hyperhomocysteinemia and venous thrombosis. This chapter gives an overview on the relation between classical homocystinuria and venous thrombosis and the relation between moderate hyperhomocysteinemia and venous thrombosis. Furthermore the relation between genetic and environmental causes of hyperhomocysteinemia with respect to venous thrombosis will be discussed as will the relation with other risk factors for venous thrombosis. Finally, some possible pathophysiologic mechanisms and the need for clinical intervention studies will be discussed.

## CLASSICAL HOMOCYSTINURIA

Because of the low incidence of classical homocystinuria, the data on the relation with vascular disease, especially venous thrombosis, are largely restricted to anecdotal case reports. In 1985 Mudd et al published an overview of 629 patients with homozygous homocystinuria due to cystathionine-β-synthase.[3] In this group, a total of 253 thromboembolic events were observed in 158 patients (25%). Of these 253 events, 130 concerned peripheral veins (51%) and 32 were accompanied by pulmonary embolism. Of those who suffered from thromboembolic complications more than 50 percent were affected before the age of thirty. Although no definite conclusion could be made, vitamin-$B_6$-responsive patients showed an incidence rate of thromboembolic complications lower than expected, when they were treated with pyridoxine with or without folate, suggesting that vitamin supplementation in this severe hyperhomocysteinemic group might be clinically effective.

In 1996 Mandel et al reported seven highly consanguineous families with homozygous homocystinuria, either due to cystathionine-β-synthase or methylenetetrahydrofolate reductase deficiency or cobalamin C/D defects.[4] Of the 11 persons with homocystinuria 6 suffered from venous thrombosis also had factor V Leiden (homozygous or heterozygous), while those without thrombosis were not carriers for factor V Leiden, suggesting that venous thrombosis in homocystinuric patients only occur in combination with activated protein C deficiency. However, these findings could not be confirmed by Quéré et al and Kluijtmans et al. Quéré et al reported 5 patients with venous thrombosis in 15 patients with cystathionine-β-synthase, of whom only 2 had factor V Leiden[5] and Kluijtmans et al reported 6 patients with venous thrombosis among 24 patients with homocystinuria due to cystathionine-β-synthase deficiency, of whom only one carried factor V Leiden.[6]

## MODERATE HYPERHOMOCYSTEINEMIA

### Venous thrombosis in general

The first studies on the relation between mild hyperhomocysteinemia and venous thrombosis were published by Bienvenu et al[7,8] and Brattstrom et al.[9] Bienvenu found elevated homocysteine levels in a group of 17 patients with venous thrombosis compared to 49 control subjects.[7] An extension of this study was published in 1993 with 23 patients with venous thrombosis (including Budd-Chiari syndrome, central retinal vein occlusion and mesenteric venous thrombosis) and 49 control subjects with the same conclusion.[8] In contrast, Brattström et al reported no significant difference in mean plasma homocysteine between patients with venous thrombosis and controls in a small series of 42 patients and 42 controls.[9] So, on the basis of these two contradictory papers no clear conclusion could be made about the relation between homocysteine and venous thrombosis.

From 1994 several studies were published. Falcon et al reported hyperhomocysteinemia as a risk factor for thrombosis occurring before the age of forty.[10] He studied patients with one or more episodes of venous thrombosis including cerebral vein thrombosis (and excluding other thrombophilic disorders), and healthy control subjects from the hospital staff. They reported a difference in homocysteine level between cases and controls particularly after methionine loading. In 1995 we published a study in patients with recurrent venous thrombosis between 20 and 70 years of age and controls from the general population.[11] In this study we found a risk estimate between 2 and 3 for homocysteine levels before and after methionine loading above the 90th percentile of the control group. Other studies published in 1995 were the study of Amundsen et al who found no significant difference in mean homocysteine in a

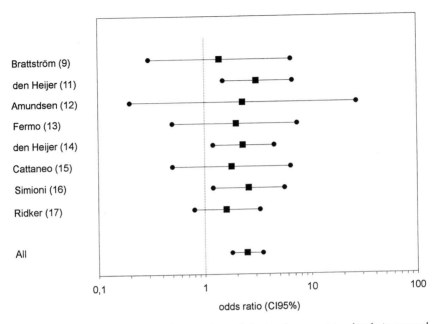

Figure 1. The odds ratios according to elevated fasting homocysteine levels in several case-control studies on venous thrombosis.[18]

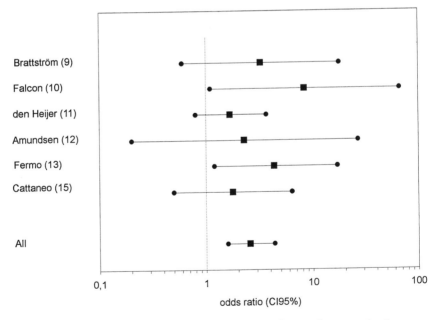

Figure 2. The odds ratios according to elevated post-methionine homocysteine increase in several case-control studies on venous thrombosis.[18]

small group of 35 patients (age less than 56) with deep-vein thrombosis and 39 controls[12] and the study of Fermo et al who found significantly higher prevalence of hyperhomocysteinemia in 107 patients with venous thrombosis before the age of 45 compared with 60 healthy persons[13]. Fermo also found an increased recurrence rate in patients with hyperhomocysteinemia.

In 1996, we reported a population based case-control study in 269 patients with a first, objectively confirmed, episode of deep-vein thrombosis and 269 matched control subjects of the general population[14]. We found a general risk estimate of 2.5 for a non-fasting homocysteine concentration above the 95th percentile of the control group. In this study women had a higher risk than men and the risk increased with age. Another population based study was published by Cattaneo et al who studied 89 patients with a first episode of deep-vein thrombosis and 89 age and sex matched controls[15]. They found similar risks for fasting and postloading hyperhomocysteinemia, and an increased risk for those who had both fasting and postloading hyperhomocysteinemia. Simioni et al published a study in 60 patients with proven deep-vein thrombosis and patients who were referred to the hospital because of clinically suspected deep-vein thrombosis but had normal venograms as control subjects; they found an odds ratio of 2.6. [16] Ridker et al presented the first prospective study on homocysteine levels in the Physicians' Health Study in 145 men who subsequently developed venous thromboembolism and 646 men free of cardiovascular disease. [17] They found hyperhomocysteinemia was associated with idiopathic venous thrombosis (odds ratio 3.4 [95%CI1.6 to 7.3] for homocysteine levels above the 95th percentile of the control group) but not with venous thrombosis of any cause (odds ratio 1.6 [95%CI 0.8 tp 3.3]).

Recently we performed a meta-analysis on ten case-control studies. [18] An overview of the risk estimates of these studies is shown in figure 1 (fasting homocysteine levels) and in figure 2 (post-methionine increase). The pooled estimate for the fasting homocysteine levels of all was 2.5 (95%CI 1.8-3.5) and for the post-methionine increase in homocysteine concentration 2.6 (95%CI 1.6-4 ). Interestingly, from both studies who reported no relation between homocysteine and venous thrombosis because they did not found a significant difference in mean plasma homocysteine levels, we could calculate an odds ratios of 1.4 and above. So, all published studies have point estimates which are in favor of the hypothesis that hyperhomocysteinemia is associated with venous thrombosis.

## Prospective data

Two studies have been published which provide prospective data. The above mentioned study of Ridker et al showed that (male) subjects with increased homocysteine levels are at increased risk for future idiopathic venous thromboembolism.[17] Kyrle et al studied 264 patients with a history of venous thrombosis.[19] Of the 66 patients with elevated homocysteine levels 12 suffered from recurrent venous thrombosis, compared with 16 out of the 198 patients with normal homocysteine levels. This implies a risk ratio of 2.7 (95%CI 1.3 to 5.8). These two studies strengthen the hypothesis that homocysteine is causally associated with venous thrombosis.

## Rare forms and special subgroups

Most studies mentioned above concerned the more common forms of venous thrombosis as deep-vein thrombosis of the legs and pulmonary embolism. There are several reports of more rare forms of venous thrombosis (cerebral venous thrombosis, portal vein thrombosis) occurring in patients with moderate hyperhomocysteinemia.[20-22] From these case-reports it is difficult to conclude that homocysteine is really involved in the causation of these rare forms of venous thrombosis. In a more systematic study of Martinelli et al in 36 patients with deep-vein thrombosis of the upper extremity and 108 control subjects they found no increased risk due to hyperhomocysteinemia (OR 0.8 [95%CI 0.1 to 7.9]).[23]

Apart from rare forms of thrombosis, several authors reported the relation between homocysteine and venous thrombosis in special groups. Beaumont reported the prevalence of hyperhomocysteinemia in 100 healthy women on oral contraceptives and 100 women with documented vascular disease (36 cases with venous thrombosis).[24] They found also in this group elevated homocysteine levels ($11.1\pm6.1$ $\mu$mol/L in patients with venous thrombosis compared with $7.8\pm2.7$ $\mu$mol/L in healthy women on oral contraceptives).

Petri et al[25] and Fijnheer et al[26] studied the relation between homocysteine and arterial and venous thrombosis in patients with systemic lupus erythematosus. Homocysteine concentrations were higher in patients than in healthy control subjects. They also found a weak association between homocysteine and the occurrence of venous thrombosis in patients with this disorder.

Gonera et al reported a patient with active ulcerative colitis and elevated postloading homocysteine levels with two thrombotic complications.[27] This finding of elevated homocysteine levels in patients with inflammatory bowel disease was confirmed by Cattaneo et al who found elevated mean homocysteine levels in 61 patients with inflammatory bowel disease compared with 183 age- and sex-matched controls.[28] These findings indicate that elevated homocysteine concentrations might contribute to the increased risk of venous thrombosis in women on oral contraceptives and in patients with SLE and patients with inflammatory bowel disease.

# DETERMINANTS OF HOMOCYSTEINE AND THE RISK OF VENOUS THROMBOSIS

Homocysteine concentration in blood is influenced by various genetic and environmental factors (as is reviewed by Refsum and Ueland in chapter 5 and 16-18 of this book). In this paragraph we will look at the effect of these factors on the risk for venous thrombosis.

## Methylenetetrahydrofolate reductase (MTHFR)

One of the determinants at the centre of interest is the common polymorphism C677T in the MTHFR gene, leading to a decreased enzym activity, especially after heating (thermobability).[29] In the homozygous state this mutation account for about 25% of elevated homocysteine levels, so it is one of the most important determinants of elevated homocysteine concentration.[30] Several authors published about the effect of this novel mutation on the risk of venous thrombosis.

The first publication on the thermolabile MTHFR mutation and venous thrombosis was of Arruda et al who looked at the prevalence of the C677T genotype in 127 patients with venous thrombosis and 296 control subjects. They found 14% patients homozygous for the C677T transition compared with 11% in the control group (odds ratio 2.9 [95%CI 1.2 to 7.0]).[31]

This finding could not be confirmed by two other studies. Cattaneo et al found 16 (20.8%) out of 77 patients with deep-vein thrombosis being homozygous for the C677T polymorphism compared with 35 (22.7%) out of 154 control subjects (odds ratio 0.8 [95%CI 0.4 to 2.0]).[32] Also Kluijtmans et al did not find any effect of the mutation on the risk of venous thrombosis in the Leiden Thrombophilia Study.[33] In his paper he also presented a summary estimate on the total of 810 patients with venous thrombosis and 870 control subjects and found an odds ratio of 1.0 (95%CI 0.8 to 1.4).

So, there is little evidence that the C677T polymorphism is a risk factor for venous thrombosis. This is remarkable, since the latter two studies found hyperhomocysteinemia being a risk factor for venous thrombosis in the same populations. Although the C677T polymorphism is a major determinant of homocysteine concentration it does not seem to affect the risk of thrombosis. However, because of the differences in prevalence of this polymorphism in different populations[34], we should wait for larger studies for definite conclusions.

*Martin den Heijer*

**Vitamins**

Besides genetic factors there are several other factors that influence homocysteine levels. The most important are creatinine concentration as a measure of renal function and the concentrations of folate and - to lesser extent - vitamin $B_6$ and vitamin $B_{12}$. Despite the relatively strong influence of these factors on homocysteine concentrations only four of the above mentioned studies reported data on B-vitamin concentrations.[9,11,12,16,35] Of these four studies, three found higher levels of B-vitamins in patients than in controls.[9,11,16,35]

None of the studies mentioned above reported on creatinine concentrations in their study populations. This should be however taken in account in future studies, because creatinine clearance is an strong determinant of homocysteine especially in the fasting state.[30]

In conclusion, although almost all studies found an increased risk of venous thrombosis due to hyperhomocysteinemia, most studies fail to find an elevated risk due to determinants of homocysteine. One should bear in mind that there might be some methodological limitations in these studies on determinants of homocysteine as risk factors of venous thrombosis. Most studies were not designed to study this relation (which requires large sample sizes, because the suspected risk estimates are lower than those of hyperhomocysteinemia itself). So far, there are no studies on the interaction between MTHFR mutation and environmental factors like folate-status. However, if larger, properly designed studies show no effect of determinants of homocysteine on the risk of venous thrombosis, this would speak strongly against the causality hypothesis of homocysteine and venous thrombosis.[35]

## INTERACTION WITH OTHER RISK FACTORS FOR VENOUS THROMBOSIS

**Homocysteine and other risk factors**

The common belief on the causation of venous thrombosis is that it has a multifactorial origin. The question arises whether the effect of hyperhomocysteinemia on the risk of venous thrombosis is independent of other known risk factors of venous thrombosis and whether hyperhomocysteinemia influences the effects of other risk factors (interaction). Several above mentioned studies dealt with this question.

From the above mentioned studies some included patients with other risk factors (such as protein C, protein S and antithrombin deficiency)[7,13,14] and others excluded these patients [10]. In our study in first time deep-vein thrombosis we found a risk of 2.6 after exclusion compared with 2.5 before.[14] Legnani did not find an increased prevalence of hyperhomocysteinemia and mutated MTHFR in patients with inherited thrombophilic coagulation defects and previous thrombosis which also suggests that there is no apparent interaction.[36]

## Activated protein C deficiency or factor V Leiden

In 1994 Dalhback described resistance to activated protein C.[37] This abnormality is one the most prevalent and strongest genetic risk factors for venous thrombosis[38] and is caused by a single adenine-for-guanine point mutation in the factor V gene (factor V Leiden).[39] Two studies investigated the interaction between hyperhomocysteinemia and activated protein C resistance or its genetic equivalent.

In our study on first-time venous thrombosis 47 out of 269 patients carried the factor V Leiden mutation, as compared with 7 out of 269 controls. The combined risk for hyperhomocysteinemia and factor V Leiden was 3.5, suggesting that both factors do not potentiate each other.[14] In contrast to this were the results of the study of Ridker who found an increased risk for subjects with both abnormalities up to 22 for idiopathic thrombosis.[17] However, both risk estimates have wide confidence intervals since they are not large enough for interaction analysis.

## MTHFR 677TT polymorphism and factor V Leiden

Although the 677TT polymorphism in the MTHFR gene is not a risk factor for venous thrombosis, several authors studied its interaction with factor V Leiden. Cattaneo et al did not find an elevated risk due to mutated MTHFR alone, but reported a risk of 13.7 for the combination of mutated MTHFR and factor V leiden, which was 65% to 75 % higher than the expected joint effect.[32] However this risk estimate depended on one control subject with both abnormalities. Kluijtmans et al did not find any interactive effects of mutated MTHFR and factor V Leiden.[33]

In a meta-analysis on 810 cases with venous thrombosis and 870 control subjects mutated MTHFR did not modify the risk in individuals with factor V Leiden genotype.[33]

## PATHOPHYSIOLOGY

Despite the epidemiological evidence for the relationship between hyperhomo-cysteinemia and venous thrombosis, little is known about its pathophysiology. A magnitude of possible mechanisms is proposed with respect to vascular disease, which have been recently reviewed.[40,41] Some of these proposed mechanisms with respect to arterial vascular disease may be applied to venous thrombosis as well. There are several reports that homocysteine may inhibit antithrombotic features of the endothelium through for instance increasing factor V [42] and tissue factor[43] and through inhibiting activity of protein C [44,45], thrombomodulin[46] and heparan sulfate[47]. However, all these associations are based on in-vitro experiments that used unphysiologic high concentrations of homocysteine. Therefore, it might be questioned whether these effects reflects the in-vivo effects of homocysteine.

Several clinical studies investigated the relation between homocysteine concentrations and those of thrombotic and antithrombotic factors. Others have looked at these factors before and after homocysteine lowering by vitamin supplementation. Bienvenu looked in 50 patients with venous or arterial thrombosis at protein C, protein S, antithrombin, plasminogen activator inhibitor (PAI), plasminogen and tissue plasminogen levels and found only a correlation between PAI and homocysteine.[8] We could not confirm this in a study in 114 healthy subjects.[48] Van den Berg et al looked at the relation with von Willebrand factor and found only a correlation between homocysteine and von Willebrand factor after vitamin supplementation.[49] We could also not confirm this in our study of 114 healthy subjects. [48]

Two studies investigated the relation between homocysteine and factors which are believed to be measures of clotting activity. Kyrle investigated the relation between homocysteine and fibrin degradation products F1+2. They found increased F1+2 levels in the hyperhomocysteinemic group, but the differences did not reach significance.[50] Cattaneo et al used the ratio between activated protein C and the protein C concentration as a measure of hemostatic system activation. [51] They found no correlation with homocysteine concentration in 98 healthy control subjects and only a weak correlation in patients with previous venous thrombosembolism. Very recently, we looked at the relation between homocysteine and thrombin activation potential (a measure of activity of the clotting system).[52] This measurement is reported to be elevated in subjects who have certain risk factors for venous thrombosis as, for instance, subjects with factor V Leiden or contraceptive use.[53] However, we did not find any association with homocysteine. So, in conclusion, there is yet no satisfying theory which explain the higher risk on venous thrombosis in subjects with hyperhomocysteinemia.

## TREATMENT OF HYPERHOMOCYSTEINEMIA AND VENOUS THROMBOSIS

The clinical relevance of the finding that hyperhomocysteinemia is a risk factor for venous thrombosis depends mainly on its treatability by vitamin supplementation. More than ten studies are published on the effects of several vitamins on lowering of the homocysteine concentration, which are reviewed in a meta-analysis.[54] One of these studies was performed in patients with venous thrombosis. In this study the vitamin supplementation caused a 30% decrease of plasma homocysteine levels, comparable to the effect in healthy volunteers.[55] A relevant observation in the homocysteine lowering trials is that also levels in the normal range could be further lowered with vitamin supplementation. The crucial question is whether the homocysteine lowering effect lead to lowering of the risk of thrombosis. Results of intervention studies with clinical endpoints are not awaited before 2002.

## ACKNOWLEDGEMENTS

I wish to thank my colleagues Henk Blom, Gerard Bos and Huub Willems for their valuable comments on a previous version of this chapter.

## REFERENCES

1.  Harker LA, Slichter SJ, Scott CR, Ross R. Homocystinemia. Vascular injury and arterial thrombosis. N Engl J Med 1974; 291:537-543.
2.  McCully KS, Wilson RB. Homocysteine theory of arteriosclerosis. Atherosclerosis 1975; 22:215-227.
3.  Mudd SH, Skovby F, Levy HL, et al. The natural history of homocystinuria due to cystathionine beta-synthase deficiency. Am J Hum Genet 1985; 37:1-31.
4.  Mandel H, Brenner B, Berant M, et al. Coexistence of hereditary homocystinuria and factor V Leiden - effect on thrombosis. N Engl J Med 1996; 334:763-768.
5.  Quere I, Lamarti H, Chadefaux Vekemans B. Thrombophilia, homocystinuria, and mutation of the factor V gene [letter]. N Engl J Med 1996; 335:289
6.  Kluijtmans LA, Boers GH, Verbruggen B, Trijbels FJ, Novakova IR, Blom HJ. Homozygous cystathionine β-synthase deficiency, combined with factor V Leiden or thermolabile methylenetetrahydrofolate reductase in the risk of venous thrombosis. Blood 1998; 91:2015-2018.
7.  Bienvenu T, Ankri A, Chadefaux B, Kamoun P. [Plasma homocysteine assay in the exploration of thrombosis in young subjects] Dosage de l'homocysteine plasmatique dans l'exploration des thromboses du sujet jeune. Presse Med 1991; 20:985-988.

8.  Bienvenu T, Ankri A, Chadefaux B, Montalescot G, Kamoun P. Elevated total plasma homocysteine, a risk factor for thrombosis. Relation to coagulation and fibrinolytic parameters. Thromb Res 1993; 70:123-129.

9.  Brattström L, Tengborn L, Lagerstedt C, Israelsson B, Hultberg B. Plasma homocysteine in venous thromboembolism. Haemostasis 1991; 21:51-57.

10. Falcon CR, Cattaneo M, Panzeri D, Martinelli I, Mannucci PM. High prevalence of hyperhomocyst(e)inemia in patients with juvenile venous thrombosis. Arterioscler Thromb 1994; 14:1080-1083.

11. den Heijer M, Blom HJ, Gerrits WBJ, et al. Is hyperhomocysteinemia a risk factor for recurrent venous thrombosis? Lancet 1995; 345:882-885.

12. Amundsen T, Ueland PM, Waage A. Plasma homocysteine levels in patients with deep venous thrombosis. Arterioscler Thromb Vasc Biol 1995; 15:1321-1323.

13. Fermo I, Vigano' D, Paroni R, Mazzola G, Calori G, D'Angelo A. Prevalence of moderate hyperhomocysteinemia in patients with early-onset venous and arterial occlusive disease. Ann Intern Med 1995; 123:747-753.

14. den Heijer M, Koster T, Blom HJ, et al. Hyperhomocysteinemia as a risk factor for deep-vein thrombosis. N Engl J Med 1996; 334:759-762.

15. Cattaneo M, Martinelli I, Mannucci PM. Hyperhomocysteinemia as a risk factor for deep-vein thrombosis [letter]. N Engl J Med 1996; 335:974-975.

16. Simioni P, Prandoni P, Burlina A, et al. Hyperhomocysteinemia and deep-vein thrombosis. A case-control study. Thromb Haemost 1996; 76:883-886.

17. Ridker PM, Hennekens CH, Selhub J, Miletich JP, Malinow MR, Stampfer MJ. Interrelation of hyperhomocyst(e)inemia, factor V Leiden, and risk of future venous thromboembolism. Circulation 1997; 95:1777-1782.

18. den Heijer M, Rosendaal FR, Blom HJ, Gerrits WBJ, Bos GMJ. Hyperhomocysteinemia and venous thrombosis: a meta-analysis. Thromb Haemost 1998; 80:874-7.

19. Eichinger S, Stümpflen A, Hirschl M et al. Hyperhomocysteinemia is a risk factor of recurrent venous thrombosembolism. Thromb Haemost 1998;80:566-9.

20. Schwab FJ, Peyster RG, Brill CB. CT of cerebral venous sinus thrombosis in a child with homocystinuria. Pediatr Radiol 1987; 17:244-245.

21. Mohamed A, McLeod JG, Hallinan J. Superior sagittal sinus thrombosis. Clin Exp Neurol 1991; 28:23-36.

22. Hong HS, Lee HK, Kwon KH. Homocystinuria presenting with portal vein thrombosis and pancreatic pseudocyst: a case report. Pediatr Radiol 1997; 27:802-804.

23. Martinelli I, Cattaneo M, Panzeri D, Taioli E, Mannucci PM. Risk factors for deep venous thrombosis of the upper extremities. Ann Intern Med 1997; 126:707-711.

24. Beaumont V, Malinow MR, Sexton G, et al. Hyperhomocyst(e)inemia, anti-estrogen antibodies and other risk factors for thrombosis in women on oral contraceptives. Atherosclerosis 1992; 94:147-152.

25. Petri M, Roubenoff R, Dallal GE, Nadeau MR, Selhub J, Rosenberg IH. Plasma homocysteine as a risk factor for atherothrombotic events in systemic lupus erythematosus. Lancet 1996;348:1120-1124.

26. Fijnheer R, Roest M, Haas FJLM, de Groot PG, Derksen RHWM. Homocysteine, methylenetertahydrofolate reductase polymorphism, antiphospholipid antibodies and

thrombo-embolic events in Systemic Lupus Erythematosus: a retrospective cohort study. J Rheum 1998;25:1737-42.

27. Gonera RK, Timmerhuis TPJ, Leyten ACM, van der Heul C. Two thrombotic complications in a patient with active ulcerative colitis. Neth J Med 1997;50:88-91.

28. Cattaneo M, Vecchi M, Zighetti ML et al. High prevalence of hyperhomocysteinemia in patients with inflammatory bowel disease: a pathogenetic link with thromboembolic complications? Thromb Haemost 1998;80:542-5.

29. Frosst P, Blom HJ, Milos R, et al. A candidate genetic risk factor for vascular disease: a common mutation in methylenetetrahydrofolate reductase [letter]. Nat Genet 1995; 10:111-113.

30. den Heijer M. Hyperhomocysteinemia and venous thrombosis. Dissertation, Leiden 1997.

31. Arruda VR, von Zuben PM, Chiaparini LC, Annichino Bizzacchi JM, Costa FF. The mutation Ala677-->Val in the methylene tetrahydrofolate reductase gene: a risk factor for arterial disease and venous thrombosis. Thromb Haemost 1997; 77:818-821.

32. Cattaneo M, Tsai MY, Bucciarelli P, et al. A common mutation in the methylenetetrahydrofolate reductase gene (C677T) increases the risk for deep-vein thrombosis in patients with mutant factor V (factor V:Q506). Arterioscler Thromb Vasc Biol 1997; 17:1662-1666.

33. Kluijtmans LA, den Heijer M, Reitsma PH, Heil SG, Blom HJ, Rosendaal FR. Thermolabile Methylenetetrahydrofolate Reductase and Factor V Leiden in the Risk of Deep-Vein Thrombosis. Thromb Haemost 1998; 79:254-258.

34. Franco RF, Araújo AG, Gueerreiro JF, Elion J, Zago MA. Analysis of the 677 C→T mutation of the methylenetetrahydrofolate reductase gene in different ethnic groups. Thromb Haemost 1998; 79:119-21.

35. den Heijer M, Bos GM, Gerrits WB, Blom HJ. Will a Decrease of Blood Homocysteine by Vitamin Supplementation Reduce the Risk for Vascular Disease? Fibrinolysis 1994; 8, Suppl 2:91-92.

36. Legnani C, Palareti G, Grauso F, Sassi S, Grossi G, Piazzi S, et al. Hyperhomocyst(e)inemia and a common methylenetetrahydrofolate reductase mutation (Ala223Val MTHFR) in patients with inherited thrombophilic coagulation defects. Arterioscler Thromb Vasc Biol 1997; 17:2924-2929.

37. Dahlback B, Carlsson M, Svensson PJ. Familial thrombophilia due to a previously unrecognized mechanism characterized by poor anticoagulant response to activated protein C: prediction of a cofactor to activated protein C. Proc Natl Acad Sci U S A 1993; 90:1004-1008.

38. Koster T, Rosendaal FR, de Ronde H, Briet E, Vandenbroucke JP, Bertina RM. Venous thrombosis due to poor anticoagulant response to activated protein C: Leiden Thrombophilia Study. Lancet 1998; 342:1503-1506.

39. Bertina RM, Koeleman B, Koster T, et al. Mutation in blood coagulation factor V associated with resistance to activated protein C. Nature 1994; 64-67.

40. Rees MM, Rodgers GM. Homocysteinemia: association of a metabolic disorder with vascular disease and thrombosis. Thromb Res 1993; 71:337-359.

41. Welch GN, Loscalzo J, Hyperhomocysteinemia and atherothrombosis. N Engl J Med 1998; 338:1043-50.

42. Rodgers GM, Kane WH. Activation of endogenous factor V by a homocysteine-induced vascular endothelial cell activator. J Clin Invest 1986; 77:1909-1916.

43. Fryer RH, Wilson BD, Gubler DB, Fitzgerald LA, Rodgers GM. Homocysteine, a risk factor for premature vascular disease and thrombosis, induces tissue factor activity in endothelial cells. Arterioscler Thromb 1993; 13:1327-1333.

44. Rodgers GM, Conn MT. Homocysteine, an atherogenic stimulus, reduces protein C activation by arterial and venous endothelial cells. Blood 1990; 75:895-901.

45. Lentz SR, Sadler JE. Inhibition of thrombomodulin Surface Expression and protein C activation by the thrombogenic agent homocysteine. J Clin Invest 1991;88:1906-1914.

46. Hayashi T, Honda G, Suzuki K. An atherogenic stimulus homocysteine inhibits cofactor activity of thrombomodulin and enhances thrombomodulin expression in human umbilical vein endothelial cells. Blood 1992; 79:2930-2936.

47. Nishinaga M, Ozawa T, Shimada K. Homocysteine, a thrombogenic agent, suppresses anticoagulant heparan sulfate expression in cultured porcine aortic endothelial cells. J Clin Invest 1993; 92:1381-1386.

48. van der Molen EF, den Heijer M, Postma J, Kluft C, Blom HJ. The relation between hyperhomocysteinemia, coagulation/fibrinolysis and 677C→Tmutation in the methylenetetrahydrofolate reductase (MTHFR) gene in healthy persons. Neth J Med 1998;52:S49.

49. van den Berg M, Boers GH, Franken DG, et al. Hyperhomocysteinemia and endothelial dysfunction in young patients with peripheral arterial occlusive disease. Eur J Clin Invest 1995; 25:176-181.

50. Kyrle PA, Stumpflen A, Hirschl M, et al. Levels of prothrombin fragment F1+2 in patients with hyperhomocysteinemia and a history of venous thromboembolism. Thromb Haemost 1997; 78:1327-1331.

51. Cattaneo M, Franchi F, Zighetti ML, Martinelli I, Asti D, Mannucci PM. Plasma levels of activated protein C in healthy subjects and patients with previous venous thromboembolism. Relationships with plasma homocysteine levels. Arterioscler Thromb Vasc Biol 1998;18:1371-1375.

52. Bos GMJ, Rijkers DTS, Willems H, den Heijer M, Gerrits WBJ, Hemker HC. Can an elevated endogenous thrombin potential explain the elevated risk for venous thrombosis in case of hyperhomocysteinemia? [Letter] Thromb Haemost 1999;81;467-8.

53. Rosing J, Tans G, Nicolaes GAF, et al. Oral contraceptives and venous thrombosis: different sensitivities to activated protein C in women using second- and third-generation oral contraceptives. Br J Haematol 1997:97:233-238.

54. Homocysteine Lowering Trialists' Collaboration. Lowering blood homocysteine with folic acid based supplements: meta-analysis of randomized trials. BMJ 1998;316:894-898.

55. den Heijer M, Brouwer IA, Bos GMJ, et al. Vitamin Supplementation reduces blood homocysteine levels. A Controlled Trial in Patients With Venous Thrombosis and Healthy Volunteers. Arterioscler Thromb Vasc Biol 1998; 18:356-361.

# 15. HOMOCYSTEINE AND RENAL DISEASE

KILLIAN ROBINSON AND VINCENT W. DENNIS

## SUMMARY

A high plasma homocysteine concentration is often found in patients with renal failure. This disturbance of homocysteine metabolism parallels abnormalities of amino acids in general and some sulfur-containing amino acids in particular. Proposed mechanisms for the hyperhomocysteinemia include reduced elimination by either renal or non renal routes or even inhibition of essential biological reactions by the uremic milieu. Elevated levels may also be attributable to absolute or relative deficiencies of folate, vitamin $B_6$ or vitamin $B_{12}$. Inhibition of intracellular vitamin activity despite high circulating concentrations of vitamins may also be possible. The association of high circulating homocysteine concentrations with vascular disorders has led to a search for a similar association between hyper-homocysteinemia and atherothrombotic complications of renal failure. Several studies using both case control-type and prospective designs have now established that hyperhomocysteinemia is an independent risk factor for such complications in patients with end-stage renal disease on chronic dialysis. As in the general population, plasma homocysteine concentrations can be reduced by administration of folic acid although pharmacologic doses may be required. The effects of vitamin $B_{12}$ or vitamin $B_6$ are unclear. Therapeutic trials are now being planned or are underway to evaluate the effects, if any, of such reduction on vascular risk in patients with renal failure.

*K. Robinson (ed.), Homocysteine and Vascular Disease, 253-270.*

## BIOCHEMICAL FORMS OF HOMOCYSTEINE IN PLASMA IN RENAL FAILURE

Under normal conditions, about 80-90% of plasma homocysteine is protein bound (see Chapter 3). Unbound homocysteine exists as homocysteine-cysteine mixed disulfide, homocysteine-homocysteine dimer (homocystine) or as truly free homocysteine. In renal failure, the concentrations of both free and protein bound homocysteine fractions increase. A study of the different fractions of homocysteine, cysteine and cysteinylglycine in 17 patients on chronic hemodialysis, 9 patients with reduced renal function and 4 patients with nephrotic syndrome showed total plasma homocysteine, cysteine and cysteinylglycine were increased in the patients with reduced renal function and in those on chronic hemodialysis relative to 14 healthy subjects (1). The free (non-protein-bound) forms of plasma homocysteine and cysteine were significantly increased in all groups but the reduced forms of plasma homocysteine and cysteine were not increased in any. Indeed, reduced plasma homocysteine was significantly decreased in the plasma of patients with reduced renal function demonstrating that the plasma levels of reduced forms of these thiol compounds do not reflect the elevation of the disulfide forms.

## BACKGROUND AND PREVALENCE OF HYPERHOMOCYSTEINEMIA IN RENAL FAILURE.

### Chronic renal failure and hemodialysis

Although Robins et al (2) had suggested the presence of homocysteine-cysteine mixed disulfides in the presence of chronic renal failure, it remained for Wilcken et al (3) and Cohen et al (4) to establish definitively that both homocysteine and cysteine concentrations increase in patients with renal failure. Since that time, the prevalence of abnormalities of homocysteine metabolism has been measured in numerous studies of patients with renal dysfunction including those with mild degrees of renal impairment, those on hemodialysis or peritoneal dialysis and patients who have undergone renal transplantation. It is now apparent that the usual total fasting plasma homocysteine concentration which normally ranges between 10-15 $\mu$mol/L, rises even with mild degrees of renal impairment. Wilcken et al measured plasma sulfur-containing amino acids in patients with chronic renal failure and compared the findings with normal subjects. Fasting cysteine-homocysteine mixed disulfide was increased almost 3-fold in the renal patients and correlated positively with reduced renal function as assessed by serum creatinine. Levels of other sulfur-containing amino acids including homocystine, cystine, taurine but not methionine were also elevated (3). Chauveau et al (5) determined the fasting plasma level of protein-bound homocysteine in 118 adult chronic uremic patients (see Table I).

*Table 1. Relationship of homocysteine to renal function and creatinine clearance*

| Groups | 1(N=28) | 2(N=29) | 3(N=22) | 4(N=39) |
|---|---|---|---|---|
| Age *years* | 59.2 $\pm$ 14.8 | 58.7 $\pm$ 14.2 | 63.3 $\pm$ 13.1 | 43.0 $\pm$ 18.5 |
| $P_{CR}$ *(μmol/L)* | 166 $\pm$ 46 | 358 $\pm$ 154 | 729 $\pm$ 206 | 1187 $\pm$ 183 |
| Purea *(mmol/L)* | 11.3 $\pm$ 2.9 | 20.5 $\pm$ 6.7 | 33.0 $\pm$ 9.1 | 30.9 $\pm$ 5.7 |
| $C_{CR}$ *(ml/min)* | 45.0 $\pm$ 10.9 | 17.3 $\pm$ 4.9 | 6.3 $\pm$ 2.1 | <2 |
| Homocysteine *(μmol/L)* | 16.2 $\pm$ 8.1 | 23.3 $\pm$ 14.7 | 29.5 $\pm$ 14.4 | 23.5 $\pm$ 10.7 |
| % High homocysteine (>14.1 *μmol/L*) | 13/28 | 23/29 | 21/22 | 32/39 |

Adapted from Chauveau et al. 1993 (5).

Seventy nine non-dialyzed patients had various degrees of chronic renal failure and were assessed by creatinine clearance. None were receiving folate, $B_6$ or $B_{12}$ vitamin supplementation. Mean plasma homocysteine levels were 16.2 $\pm$ 8.1 μmol/L in 28 patients with mild renal failure (creatinine clearance 30 to 75 ml/min), and rose to 23.3 $\pm$ 14.7 μmol/L in 29 patients in whom creatinine clearance was between 10 and 29.9 ml/min. In 22 patients with advanced renal failure, and creatinine clearances of less than 10 ml/min, the mean homocysteine level was 29.5 $\pm$ 14.4 μmol/L. These findings have been corroborated in other studies (6, 7) and the levels in those with the most severe creatinine clearances are similar to those seen in patients on hemodialysis. In our studies, we have demonstrated a prevalence of hyperhomocysteinemia of 85% in more than 170 patients with end stage renal disease. In patients on hemodialysis, mean homocysteine concentrations were almost 30 μmol/L. In one study, there was little if any diurnal variation of plasma homocysteine in patients with varying renal function even following the intake of a protein-rich meal (8). In another, levels were stable in patients undergoing peritoneal dialysis but not hemodialysis (9). In summary, the prevalence and intensity of hyperhomocysteinemia increase in proportion to reductions in glomerular filtration rate.

*Table II. Homocysteine concentrations (μmol/L) in patients on hemodialysis and chronic ambulatory peritoneal dialysis.*

|  | CAPD | Hemodialysis |
|---|---|---|
| Hultberg et al 1993 (8) | 24 (6.7-92.4)* | 27.9 (8-41.9)* |
| Kim et al 1994 (10) | 32.7 μ 18.5** | 25.2 ± 10.9** |
| Bostom et al 1996 (21) | 21.3H | 22.5H |
| Janssen et al 1996 (9) | 50.5 ± 14.3 | 55 ±10.1 |
| Robinson et al 1996 (7) | 19.5 ± 1.7 | 29.5 ± 1.7 |

*= Range; H=Geometric mean; ** not on vitamin supplements; CAPD = Chronic ambulatory peritoneal dialysis.

## Peritoneal dialysis

The homocysteine levels in patients undergoing peritoneal dialysis have been lower than in those undergoing hemodialysis in some studies (6-8) but not others (9, 10) and there is considerable variation in the published results from different investigators (see Table II). Some of the differences may relate to the patient populations, degrees of residual renal function, length of time on dialysis or even the prevalence of supplementation with multivitamin pills.

## Renal transplantation

Homocysteine concentrations also rise following renal transplantation. This observation was first made by Wilcken et al in 1981 (11) who, using a case-control design, demonstrated elevated mean levels of homocysteine-cysteine mixed disulfide in 27 patients. Massy et al (12) demonstrated higher homocysteine levels in renal transplant subjects compared to age and sex matched controls a mean of 11 years after operation. In a study by Arnadottir et al (13), increased homocysteine levels were seen in 120 renal transplant recipients compared with both healthy controls and with patients without a transplant but with a comparable degree of renal failure (19.0 ± 6.9 vs 11.6 ± 2.8 and 16.0 ± 4.9 μmol/L respectively). As with non-transplant populations there was an inverse correlation between glomerular filtration rates and homocysteine concentrations in the recipients. In addition, transplant recipients on cyclosporine had higher plasma homocysteine concentrations than those not on cyclosporine. The authors concluded that the hyperhomocysteinemia of renal transplant recipients not treated with cyclosporine was due to renal insufficiency. In transplant recipients treated with cyclosporine, however, drug-induced interference with folate-assisted remethylation of homocysteine may be important. Bostom et al assessed the prevalence of hyperhomocysteinemia both fasting and 2 hours after methionine loading in renal transplant recipients and controls. Both values were greater in the transplant recipients as were the odds for low circulating folate or vitamin $B_6$ status (14). In another study, Fogarty et al (15) demonstrated significantly higher plasma homocysteine concentrations in renal transplant recipients compared to normal controls. In this study, however, there was no difference in the homocysteine levels between the cyclosporine treated patients and those treated with azathioprine and prednisone.

Following transplantation homocysteine levels fall. van Guldener et al studied the effect of renal transplantation on hyperhomocysteinemia in 8 dialysis patients after successful kidney transplantation and demonstrated decreasing post-transplantation homocysteine concentrations with improving renal function (16).

Notably, a high homocysteine level is also frequently seen after heart, liver and lung transplantation (17-19, unpublished observations). The relationship of these findings to the development of atherothrombotic complications in the transplant population is discussed below.

## THE METHIONINE LOADING TEST IN RENAL FAILURE

Several studies have also examined the methionine loading test in patients with renal failure. Hultberg et al (8) studied in patients with severe chronic renal failure after methionine loading and noted an abnormal increase of plasma homocysteine indicating impaired transsulfuration. Postmethionine-loading hyperhomocysteinemia has also been shown in renal transplant recipients using a two hour test (14). In this study there were significant correlations between both creatinine and folate and fasting homocysteine as well as between creatinine and pyridoxal 5'-phosphate and postmethionine-loading increase in homocysteine levels. As among patients without renal failure, the use of the methionine loading test in routine clinical practice is costly, cumbersome and remains ill-defined.

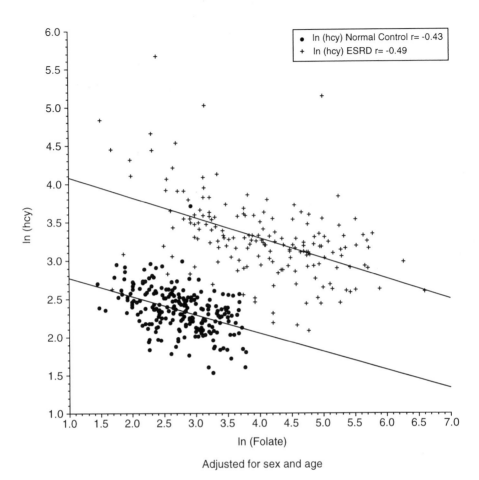

*Figure 1. Scatter plots for concentrations of plasma folate and homocysteine in patients with end-stage renal disease compared with normal subjects. Reproduced with permission from Robinson et al Circulation 1996 (7).*

## CAUSES OF HYPERHOMOCYSTEINEMIA & FACTORS AFFECTING HOMOCYSTEINE LEVELS IN RENAL FAILURE

### Genetic influences

Although age and gender contribute to the normal variation in homocysteine concentrations these influences are apparently lost with the onset of renal disease. There is no evidence that the genetic causes for homocystinuria including deficiencies of cystathionine ß-synthase, methionine synthase and the variants of methylenetetrahydrofolate reductase defects play a major role. Indeed, in a recent study the allelic frequency of the C677T transition in the MTHFR-gene mutation in hemodialysis patients was 34.7% versus 35.5% in healthy controls. Overall, the mean homocysteine level in hemodialysis patients was 28.7 ± 11.0 compared with 10.0 ± 3.0 µmol/L in controls. The mean level was 36.4 ± 13.4 µmol/L in homozygote patients and 12.2 ± 4.5 µmol/L in homozygote controls, 28.7 ± 10.8 µmol/L in heterozygote patients and 9.9 ± 2.7 µmol/L in heterozygote controls and 25.4 ± 8.5 µmol/L in wild type hemodialysis patients versus 9.7 ± 2.8 µmol/L in similar controls. There was a significant influence of the homozygote genotype, albumin and folate status on homocysteine levels in the patients (20). In another study, there was also a significant interaction between presence of the thermolabile variant and folate status on plasma homocysteine. Among patients with plasma folate below the median (< 29.2 ng/ml), mean homocysteine levels were 33% greater (29.0 compared to 21.8 µmol/L) in the thermolabile group compared to normal subjects (21). These studies suggest that there is no greater frequency of genetic abnormalities in this population than others although folate may acquire additional importance as a modulator of homocysteine levels in the presence of the thermolabile variant.

**Vitamin abnormalities**

Abnormalities of folate and related vitamins appear to be the principal cause of high homocysteine concentrations in patients with end-stage renal disease and there is ample evidence that folate is the main determinant of homocysteine levels in this setting (7, 20-22). As in normal subjects, homocysteine levels rise with falling folate concentrations (see Figure 1). In addition, although absolute deficiency is uncommon (11, 23) folic acid supplementation reduces homocysteine levels in these patients (9, 23-26). Indeed, the reduction in homocysteine may be particularly pronounced in patients with low-normal serum folate (27). Improved remethylation in tissues is suggested by an improved methionine response to homocysteine loading after folic acid administration although correction of homocysteine to normal values may be difficult (26).

While folate may be a major determinant of homocysteine concentration among patients on hemodialysis this may not be the case among those on peritoneal dialysis. Based on our studies, concentrations of homocysteine are higher, and those of folate, vitamin $B_{12}$ and vitamin $B_6$, are lower in hemodialysis patients than in peritoneal dialysis. The lower prevalence of hyperhomocysteinemia in patients on peritoneal dialysis may be due to their higher levels of plasma folate. In addition, the lower folate levels in patients on hemodialysis may be attributable to greater dialysis losses (27). Another possibility is that less folate is absorbed in hemodialysis patients due to the presence of folate conjugase inhibitors in uremia (28) which cleave dietary polyglutamate forms of folate into the more readily absorbed monoglutamates (29).

## Metabolic disturbances

The metabolism of homocysteine is covered extensively in Chapter 3. In man, the enzymes for remethylation and transsulfuration reactions are found both in the liver and the kidney. Accordingly, the hypothesis that the high homocysteine concentrations seen in patients with renal failure might be attributable to reduced renal excretion or metabolism appears attractive. Under normal circumstances, however, only tiny amounts of homocysteine are excreted in the urine (30) and diminished excretion is therefore unlikely to play a role. An alternative is that possible renal metabolism is reduced with falling renal function. Renal metabolism of homocysteine appears to be important in the rat (31). However, a recent study has demonstrated no net renal extraction of homocysteine in fasting humans. In a study of 20 patients with normal renal function, plasma total and free homocysteine concentrations were measured in arterial and renal venous blood sampled from the aorta and right-side renal vein during cardiac catheterization. There was no significant renal extraction demonstrated either for total or for free homocysteine. The loss of such uptake, therefore, cannot cause hyperhomocysteinemia in humans with renal failure (32). This may indicate important species differences in the metabolism of homocysteine. Some studies have demonstrated that all the enzymes necessary for metabolizing homocysteine are present in the human kidney (33, 34) while cystathionine β-synthase may be more abundant in the rat (35, 36).

An alternative is that homocysteine is cleared or metabolized by non-renal, metabolic processes which are impaired in renal failure. Guttormsen et al in vestigated the elimination of total homocysteine from plasma after oral and intravenous homocysteine loading. The area under the plasma concentration curve ($AUC_{0-48 h}$) was proportional to the administered dose (33.5-134 μmol/kg body wt). Plasma homocysteine showed first-order elimination kinetics and the half-life ($T_{1/2}$) was 223 ± 45 min. The transient increase in homocysteine was associated with an increase in plasma methionine reflecting remethylation of homocysteine. Less than 2% of the administered homocysteine dose was recovered in the urine (37). The authors further proposed that the 50% bioavailability could be due to hepatic transsulfuration as the $K_m$ for both methylene-

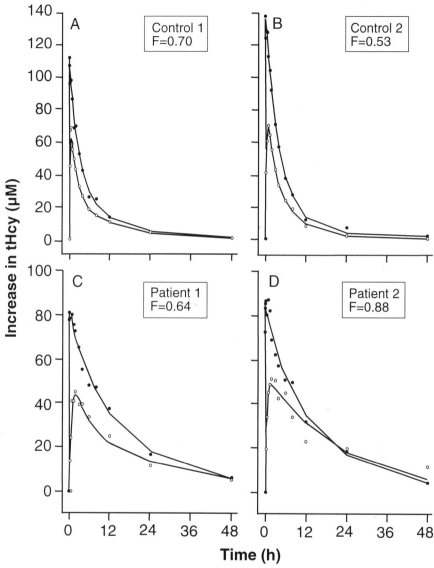

*Figure 2. Oral (B) and intravenous (X) homocysteine loading studies in 2 healthy controls and 2 patients with renal failure. Both $AUC_{0-48\ h}$ and also of $T_2$ were markedly higher than controls. Permissions obtained.*

tetrahydrofolate reductase and methionine synthase are low while that for cystathionine synthase is high. These studies were later extended to patients with chronic renal failure (38). Both $AUC_{0-48\ h}$ and $T_{1/2}$ were markedly higher than controls (see Figure 2). In addition, total clearance was reduced to $26 \pm 8$ ml/min compared to about $101 \pm 15$ ml/min for normal controls. Taken in conjunction with the findings of van Guldener et al (32) these observations suggest that inhibition of systemic ie non-renal homocysteine clearance is the likely mechanism of hyperhomocysteinemia of renal failure. Such abnormalities may be related to reduction in hepatic uptake of homocysteine bioavailability of homocysteine being similar in renal failure compared with controls (38).

In our studies of dialysis patients, the levels of homocysteine in peritoneal dialysis patients were lower than in hemodialysis patients for any given serum concentration of folate raising the possibility of incomplete conversion of folate to its metabolically active form or inhibition of normal intracellular folate function.

A further contributing factor to the high homocysteine concentrations seen in dialysis patients may be vitamin $B_6$ deficiency. We found deficiency of this vitamin in 18% of ESRD patients compared with only 2% in the controls (7). The increased prevalence of vitamin $B_6$ deficiency in patients with end-stage renal failure suggests deranged metabolism of this vitamin also. This could be due to impaired absorption, increased clearance or even uremic inhibition of pyruvate kinase which is required for production of pyridoxal 5'-phosphate (39). Functional vitamin $B_6$ deficiency could explain the abnormal methionine loading tests previously reported in ESRD patients since this may be a manifestation not only of dysfunction of cystathionine $\beta$-synthase but also of availability of this essential cofactor.

## EFFECT OF DIALYSIS ON HOMOCYSTEINE LEVELS

Wilcken et al originally reported the effect of hemodialysis on homocysteine concentrations in patients with renal failure (40). After 3-4 hours of dialysis cysteine-homocysteine mixed disulfide was decreased by about 40%. Kang et al later reported that predialysis protein bound homocysteine values decreased significantly following dialysis (41). Others have also reported that dialysis reduces homocysteine concentrations by 30-50% (42). The type of dialysis membrane may also influence homocysteine levels. Smolin et al (43) demonstrated a decline of only 11% in homocysteine concentrations using a low flux membrane but high-flux dialysis techniques may remove homocysteine in greater amounts. Differences in dialysis membranes may also explain the lower homocysteine concentrations in patients on chronic ambulatory peritoneal dialysis than hemodialysis patients (7).

# HYPERHOMOCYSTEINEMIA AND ATHEROSCLEROSIS IN RENAL DISEASE

## Chronic renal failure

Both Cohen and Wilcken hypothesized that accumulation of homocysteine could be relevant to the development of accelerated vascular disease in patients with chronic renal failure by producing endothelial damage (3, 4). In 79 patients with non-dialysis dependent chronic renal failure, Chauveau et al (5) reported higher homocysteine concentrations in 20 patients with prior histories of occlusive arterial disease compared to 59 patients who had no such history. Recently, Jungers et al (44) reported on risk factors and the incidence of atherosclerotic vascular events in 147 predialysis chronic renal failure patients followed prospectively for 9 years. In multivariate analysis, cigarette smoking, systolic blood pressure, low HDL-cholesterol and fibrinogen were independent risk factors for vascular accidents. LDL-cholesterol, triglycerides, apoB, Lp(a), and homocysteine levels were all significantly higher in those with vascular accidents. In a further study, Jungers et al (45) determined total plasma homocysteine levels in 93 consecutive chronic renal failure patients over 6 years. Homocysteine levels were higher in those with vascular accidents and logistic regression analysis identified homocysteine as an independent risk factor.

## Hemodialysis patients

In the dialysis-dependent population, Bachmann et al (46) studied 50 patients on regular hemodialysis of whom 24 had vascular occlusive disease. They demonstrated a significant association between homocysteine concentrations and occlusive arterial disease. This association was also observed for hypertension but not for lipid abnormalities, diabetes, smoking or fibrinogen. In a larger study of ESRD patients higher homocysteine concentrations were associated with an increased risk of atherosclerotic and thrombotic complications independent of other traditional risk factors and length of time on dialysis (7). Two prospective studies corroborate these observations (47, 48). Bostom et al (47) studied 73 maintenance peritoneal dialysis or hemodialysis patients and determined the incidence of nonfatal and fatal CVD. After a median follow-up of only 17.0 months homocysteine levels in the upper quartile (>27 μmol/L) versus the lower three quartiles (< 27 μmol/L) were associated with relative risk estimates ranging from 3.0 to 4.4 adjusted

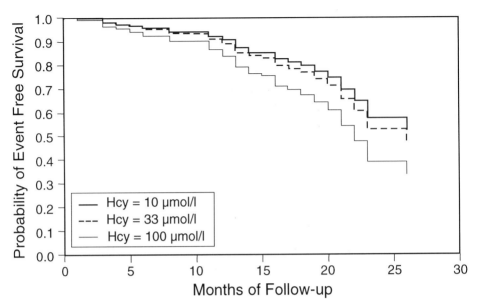

*Figure 3. Probability for event-free survival during the follow-up period for patients with mean homocysteine values of 10, 33 and 100 µmol/L. Reproduced with permission from Moustapha et al Circulation 1998 (48).*

for other established CVD risk factors. Moustapha et al (48) followed 167 patients for a mean of 17.4 ± 6.4 months. Cardiovascular events and causes of mortality were related to total homocysteine values and other cardiovascular risk factors. Fifty-five patients (33%) developed cardiovascular events and 31 (19%) died, 12 (8%) of cardiovascular causes. Total plasma homocysteine levels were higher in patients who had cardiovascular events or died of cardiovascular causes and the relative risk for cardiovascular events, including death, increased 1% per 1 µmol/L increase in total homocysteine concentration (see Figure 3). These prospective studies confirm that hyperhomocysteinemia is an independent risk factor for cardiovascular morbidity and mortality in end-stage renal disease but do not establish that this risk factor can be modified sufficiently to improve mortality or morbidity. Specific data in relation to the role of hyperhomocysteinemia, if any, in the development of vascular complications associated with peritoneal dialysis are needed.

**Renal transplantation**

Wilcken et al (11) noted that homocysteine concentrations rise following renal transplantation and similar studies have since been reported (12-14). In one, (12) recipients with cardiovascular events had higher homocysteine concentrations compared to those without a vascular event although the difference was not statistically significant. In another, (13) concentrations were higher in the renal transplant recipients with a history of atherosclerotic complications compared with those without (20.8 ± 4.4 vs. 18.5 ± 7.3 µmol/L). As noted above, homocysteine concentrations also rise in other transplantation populations (17-19). In addition, some authors (49), but not others (50) report a greater risk of vascular complications in such patients in the presence of hyperhomocysteinemia. Underlying mechanisms of the high plasma homocysteine level and a role, if any, in the development of accelerated atherosclerosis in the transplant population require further study.

MECHANISMS OF VASCULAR DAMAGE

The mechanisms by which high homocysteine concentrations might cause vascular damage in patients with (51, 52) or without (53, 54) renal failure remains unclear and have been reviewed in several other chapters in this text. Potential mechanisms include adverse effects of homocysteine on endothelial cells, on platelets and/or coagulation factors. In chronic hemodialysis patients van Guldener et al (55) used a vessel wall movement detector system to investigate endothelium-dependent, flow-mediated and endothelium-independent, glyceryl trinitrate-induced brachial arterial vasodilatation. Endothelium-dependent vasodilatation was markedly reduced (3.7 ± 1.1 vs. 9.7 ± 1.2%), and plasma total homocysteine was elevated similar to findings previously reported in subjects without renal failure (56).

TREATMENT OF HYPERHOMOCYSTEINEMIA IN RENAL FAILURE

As in patients without renal failure, folic acid remains the cornerstone of therapy for elevated homocysteine concentrations. The first studies were made by Wilcken et al (11, 23). In one study, the effect of a 5 mg daily oral dose of folic acid given for approximately 2 weeks on homocysteine levels in patients with chronic renal insufficiency was studied. Plasma homocysteine declined by 50% in proportion to the prefolate homocysteine level. Methionine concentrations were normal in the patients and did not change after folate administration. Plasma levels of serine fell about 25% and those of glycine rose by about 15%, however, suggesting enhanced activity of folate- and cobalamin-dependent remethylation. Folate levels were normal in the patients before treatment. A similar mechanism has been adduced from enhanced post-homocysteine loading methionine concentrations following administration of folic acid (38). These effects of folic acid have been confirmed in many other studies (9, 21, 24, 25).

Although patients without renal failure often respond to doses of folic acid as low as 0.2-1mg (57) those with renal failure often require much higher doses (9, 21, 24, 25). This apparent resistance to the effects of folic acid is characteristic of patients with renal failure. Indeed, even with short term (several week) courses of folic acid using as much as 5mg (58), 15 mg (26) or even 40 mg/day (unpublished observations), homocysteine values may stay well above normal in patients with end stage renal disease.

Factors which could influence the response to folic acid include the degree of renal dysfunction, the coexistence of other vitamin deficiencies or the presence of the thermolabile form of methylenetetrahydrofolate reductase. Furthermore, there are important differences in folate responsiveness which may be dependent on mode of dialysis. For example, in patients on hemodialysis, the folate/homocysteine dose response curve suggests that responsiveness to folate persists even at high circulating vitamin levels (Fig 1) although for patients on peritoneal dialysis there may be a relative lack of responsiveness to folate. The mechanisms for this difference between the groups is unclear but suggest a process which is saturated at the higher folate levels observed in peritoneal dialysis patients. In spite of this, Janssen et al (9) administered folic acid supplements to patients on peritoneal dialysis in whom folate levels were normal and demonstrated that homocysteine concentrations decreased substantially. Further work is needed in this area.

Neither pyridoxine, an essential requirement for normal transsulfuration, nor vitamin $B_{12}$ alone are effective in lowering homocysteine in these patients (11, 25). This may be because frank vitamin $B_{12}$ deficiency is rare or because increasing cofactor rather than cosubstrate concentrations might not be expected to lower homocysteine concentrations. Further study is required to evaluate the effects, if any, of vitamin $B_6$ in lowering homocysteine levels as low concentrations of pyridoxal 5'-phosphate are frequently seen in these patients. Wilcken et al (11) could not demonstrate an effect in their patients, but small numbers and patient selection may have obscured an effect. Arnadottir et al and Chauveau et al also used vitamin $B_6$ without effect on basal homocysteine concentrations (24, 25). In other studies, serine (6), betaine (59, 60) and N-acetylcysteine (61) did not lower homocysteine concentrations. Trials to assess the effects, if any, of folic acid supplementation on vascular outcomes in patients with renal failure are now being planned or carried out.

# REFERENCES

1. Hultberg B, Andersson A, Arnadottir M. Reduced, free and total fractions of homocysteine and other thiol compounds in plasma from patients with renal failure. Nephron 1995;70(1):62-7.
2. Robins AJ, Milewczyk BK, Booth EM, Mallick NP. Plasma amino acid abnormalities in chronic renal failure. Clinica Chimica Acta 1972;42(1):215-7.
3. Wilcken DE, Gupta VJ. Sulfur containing amino acids in chronic renal failure with particular reference to homocystine and cysteine-homocysteine mixed disulfide. European Journal of Clinical Investigation 1979;9(4):301-7.
4. Cohen BD, Patel H, Kornhauser RS. Alternate reasons for atherogenesis in uremia. Proceedings of the Clinical Dialysis & Transplant Forum 1977;7:178-80.
5. Chauveau P, Chadefaux B, Coude M, et al. Hyperhomocysteinemia, a risk factor for atherosclerosis in chronic uremic patients. Kidney International - Supplement 1993;41:S72-7.
6. Bostom AG, Shemin D, Lapane KL, et al. Hyperhomocysteinemia and traditional cardiovascular disease risk factors in end-stage renal disease patients on dialysis: a case-control study. Atherosclerosis 1995;114(1):93-103.
7. Robinson K, Gupta A, Dennis V, et al. Hyperhomocysteinemia confers an independent increased risk of atherosclerosis in end-stage renal disease and is closely linked to plasma folate and pyridoxine concentrations. Circulation 1996;94(11):2743-8.
8. Hultberg B, Andersson A, Sterner G. Plasma homocysteine in renal failure. Clinical Nephrology 1993;40(4):230-5.
9. Janssen MJ, van Guldener C, de Jong GM, van den Berg M, Stehouwer CD, Donker AJ. Folic acid treatment of hyperhomocysteinemia in dialysis patients. Mineral & Electrolyte Metabolism 1996;22(1-3):110-4.
10. Kim SS, Hirose S, Tamura H, et al. Hyperhomocysteinemia as a possible role for atherosclerosis in CAPD patients. Advances in Peritoneal Dialysis 1994;10:282-5.
11. Wilcken DE, Gupta VJ, Betts AK. Homocysteine in the plasma of renal transplant recipients: effects of cofactors for methionine metabolism. Clinical Science 1981;61(6):743-9.
12. Massy ZA, Chadefaux-Vekemans B, Chevalier A, et al. Hyperhomocysteinemia: a significant risk factor for cardiovascular disease in renal transplant recipients. Nephrology, Dialysis, Transplantation 1994;9(8):1103-8.
13. Arnadottir M, Hultberg B, Vladov V, Nilsson-Ehle P, Thysell H. Hyperhomocysteinemia in cyclosporine-treated renal transplant recipients. Transplantation 1996;61(3):509-12.
14. Bostom AG, Gohh RY, Tsai MY, et al. Excess prevalence of fasting and postmethionine-loading hyperhomocysteinemia in stable renal transplant recipients. Arteriosclerosis, Thrombosis & Vascular Biology 1997;17(10):1894-900.
15. Fogarty DG, Woodside J, Lightbody JH, al. e. Plasma homocysteine in renal transplant recipients. J Am Soc Nephrol 1996;7(9):3421A.
16. van Guldener C, Janssen MJ, Stehouwer CD, et al. The effect of renal transplantation on hyperhomocysteinemia in dialysis patients, and the estimation of renal homocysteine extraction in patients with normal renal function. Netherlands Journal of Medicine 1998;52(2):58-64.

17. Ambrosi P, Barlatier A, Habib G, et al. Hyperhomocysteinemia in heart transplant recipients. European Heart Journal 1994;15(9):1191-5.
18. Berger PB, Jones JD, Olson LJ, et al. Increase in total plasma homocysteine concentration after cardiac transplantation. Mayo Clinic Proceedings 1995;70(2):125-31.
19. Gupta A, Moustapha A, Jacobsen DW, et al. High homocysteine, low folate, and low vitamin $B_6$ concentrations: prevalent risk factors for vascular disease in heart transplant recipients. Transplantation 1998;65(4):544-50.
20. Fodinger M, Mannhalter C, Wolfl G, et al. Mutation (677 C to T) in the methylenetetrahydrofolate reductase gene aggravates hyperhomocysteinemia in hemodialysis patients. Kidney International 1997;52(2):517-23.
21. Bostom AG, Shemin D, Lapane KL, et al. Folate status is the major determinant of fasting total plasma homocysteine levels in maintenance dialysis patients. Atherosclerosis 1996;123(1-2):193-202.
22. Tamura T, Johnston KE, Bergman SM. Homocysteine and folate concentrations in blood from patients treated with hemodialysis. Journal of the American Society of Nephrology 1996;7(11):2414-8.
23. Wilcken DE, Dudman NP, Tyrrell PA, Robertson MR. Folic acid lowers elevated plasma homocysteine in chronic renal insufficiency: possible implications for prevention of vascular disease. Metabolism: Clinical & Experimental 1988;37(7):697-701.
24. Chauveau P, Chadefaux B, Coude M, Aupetit J, Kamoun P, Jungers P. Long-term folic acid (but not pyridoxine) supplementation lowers elevated plasma homocysteine level in chronic renal failure. Mineral & Electrolyte Metabolism 1996;22(1-3):106-9.
25. Arnadottir M, Brattstrom L, Simonsen O, et al. The effect of high-dose pyridoxine and folic acid supplementation on serum lipid and plasma homocysteine concentrations in dialysis patients. Clinical Nephrology 1993;40(4):236-40.
26. Bostom AG, Shemin D, Lapane KL, et al. High dose-B-vitamin treatment of hyperhomocysteinemia in dialysis patients. Kidney International 1996;49(1):147-52.
27. Ramirez G, Chen M, Boyce HW, Jr., et al. Longitudinal follow-up of chronic hemodialysis patients without vitamin supplementation. Kidney International 1986;30(1):99-106.
28. Jennette JC, Goldman ID. Inhibition of the membrane transport of folates by anions retained in uremia. Journal of Laboratory & Clinical Medicine 1975;86(5):834-43.
29. Halsted CH. The intestinal absorption of dietary folates in health and disease. Journal of the American College of Nutrition 1989;8(6):650-8.
30. Refsum H, Helland S, Ueland PM. Radioenzymic determination of homocysteine in plasma and urine. Clinical Chemistry 1985;31(4):624-8.
31. Bostom A, Brosnan JT, Hall B, Nadeau MR, Selhub J. Net uptake of plasma homocysteine by the rat kidney in vivo. Atherosclerosis 1995;116(1):59-62.
32. van Guldener C, Donker AJ, Jakobs C, Teerlink T, de Meer K, Stehouwer CD. No net renal extraction of homocysteine in fasting humans. Kidney International 1998;54(1):166-9.
33. Gaull GE, Von Berg W, Raiha NC, Sturman JA. Development of methyltransferase activities of human fetal tissues. Pediatric Research 1973;7(5):527-33.
34. McKeever MP, Weir DG, Molloy A, Scott JM. Betaine-homocysteine methyltransferase: organ distribution in man, pig and rat and subcellular distribution in the rat. Clinical Science 1991;81(4):551-6.

35. House JD, Brosnan ME, Brosnan JT. Characterization of homocysteine metabolism in the rat kidney. Biochemical Journal 1997;328(Pt 1):287-92.

36. Sturman JA, Rassin DK, Gaull GE. Distribution of transulfuration enzymes in various organs and species. Int J Biochem 1970;1:251-3.

37. Guttormsen AB, Mansoor AM, Fiskerstrand T, Ueland PM, Refsum H. Kinetics of plasma homocysteine in healthy subjects after peroral homocysteine loading. Clinical Chemistry 1993;39(7):1390-7.

38. Guttormsen AB, Ueland PM, Svarstad E, Refsum H. Kinetic basis of hyperhomocysteinemia in patients with chronic renal failure. Kidney International 1997;52(2):495-502.

39. Dobbelstein H, Korner WF, Mempel W, Grosse-Wilde H, Edel HH. Vitamin $B_6$ deficiency in uremia and its implications for the depression of immune responses. Kidney International 1974;5(3):233-9.

40. Wilcken DE, Gupta VJ, Reddy SG. Accumulation of sulfur-containing amino acids including cysteine-homocysteine in patients on maintenance haemodialysis. Clinical Science 1980;58(5):427-30.

41. Kang SS, Wong PW, Bidani A, Milanez S. Plasma protein-bound homocyst(e)ine in patients requiring chronic haemodialysis [letter]. Clinical Science 1983;65(3)(September):335-6.

42. Chauveau P, Chadefaux B, Coude M, et al. Increased plasma homocysteine concentration in patients with chronic renal failure. Mineral & Electrolyte Metabolism 1992;18(2-5):196-8.

43. Smolin LA, Laidlaw SA, Kopple JD. Altered plasma free and protein-bound sulfur amino acid levels in patients undergoing maintenance hemodialysis. American Journal of Clinical Nutrition 1987;45(4):737-43.

44. Jungers P, Massy ZA, Khoa TN, et al. Incidence and risk factors of atherosclerotic cardiovascular accidents in predialysis chronic renal failure patients: a prospective study. Nephrology, Dialysis, Transplantation 1997;12(12):2597-602.

45. Jungers P, Chauveau P, Bandin O, et al. Hyperhomocysteinemia is associated with atherosclerotic occlusive arterial accidents in predialysis chronic renal failure patients. Mineral & Electrolyte Metabolism 1997;23(3-6):170-3.

46. Bachmann J, Tepel M, Raidt H, et al. Hyperhomocysteinemia and the risk for vascular disease in hemodialysis patients. Journal of the American Society of Nephrology 1995;6(1):121-5.

47. Bostom AG, Shemin D, Verhoef P, et al. Elevated fasting total plasma homocysteine levels and cardiovascular disease outcomes in maintenance dialysis patients. A prospective study. Arteriosclerosis, Thrombosis & Vascular Biology 1997;17(11):2554-8.

48. Moustapha A, Naso A, Nahlawi M, et al. Prospective study of hyperhomocysteinemia as an adverse cardiovascular risk factor in end-stage renal disease [published erratum appears in Circulation 1998 Feb 24;97(7):711]. Circulation 1998;97(2):138-41.

49. Ambrosi P, Garcon D, Riberi A, et al. Association of mild hyperhomocysteinemia with cardiac graft vascular disease. Atherosclerosis 1998;138:347-350.

50. Nahlawi M, Naso A, Boparai N, et al. Low vitamin $B_6$: an independent predictor of cardiovascular morbidity and mortality in heart transplant recipients. Circulation 1998;98(Suppl I):690.

51. Dennis VW, Robinson K. Homocysteinemia and vascular disease in end-stage renal disease. Kidney International - Supplement 1996;57:S11-7.
52. Bostom AG, Lathrop L. Hyperhomocysteinemia in end-stage renal disease: prevalence, etiology, and potential relationship to arteriosclerotic outcomes. Kidney International 1997;52(1):10-20.
53. Mayer EL, Jacobsen DW, Robinson K. Homocysteine and coronary atherosclerosis. Journal of the American College of Cardiology 1996;27(3):517-27.
54. Ueland PM, Refsum H. Plasma homocysteine, a risk factor for vascular disease: plasma levels in health, disease, and drug therapy. Journal of Laboratory & Clinical Medicine 1989;114(5):473-501.
55. van Guldener C, Lambert J, Janssen MJ, Donker AJ, Stehouwer CD. Endothelium-dependent vasodilatation and distensibility of large arteries in chronic haemodialysis patients. Nephrology, Dialysis, Transplantation 1997;12(Suppl 2):14-8.
56. Tawakol A, Omland T, Gerhard M, Wu JT, Creager MA. Hyperhomocyst(e)inemia is associated with impaired endothelium-dependent vasodilation in humans. Circulation 1997;95(5):1119-21.
57. Anonymous. Lowering blood homocysteine with folic acid based supplements: meta-analysis of randomized trials. Homocysteine Lowering Trialists' Collaboration. BMJ 1998;316(7135):894-8.
58. van Guldener C, Janssen MJ, Lambert J, ter Wee PM, Donker AJ, Stehouwer CD. Folic acid treatment of hyperhomocysteinemia in peritoneal dialysis patients: no change in endothelial function after long-term therapy. Peritoneal Dialysis International 1998;18(3):282-9.
59. Bostom AG, Shemin D, Nadeau MR, et al. Short term betaine therapy fails to lower elevated fasting total plasma homocysteine concentrations in hemodialysis patients maintained on chronic folic acid supplementation [letter]. Atherosclerosis 1995;113(1):129-32.
60. van Guldener C, Janssen MJ, Lambert J, et al. No change in impaired endothelial function after long-term folic acid therapy of hyperhomocysteinemia in haemodialysis patients. Nephrology, Dialysis, Transplantation 1998;13(1):106-12.
61. Bostom AG, Shemin D, Yoburn D, Fisher DH, Nadeau MR, Selhub J. Lack of effect of oral N-acetylcysteine on the acute dialysis-related lowering of total plasma homocysteine in hemodialysis patients. Atherosclerosis 1996;120(1-2):241-4.

# 16. MOLECULAR BIOLOGY OF METHYLENETETRAHYDROFOLATE REDUCTASE (MTHFR): INTERRELATIONSHIPS WITH FOLIC ACID, HOMOCYSTEINE AND VASCULAR DISEASE

RIMA ROZEN

## SUMMARY

Methylenetetrahydrofolate reductase (MTHFR) is required for the synthesis of 5-methyltetrahydrofolate, a methyl donor for homocysteine remethylation to methionine. Severe deficiency of MTHFR is associated with the inborn error of metabolism, homocystinuria, whereas a milder deficiency of the enzyme is associated with mild to moderate hyperhomocysteinemia. The isolation of the cDNA and gene for human MTHFR has made it possible to study MTHFR deficiency at the molecular level. Eighteen rare MTHFR mutations have been identified in patients with homocystinuria. Five common variants in MTHFR have been reported, but only one, 677 C→T (an alanine to valine substitution), has been consistently demonstrated to influence homocysteine levels. Individuals with the homozygous mutant genotype can overcome the effect of the mutation by maintaining adequate folate levels. The frequency of the homozygous mutant genotype ranges from 11% - 15% of North Americans and 5% - 23% of Europeans. Several, but not all, studies have reported an increased risk of vascular disease for individuals with the homozygous mutant genotype. The influence of the genotype on disease risk is dependent on nutritional status (folate level), as well as on the number of other more traditional risk factors present in the study group, supporting the multifactorial nature of cardiovascular disease.

*K. Robinson (ed.), Homocysteine and Vascular Disease, 271-289.*
© 2000 *Kluwer Academic Publishers. Printed in the Netherlands.*

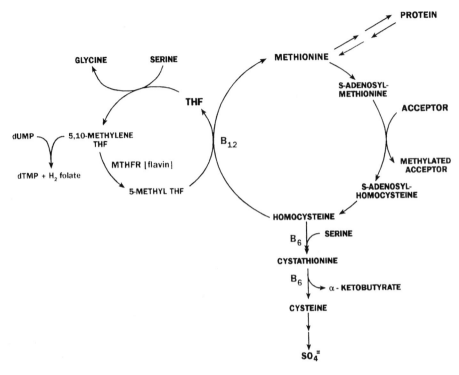

*Figure 1. MTHFR in metabolism of homocysteine and methionine. The vitamins involved in homocysteine metabolism are indicated where appropriate. 5-Methyltetrahydrofolate is a substrate for methionine synthase. The other 3 vitamins indicated in the figure – flavin, $B_{12}$, $B_6$ (or their derivatives) – are cofactors for MTHFR, methionine synthase and cystathionine synthase/cystathionase, respectively.*

## INTRODUCTION

Homocysteine can be metabolized through two major pathways: 1) remethylation to methionine or 2) transsulfuration to cysteine with ultimate degradation to inorganic sulfate. Genetic defects in the enzymes that metabolize homocysteine can contribute to mild, moderate or severe hyperhomocysteinemia, depending on the nature of the gene product and the level of residual enzyme activity. Several enzymatic defects can give rise to severe hyperhomocysteinemia and homocystinuria, an inborn error of metabolism with a wide variety of clinical features including thrombosis. These defects include mutations in the genes encoding cystathionine synthase, methylenetetrahydrofolate reductase, and methionine synthase. These types of mutations are relatively rare and do not significantly contribute to the mild or moderate hyperhomocysteinemia that is associated with vascular disease in the general population. However, methylenetetrahydrofolate reductase (MTHFR) is an interesting example of a gene involved in both types of disorders: homocystinuria and mild hyperhomocysteinemia. Multiple, but rare, mutations in MTHFR are associated with homocystinuria while a single, but common, variant is associated with mild hyperhomocysteinemia.

Since vascular disease with mild hyperhomocysteinemia is a multifactorial disorder, with genetic and environmental components, the contribution of a single genetic factor, such as a mutation in MTHFR, may be highly dependent on nutritional factors or on other genetic determinants, to manifest the clinical phenotype. This chapter will cover the biochemical and molecular genetic aspects of MTHFR, with an emphasis on the common variant as a component of vascular disease.

## MTHFR STRUCTURE AND FUNCTION

MTHFR (EC.1.5.1.20) catalyzes the NAD(P)H-dependent reduction of 5,10-methylenetetrahydrofolate to 5-methyltetrahydrofolate, a methyl donor for homocysteine remethylation to methionine [1]. The folate-dependent remethylation reaction, a component of the methionine cycle, is catalyzed by methionine synthase which utilizes methylcobalamin ($B_{12}$) as a cofactor (Figure 1). Methionine is converted to S-adenosylmethionine (SAM), which can donate its methyl group in over 100 biologic reactions, to yield S-adenosylhomocysteine (SAH) and the appropriate methylated acceptors. SAH can then be hydrolyzed to reform homocysteine. The second pathway for homocysteine metabolism, the transsulfuration pathway [2], is utilized for synthesis of cysteine (and other sulfur compounds including glutathione and taurine) as well as for the final degradation of the sulfur atom to inorganic sulfate. The first two enzymes in the transsulfuration pathway, cystathionine synthase and cystathionase, are pyridoxal phosphate ($B_6$)-dependent proteins. The outflow of homocysteine through these 2 major pathways is controlled by SAM, which is an allosteric inhibitor of MTHFR and an activator of cystathionine synthase. When dietary protein intake is high and methionine/SAM are readily available, the remethylation of homocysteine to methionine will be decreased, because of the inhibition of MTHFR by SAM, while homocysteine degradation through the transsulfuration pathway will be stimulated through the SAM-dependent activation of cystathionine synthase.

MTHFR is a homodimer of 77 kDa subunits with one equivalent of non-covalently bound FAD per subunit. The 77 kDa monomer can be cleaved by trypsin into 2 domains: a 40 kDa N-terminal catalytic domain and a 37 kDa C-terminal regulatory domain which contains the binding site for SAM [4]. Western blotting has demonstrated that the major subunit in most human tissues is also 77 kDa but a second isozyme of approximately 70 kDa was also observed in some tissues, including human fetal liver and porcine liver [5].

The deduced amino acid sequence of human MTHFR, based on the cDNA sequence (see below), has revealed strong homologies to the amino acid sequence of 10 porcine peptides localized to both the catalytic and regulatory domains, suggesting conservation of domains for the human enzyme [6]. MTHFRs in yeast and in the roundworm *C. elegans* are also believed to contain the C-terminal regulatory domain, based on sequence similarity to the human enzyme [7]. Yeast has 2 isozymes of MTHFR (proteins of 657 and 599 amino acids) which have approximately 35% identity to the human enzyme [8]. In contrast to the aforementioned species, bacterial MTHFRs do not contain the C-terminal regulatory domain. The enzyme from *E. coli* is a tetramer of 33 kDa subunits, which has approximately 30% identity to the human enzyme in the catalytic domain only. The purified *E. coli* enzyme is also a flavoprotein, but the enzyme-bound flavin is reduced more readily by NADH, unlike the mammalian enzymes which utilize NADPH [7].

## MTHFR CDNA AND GENE

A cDNA for human MTHFR was first isolated by PCR-based methods, using degenerate oligonucleotides that were synthesized on the basis of the amino acid sequence of a large porcine peptide [6]. The available cDNA sequence of 2.2 kb [5] contains coding information for a protein of 656 amino acids (GenBank accession number U09806). The cDNA has been expressed in bacterial extracts to generate a catalytically-active enzyme which migrates to the same position on gel electrophoresis as the smaller human isozyme (approximately 70 kDa) [5]. The missing coding sequences (approximately 7 kDa) required to encode the larger human isozyme of 77 kDa are presumed to be at the 5'end of the protein since sequences homologous to the N-terminal peptide of the porcine liver enzyme have not yet been identified in human MTHFR. The deduced amino acid sequence of the human cDNA has demonstrated homologies to MTHFR in many species, as mentioned above. Inspection of the human sequence has also revealed a stretch of hydrophilic amino acids that has been predicted to be the site of proteolytic cleavage into the 2 domains. The predicted site of SAM binding is at one end (N-terminal) of the 37 kDa regulatory domain [6].

Two mRNAs for human MTHFR (approximately 7.5 and 8.5 kb) have been seen in many human tissues on Northern blots, indicating very large untranslated regions. A complicated pattern of alternative splicing into exon 1 has also been observed. The long untranslated regions and the alternative splicing events suggest that regulation of MTHFR may be quite complex [9].

The genomic structure for human MTHFR has been reported [10]. The cDNA sequence of 2.2 kb is contained in a single genomic clone of approximately 17 kb, with 11 exons ranging in size from approximately 100 bp – 400 bp. The mouse cDNA and gene structure is very similar to that of the human counterpart, with 90% identity in the coding sequences.

Human MTHFR has been mapped by in situ hybridization to chromosomal region 1p36.3 [6] while mouse MTHFR has been mapped to the homologous region of the mouse genome, distal Chromosome 4 [11].


## MTHFR AND HOMOCYSTINURIA

Homocystinuria is an inborn error of metabolism caused by disruption of the remethylation or transsulfuration pathways of homocysteine metabolism. An important biochemical distinction between homocystinuria due to remethylation defects and homocystinuria due to transsulfuration defects is that the latter is associated with high levels of both homocysteine and methionine, while the former has normal or low plasma methionine levels [1,2].

In the remethylation pathway, severe deficiency of MTHFR is the most common genetic cause of homocystinuria. Nonetheless, this type of MTHFR deficiency is relatively rare, with approximately 50 cases reported worldwide. Patients present in infancy or adolescence with a wide variety of neurological and vascular complications, including developmental delay, motor and gait abnormalities, seizures, hypotonia, thrombosis and psychiatric manifestations. Enzyme activity is usually less than 15% of control levels, resulting in a dramatic elevation of homocysteine in plasma and urine due to the decreased levels of 5-methyltetrahydrofolate, the product of the MTHFR reaction [1].

Eighteen different mutations have been identified in homocystinuric patients with severe MTHFR deficiency (Table 1) [6,12,13,14]. Each of these mutations has been seen in only 1 or 2 families of various ethnic backgrounds. The mutations are therefore deemed to be non-polymorphic since they have been observed only in these rare patients and not in panels of control individuals.

*Table 1. Non-polymorphic mutations in methylenetetrahydrofolate reductase (MTHFR)*

| Mutation | Change in amino acid or splice site | Exon or intron | Reference |
|----------|-------------------------------------|----------------|-----------|
| 164 G→C | R→P | exon 1 | 13 |
| 167 G→A | R→Q | exon 1 | 12 |
| 249-1 G→T | 3'splice site | intron 1 | 13 |
| 458 GC → TT | G→V | exon 2 | 13 |
| 482 G→A | R→Q | exon 2 | 6 |
| 559 C→T | R→X | exon 3 | 6 |
| 692 C→T | T→M | exon 4 | 12 |
| 764 C→T | P→L | exon 4 | 12 |
| 792+1 G→A | 5'splice site | intron 4 | 12 |
| 980 T→C | L→P | exon 5 | 13 |
| 983 A→G | N→S | exon 5 | 14 |
| 985 C→T | R→C | exon 5 | 12 |
| 1015 C→T | R→C | exon 5 | 12 |
| 1027 T→G | W→G | exon 5 | 14 |
| 1081 C→T | R→C | exon 6 | 12 |
| 1084 C→T | R→X | exon 6 | 14 |
| 1141 C→T | R→C | exon 6 | 13 |
| 1711 C→T | R→X | exon 10 | 14 |

Sequence numbering is based on the cDNA sequence reported in Goyette et al (6), GenBank accession number U09806. Exon designations are based on Goyette et al (10).

Most of these substitutions (13/18) are missense mutations with 3 nonsense mutations and 2 splice site mutations. The mutations are assumed to be deleterious but expression studies are required to confirm their effect on enzyme function. Some of the mutations occur in residues in the catalytic domain that are conserved in the *E. coli* enzyme; consequently site-directed mutagenesis of the bacterial and human MTHFR sequences, with expression of the mutagenized constructs, can be performed in parallel. These types of studies are in progress [7,15].

Although all patients with homocystinuria and severe MTHFR deficiency have elevated plasma homocysteine, vascular symptoms have not been reported in all patients. Some of the children die in the first few years of life due to their neurological complications or are too young at diagnosis to have developed clinically significant manifestations of vascular disease. It is also possible that other genetic factors, such as Factor V Leiden, may contribute to the risk of thrombosis in these patients. In a study of 4 patients with severe MTHFR deficiency, Mandel et al. suggested that only the patients with the Factor V Leiden mutation had developed thromboses [16]. In our series of 32 patients, 3 patients and 2 obligate heterozygous parents were carriers or homozygotes of this Factor V mutation [17]. Two of the 3 patients and both parents had evidence of thrombosis while the third patient was still quite young.

## MTHFR POLYMORPHISMS

In a study of coronary artery disease patients in North America, Kang et al reported that 17% of these patients (compared to 5% of controls) carried a distinct MTHFR variant, which had reduced specific activity at 37°C and increased thermolability after heating lymphocyte extracts for 5 minutes at 46° C [18]. Similar findings were later reported in a study of Dutch patients with cardiovascular disease [19].

Frosst et al identified a sequence change in MTHFR, 677 C→T, which converted an alanine to a valine codon [5]. This mutation can be easily detected by PCR and restriction digestion since the mutation creates a HinfI and a TaqI restriction enzyme recognition sequence, although several other diagnostic methods have been reported. Because this change was frequently observed in control individuals [5], as well as in patients with homocystinuria [13], this mutant sequence was suspected of encoding the thermolabile MTHFR variant. Confirmation was achieved after site-directed mutagenesis and expression of the wild-type and mutagenized constructs in bacterial extracts; the recombinant enzyme with the valine substitution was clearly more thermolabile than the recombinant enzyme with the alanine codon [5]. Similar results have been observed with the two forms of the enzyme in *E.coli* [7].

The 677 C→T variant is extremely common in North America, with allele frequencies of approximately 0.35 and homozygosity frequencies of 11% - 15% (Table 2). European frequencies of this variant are population-dependent with an increasing gradient of the mutation from Northern to Southern Europe. The highest frequencies of this mutation reported thus far have been in the Mediterranean countries and in Hispanic Americans.

*Table 2. Frequency of MTHFR 677C→T variant in control populations*

|  | % (V/V) | Reference |
|---|---|---|
| **North America** | | |
| Canada and U.S. | 11%–15% | 5,20,21,22 |
| Hispanic Americans | 25% | 23 |
| African Americans | 0–1% | 24,25 |
| **South America** | | |
| Brazil | 4% | 26 |
| **Europe** | | |
| Finland | 5% | 24 |
| Norway | 10% | 27 |
| U.K | 13% | 28 |
| Ireland | 8% | 29 |
| France | 10% | 30 |
| Netherlands | 8% | 31 |
| Austria | 10% | 32 |
| Russia | 8% | 33 |
| Italy | 15%-23% | 34,35,36 |
| **Asia** | | |
| Japan | 10% -12% | 37,38 |
| **Australia** | 11% | 39 |

The mutant homozygous genotype (V/V) is consistently associated with reduced specific activity and increased thermolability in lymphocyte extracts, in control individuals, as well as in individuals with cardiovascular disease [5,40,41]. The specific activity at 37°C in homozygous mutant individuals is usually 25% - 35% of control values, while heterozygotes have values that are intermediate between controls and homozygous mutants. The residual activities after heating at 46°C are approximately 30% of control values in homozygous mutant individuals while heterozygotes have intermediate values.

The correlation between the homozygous V/V genotype and enzyme activity and thermolability have been very good, suggesting that other MTHFR polymorphisms, if present in the general population, are not likely to have dramatic effects on enzyme activity. This hypothesis has held up thus far. Although other MTHFR polymorphisms have been identified (Table 3), either their effects on enzyme activity have not been demonstrated or the effect is

*Table 3. Polymorphic mutations in methylenetetrahydrofolate reductase (MTHFR)*

| Mutation | Change in amino acid | Exon or intron | Reference |
|---|---|---|---|
| 677 C/T | A/V | exon 4 | 5 |
| 1068 T/C | S/S | exon 6 | 12 |
| 1178 + 31 T/C | 5'splice site | intron 6 | 13 |
| 1298 A/C | E/A | exon 7 | 42,43,44 |
| 1317 T/C | F/F | exon 7 | 44 |

Sequence numbering is based on the cDNA sequence reported in Goyette et al (6), GenBank accession number U09806. Exon designations are based on Goyette et al (10).

clearly less than that of the 677 C→T polymorphism. Only one other common MTHFR variant has been reported to affect activity, the 1298 A→ C substitution, which converts a glutamate to an alanine codon [42,43,44]. The frequency of this variant is similar to that of the 677 C→T variant, but the specific activity at 37°C of individuals who are homozygous for the 1298 A→C variant is approximately 60% of control levels; thermolability has not been observed for this variant. The levels of specific activity for 1298 A→C homozygotes are clearly higher than those observed for homozygotes of the 677 C→T polymorphism and are within the ranges seen for 677 C→T heterozygotes. Interestingly, homozygotes for both polymorphisms have not been observed and the 2 mutations have not been seen on a single haplotype except for 1 individual [43,44]. This finding suggests that the two mutations occurred independently on a 677C/1298A (alanine/glutamate) haplotype and recombination is rare.


## MTHFR 677 C→T POLYMORPHISM – EFFECTS ON FOLATE AND HOMOCYSTEINE

Since MTHFR is required to synthesize 5-methyltetrahydrofolate, the primary folate in plasma, deficient MTHFR activity might be expected to lower plasma folate levels. Decreased plasma folate in individuals with the homozygous mutant genotype for the 677 C→T polymorphism has been demonstrated in several studies [22,40,45]. As a consequence of the decreased methylfolate levels, homocysteine levels are increased in homozygous mutant individuals.

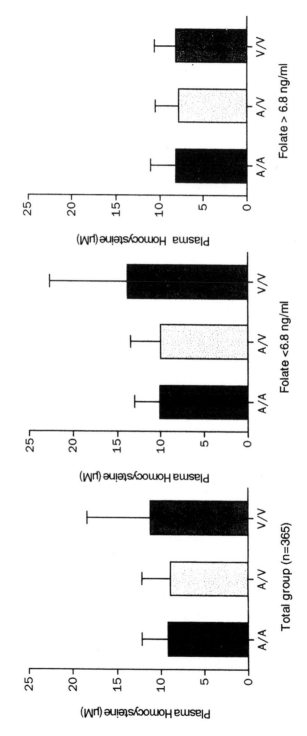

280    *Rima Rozen*

Figure 2. Plasma homocysteine levels and MTHFR genotypes in 365 individuals from the NHLBI Family Heart Study (data obtained from Jacques et al. [20]). The left panel illustrates the values of the entire group, while the middle and right panels illustrate the results in individuals with folates below and above the median value, respectively.

Homocysteine levels are not elevated in individuals who are homozygous for the 1298 A→C mutation since enzyme activity is only slightly compromized by the mutation [43,44]. One report suggests that homocysteine levels may be somewhat elevated in individuals who are heterozygous for both the 677 C→T and the 1298 A→C mutations, but the clinical significance is likely to be limited with such a small increase [43].

Although there is general agreement about the effect of the 677 C→T mutation on plasma folate, the effect on red blood cell (RBC) folate is not as clear. Some studies have demonstrated increased RBC folates in mutant individuals [40] and have attributed this finding to the increased levels of 5,10-methylenetetrahydrofolate, which is a better substrate for polyglutamylation; folate polyglutamates are the preferred intracellular storage forms of folate. One group has reported decreased RBC folates in homozygous mutant individuals [46]. The different methodologies used in the measurement of folates may have contributed to the discrepancies in the literature.

The 677 C→T polymorphism has been shown to be associated with mild to moderate hyperhomocysteinemia in numerous studies. Manifestation of hyperhomocysteinemia is largely dependent on plasma folate, as first shown in Jacques et al. [20] and illustrated in Figure 2. In this study of 365 individuals, the mutant genotype was associated with hyperhomocysteinemia when the entire group of control individuals was examined. When the group was divided by the median folate value, hyperhomocysteinemia was not observed in homozygous mutant individuals when their plasma folate was above the median value. The mutant genotype was associated with elevated homocysteine only in the individuals with the lower folate status. It is important to note that these folate values are not considered to be in the deficient range, but, rather, in the lower end of the normal range. Studies have shown that the negative correlation between homocysteine and folate is greatest in individuals who are homozygous mutant, suggesting that they are particularly sensitive to folate levels [27,47], compared to individuals without the mutation.

The risk for hyperhomocysteinemia conferred by the mutant genotype has been examined in several studies. In a population of Norwegian individuals selected for high homocysteine levels (greater than 40 μM), the odds ratios (O.R.) for the mutant genotype, compared to the wild-type genotype, were 10.1 for individuals with folate ≥ 3.7 nmol/l and 175 for individuals with folate < 3.7 nmol/l [27]. Heterozygotes with low folate also had a highly significant O.R. (55.1). In an unselected population of males from Northern Ireland, the risks conferred by the mutant genotype (O.R.) were 9.7, 5.7, 2.6 and 1.7 for being in the top 5, 10, 20 and 50% of individuals, respectively, ranked by homocysteine levels (Table 4) [45].

Table 4 Mild hyperhomocysteinemia in a working male population in Belfast (n=625). tHcy = total plasma homocysteine

**4a.** Homocysteine and folate levels stratified by MTHFR genotype

|  | A/A | A/V | V/V |
|---|---|---|---|
| Mean tHcy (μM) | 6.8 | 7.1 | 9.5* |
| Mean tHcy in men with folate < median | 7.4 | 7.9 | 11.2* |
| Mean tHcy in men with folate > median | 6.3 | 6.5 | 6.8 |
| Serum folate (nM) | 12.3 | 10.8 | 9.3** |

* $p<0.003$ between V/V genotype and the other two genotypes

** all 3 genotypes are significantly different from each other ($p<0.001$).

**4b.** Relative risk of mild hyperhomocysteinemia conferred by MTHFR genotype

| tHcy Rank | V/V relative to A/A |
|---|---|
| top 5% | 9.7 (3.9-24.2) |
| top 10% | 5.7 (3.1-10.4) |
| top 20% | 2.6 (1.8-3.9) |
| top 50% | 1.7 (1.4-2.1) |

Data obtained from Harmon et al. (45)

The influence of folate status on the impact of the mutation could be explained by folate-dependent stabilization of the enzyme. Regardless of the mechanism, however, this genetic-nutrient interactive effect suggests that folate supplementation should overcome the effect of the mutation and prevent hyperhomocysteinemia in mutant individuals. The folate responsiveness of mutant individuals, with respect to homocysteine lowering, has been demonstrated [27,48].

## MTHFR 677 C→T POLYMORPHISM AND CARDIOVASCULAR DISEASE

Since hyperhomocysteinemia increases the risk for cardiovascular disease, many studies have examined the MTHFR 677 C→T polymorphism as a genetic risk factor for cardiovascular disease. It is not the intention of this chapter to review the published literature on this topic, but rather to illustrate some salient points after discussing a few relevant publications.

Homozygosity for the MTHFR variant has been positively correlated with risk for several different types of cardiovascular disease. Some of the studies with large numbers of participants included a report of 362 Japanese males with coronary artery disease and 778 male controls; a significant increase in frequency of the homozygous mutant genotype in patients, compared to controls, was observed. The association with the mutant genotype was further increased in patients with > or = 99% stenosis and in those with triple-vessel disease compared to single- or double-vessel disease [38]. The mutant allele, in one or two copies, has been associated with increased risk of cerebral infarction in a different Japanese study of 256 stroke patients and 325 controls [49]. The risk of venous thrombosis in an Italian study of 277 patients and 431 controls was significantly increased for carriers and homozygous mutant individuals [35]. A study of venous thrombosis in Brazil (127 patients and 296 controls) also reported a positive association between the genotype and risk of thrombosis [26].

In contrast, several studies have not found the MTHFR genotype to be a significant factor in cardiovascular disease risk. A study of American physicians (293 cases of myocardial infarction and 290 controls) did not find a significant increase in frequency of the genotype in cases compared to controls [22]. Similar conclusions were obtained in a Dutch study of coronary artery disease (735 patients and 1250 population-based controls) [50], in a British study of cerebrovascular disease (345 cases and 161 controls) [28], and in a Dutch study of venous thrombosis (471 patients and 474 controls) [51].

The issue of appropriate controls is relevant for all studies of vascular disease, but there are several unique properties of the MTHFR polymorphism that require consideration. The variant is so common in the general population that large numbers of patients and careful selection of controls are required to adequately address the issue of risk. In addition, since the genotype is dependent on folate status for manifestation of hyperhomocysteinemia, the nutritional status of the study group is an important consideration. Most of the aforementioned studies did not assess folate status in conjunction with the genotype in the assessment of risk. Despite the different results in various reports, a meta-analysis of 8 studies concluded that the MTHFR polymorphism was a modest but significant risk factor for cardiovascular disease, but, again, this analysis did not examine folate status [50].

Other influences that have affected outcome include the selection criteria for patients. When patients with other conventional risk factors (such as hyperlipoproteinemia and hypertension) are excluded, the risk for the MTHFR genotype can become significant [26,52]. Finally, since cardiovascular disease is a multifactorial disorder, the influence of any one genetic determinant may be small, but in combination with other genetic or nongenetic predisposing factors, it could have a greater impact. For example, the Factor V Leiden mutation in combination with the MTHFR genotype may be a greater risk factor for thrombosis than MTHFR alone [35,36]. Similarly, the MTHFR genotype has been associated with increased risk of myocardial infarction in non-insulin dependent diabetics [53]. In a study of children with familial hypercholesterolemia, the MTHFR mutant genotype was found more frequently in the group with parental history of cardiovascular disease [54]. In summary, the complex interplay between multiple genetic determinants and nutritional status may result in different outcomes in ethnically-distinct populations.

## MTHFR 677 C→T POLYMORPHISM AND OTHER DISORDERS

The MTHFR 677 C→T polymorphism is also a genetic risk factor for neural tube defects, as first suggested in 1995 [40,55], and recently confirmed in a meta-analysis [31]. It has been known for some time that these birth defects are multifactorial disorders which are folate-responsive in 60% - 70% of cases. The identification of a genetic risk factor in homocysteine/folate metabolism, which is dependent on folate status, is consistent with the multifactorial basis of neural tube defects and with the earlier observations of mild hyperhomocysteinemia in the mothers of children with spina bifida [56,57].

This polymorphism has also been proposed as a risk factor for several other complex traits; some of these traits are associated with vasculopathies. However, since the association has been reported in only 1 or 2 studies, these reports require confirmation. These disorders include pre-eclampsia [58], recurrent early pregnancy loss [59], schizophrenia [60], retinal vein occlusion [61], varicose veins [33], and diabetic retinopathy [62].

The high prevalence of a common mutation in many populations around the world can be indicative of a selective advantage, as proposed for mutations in the hemoglobin genes and selective advantage for heterozygotes against malaria [63]. The only disorder in which the MTHFR polymorphism has been shown to be protective, thus far, is colon cancer. Two studies have demonstrated a 2-fold reduction in risk for colon cancer for individuals who are homozygous mutant [64]. However, when the study group was stratified by folate levels and alcohol intake, the protective effect was seen only in mutant individuals who were folate-sufficient or who had low alcohol intake. The proposed mechanisms include decreased DNA methylation and increased conversion of dUMP to thymidine. Although colon cancer is a late-onset disorder and is therefore unlikely to affect reproductive fitness, the enhanced thymidine and DNA synthesis may offer a selective advantage in other circumstances, such as fetal development. One recent report has suggest heterozygote advantage of the MTHFR mutation in families with neural tube defects [65].

## CONCLUSIONS

The MTHFR 677 C→T variant is the first common genetic determinant of mild hyperhomocysteinemia. Homozygous mutant individuals are found in 11% - 15% of North Americans and in 5%-23% of Europeans. Since hyperhomocysteinemia is not observed when these mutant individuals are folate replete, folate supplementation is an effective means of regulating plasma homocysteine in this group and, presumably, in lowering their risk of cardiovascular disease. The identification of genetically-predisposed individuals at a younger age, before onset of disease, offers a strategy for prevention of hyperhomocysteinemia in a large segment of the population.

The cardiovascular disease risk attributable to this polymorphism will depend on the genetic background and the nutritional status of the population. Since the nutritional determinants of mild hyperhomocysteinemia are relatively well-established compared to the genetic determinants, further work is required to identify other genetic variants in the pathways regulating homocysteine and folate metabolism. Equally important is an understanding of how other common risk factors for cardiovascular disease (hyperlipoproteinemia, mutations in the coagulation cascade, etc.) might interact with the MTHFR polymorphism to increase disease risk.

## REFERENCES

1.  Rosenblatt DS. Inherited disorders of folate transport and metabolism. In : Scriver CR, Beaudet AL, Sly WS, Valle D, editors. The metabolic and molecular bases of inherited disease , 7th edition, New York : McGraw-Hill, 1995 : 3111-3128.
2.  Mudd SH, Levy HL, Skovby B. Disorders of transsulfuration. In : Scriver CR, Beaudet AL, Sly WS, Valle D, editors. The metabolic and molecular bases of inherited disease, 7th edition., New York :McGraw Hill, 1995 :1279-1327.

3.  Daubner SC, Matthews, R.G. Purification and properties of methylenetetrahydrofolate reductase from pig liver. J Biol Chem 1982;57 :140-145.

4.  Matthews RG, Vanoni MA, Hainfeld JF, Wall J. Methylenetetrahydrofolate reductase. Evidence for spatially distinct subunit domains obtained by scanning transmission electron microscopy and limited proteolysis. J Biol Chem 1984;259 :11647-11640.

5.  Frosst P, Blom HJ, Milos R et al. A candidate genetic risk factor for vascular disease: a common mutation in methylenetetrahydrofolate reductase. Nature Genet 1995;10:111-113.

6.  Goyette P, Sumner JS, Milos R et al. Human methylenetetrahydrofolate reductase: isolation of cDNA, mapping and mutation identification. Nature Genet 1994;7:195-200.

7.  Matthews RG, Sheppard C, Goulding C. Methylenetetrahydrofolate reductase and methionine synthase : biochemistry and molecular biology. Eur J Pediatr 1998;157 :S54-S59.

8.  D. Appling, personal communication.

9.  Goyette P, Chan M, Tran P and Rozen R, unpublished data.

10. Goyette P, Pai A, Milos R, et al. Gene structure of human and mouse methylenetetrahydrofolate reductase (MTHFR). Mamm Genome 1998;9:652-656.

11. Frosst P, Zhang Z-X, Pai A, Rozen R. The methylenetetrahydrofolate reductase (MTHFR) gene maps to distal mouse chromosome 4. Mamm Genome 1996;7:864-865.

12. Goyette P, Frosst P, Rosenblatt DS, Rozen R. Seven novel mutations in the methylenetetrahydrofolate reductase gene and genotype/phenotype correlations in severe MTHFR deficiency. Am J Hum Genet 1995;56:1052-1059.

13. Goyette P, Christensen B, Rosenblatt DS, Rozen R. Severe and mild mutations in cis for the methylenetetrahydrofolate reductase (MTHFR) gene, and description of 5 novel mutations in MTHFR. Am J Hum Genet 1996;59:1268-1275.

14. Kluijtmans LAJ, Wendel U, Stevens EMB, van den Heuvel LPWJ, Trijbels FJM, Blom H. Identification of four novel mutations in severe methylenetetrahydrofolate reductase deficiency. Eur J Hum Genet 1998;6 :257-265.

15. Goyette P. Molecular characterization of methylenetetrahydrofolate reductase deficiency [dissertation]. Montreal (Que) : McGill University, 1997.

16. Mandel, H, Brenner B, Berant M et al. Coexistence of hereditary homocystinuria and factor V Leiden – effect on thrombosis. N Engl J Med 1996;334 :763-768.

17. Goyette P, Rosenblatt D, Rozen R. Homocystinuria (Methylenetetrahydrofolate Reductase Deficiency) and mutation of factor V gene. J Inher Metab Dis 21;1998:690-691.

18. Kang S-S, Wong PWK, Susmano A, Sora J, Norusis M, Ruggie N. Thermolabile methylenetetrahydrofolate reductase: an inherited risk factor for coronary disease. Am J Hum Genet 1991; 48:536-545.

19. Engbersen AMT, Franken DG, Boers GHJ, Stevens EMB, Trijbels FJM, Blom HJ. Thermolabile 5,10-methylenetetrahydrofolate reductase as a cause of mild hyperhomocysteinemia. Am J Hum Genet 1995;56:142-150.

20. Jacques PF, Bostom AG, Williams RR et al. Relation between folate status, a common mutation in methylenetetrahydrofolate reductase, and plasma homocysteine concentrations. Circulation 1996;93:7-9.

21. Chen J, Giovannucci E, Kelsey K et al. A methylenetetrahydrofolate reductase polymorphism and the risk of colorectal cancer. Cancer Res 1996; 56:4862-4864.

22. Ma J, Stampfer MJ, Hennekens CH et al. Methylenetetrahydrofolate reductase polymorphism, plasma folate, homocysteine, and risk of myocardial infarction in U.S. physicians. Circulation 1996;94:2410-2416.

23. Shaw GM, Rozen R, Finnell RH, Wasserman CR, Lammer EJ. Maternal vitamin use, genetic variation of infant methylenetetrahydrofolate reductase and risk for spina bifida. Amer J Epidem 1998; 148:30-37.

24. Motulsky AG. Nutritional Ecogenetics: Homocysteine-related arteriosclerotic vascular disease, neural tube efects, and folic acid. Am J Hum Genet 1996;58:17-20.

25. Stevenson RE, Schwartz CE, Du YZ, Adams MJ. Differences in methylenetetrahydrofolate reductase genotype frequencies, between whites and blacks. Am J Hum Genet 1997;60 :230-233.

26. Arruda VR, von Zuben PM, Chiaparini LC, Annichino-Bizzacchi JM, Costa FF. The mutation Ala677→Val in the methylenetetrahydrofolate reductase gene : A risk factor for arterial disease and venous thrombosis. Thromb Haemost 1997;77 :818-821.

27. Guttormsen AB, Ueland PM, Nesthus I et al. Determinants and vitamin responsiveness of intermediate hyperhomocysteinemia ($\geq$ 40 μmol/liter) J Clin Invest 1996;98 :2174-2183.

28. Markus HS, Ali N, Swaminathan R, Sankaralingam A, Molloy J, Powell J. A common polymorphism in the methylenetetrahydrofolate reductase gene, homocysteine, and ischemic cerebrovascular disease. Stroke 1997:28:1739-1743.

29. Kirke PN, Mills JL, Whitehead AS, Molloy A, Scott JM. Methylenetetrahydrofolate reductase mutation and neural tube defects. Lancet 1996;348:1037-1038.

30. Mornet E, Muller F, Lenvoisé-Furet A et al. Screening of the C677T mutation in the methylenetetrahydrofolate reductase gene in French patients with neural tube defects. Human Genet 1997;100 :512-514.

31. van der Put NMJ, Eskes TKAB, Blom HJ. Is the common 677C→T mutation in the methylenetetrahydrofolate reductase gene a risk factor for neural tube defects? A meta-analysis. Q J Med 1997;90 :111-115.

32. Födinger M, Mannhalter C, Wölfli G et al. Mutation (677 C to T) in the methylenetetrahydrofolate reductase gene aggravates hyperhomocysteinemia in hemodialysis patients. Kidney International 1997;52 :517-523.

33. Sverdlova AM, Bubnova NA, Baranovskaya SS. Vasina VI, Avitisjan AO, Schwartz EI. Prevalence of the methylenetetrahydrofolate reductase (MTHFR) C677T mutation in patients with varicose veins of lower limbs. Molec Genet Metab 1998;63 :35-36.

34. de Franchis R, Mancini FP, D'Angelo A et al. Elevated total plasma homocysteine and 677C→T mutation of the 5,10-methylenetetrahydrofolate reductase gene in thrombotic vascular disease. Am J Hum Genet 1996;59 :262-264.

35. Margaglione M, D'Andrea G, d'Addedda M, et al. The methylenetetrahydrofolate reductase TT677 genotype is associated with venous thrombosis independently of the coexistence of the FV Leiden and the prothrombin A20210 mutation. Thromb Haemost 1998;79 :907-911.

36. Cattaneo M, Tsai MY, Bucciarelli P et al. A common mutation in the methylenetetrahydrofolate reductase gene (C677T) increases the risk for deep-vein thrombosis in patients with mutant factor V (factor V :Q506). Arterioscler Thromb Vasc Biol 1997;17 :1662-1666.

37. Izumi M, Iwai N, Ohmichi N, Nakamura Y, Shimoike H, Kinoshita M. Molecular variant of 5,10-methylenetetrahydrofolate reductase is a risk factor of ischemic heart disease in the Japanese population. Atherosclerosis 1996;121: 293-294.

38. Morita H, Taguchi J-I, Kurihara H, et al. Genetic polymorphism of 5,10-methylenetetrahydrofolate reductase (MTHFR) as a risk factor for coronary artery disease. Circulation 1997;95 :2032-2036.

39. Wilcken DEL, Wang XL, Sim AS, McCredie RM. Distribution in healthy and coronary populations of the methylenetetrahydrofolate reductase (MTHFR) $C_{677}$ T mutation. Arterioscler Thromb Vasc Biol 1996;16 :878-882.

40. van der Put NMJ, Steegers-Theunissen RPM, Frosst P.et al. Mutated methylenetetrahydrofolate reductase as a risk factor for spina bifida. Lancet 1995;346:1070-1071.

41. Christensen B, Frosst P, Lussier-Cacan S et al. Correlation of a common mutation in the methylenetetrahydrofolate reductase (MTHFR) gene with plasma homocysteine in patients with premature coronary artery disease. Arterioscler. Thromb. Vasc. Biol. 1997;17:569-573.

42. Viel A, Dall'Agnese L, Simone F et al. Loss of heterozygosity at the 5,10-methylenetetrahdyrofolate reductase locus in human ovarian carcinomas. Br J Cancer 1997; 75 :1105-1110.

43. van der Put NMY, Gabreels F, Stevens EMB, et al.. A second common mutation in the methylenetetrahydrofolate reductase gene : An additional risk factor for neural-tube defects? Am J Hum Genet 1998;62 :1044-1051.

44. Weisberg I, Tran P, Christensen B, Sibani S, Rozen R. A second genetic polymorphism in methylenetetrahydofolate reductase (MTHFR) associated with decreased enzyme activity. Molec. Genet. Metab.1998;64 :169-172.

45. Harmon DL, Woodside JV, Yarnell JWG, et al. The common'thermolabile' variant of me-thylene tetrahydrofolate reductase is a major determinant of mild hyperhomocysteinemia. Q J Med 1996; 89 :571-577.

46. Molloy AM, Daly S, Mills JL et al. Thermolabile variant of 5,10-methylenetetrahydrofolate reductase associated with low red-cell folates: implications for folate intake recommendations. Lancet 1997: 349:1591-1593.

47. Deloughery TG, Evans A, Sadeghi A et al. Common mutation in methylenetetrahydrofolate reductase. Correlation with homocysteine metabolism and late-onset vascular disease. Circulation 1996; 94 :3074-3078.

48. Malinow MR, Nieto FJ, Kruger WD et al. The effects of folic acid supplementation on plasma total homocysteine are modulated by multivitamin use and methylenetetrahydrofolate reductase genotypes. Arterioscler Thromb Vasc Biol 1997; 17 :1157-1162.

49. Morita H, Kurihara H, Tsubaki S et al. Methylenetetrahydrofolate reductase gene polymorphism and ischemic stroke in Japanese. Arterioscler Thromb Vasc Bio 1998;18 :1465-1469.

50. Kluijtmans LAJ, Kastelein JJ, Lindemans J, et al. Thermolabile methylenetetrahydrofolate reductase in coronary artery disease. Circulation 1997;96 :2573-2577.

51. Kluijtmans LA, den Heijer M, Reitsma PH, Heil SG, Blom HJ, Rosendaal FR. Thermolabile methylenetetrahydrofolate reductase and factor V Leiden in the risk of deep-vein thrombosis. Thromb Haemost 1998;79 :254-258.
52. Kluijtmans LAJ, van den Heuvel LP, Boers GHJ. Molecular genetic analysis in mild hyperhomocysteinemia: A common mutation in the methylenetetrahydrofolate reductase gene is a genetic risk factor for cardiovascular disease. Am J Hum Genet 1996;58:35-41.
53. Arai K, Yamasaki Y, Kajimoto Y et al. Association of methylenetetrahydrofolate reductase gene polymorphism with carotid arterial wall thickening and myocardial infarction risk in NIDDM. Diabetes 1997;46 :2102-2104.
54. Tonstad S, Refsum H, Ueland PM. Association between plasma total homocysteine and parental history of cardiovascular disease in children with familial hypercholesterolemia. Circulation 1997;96 :1803-1808.
55. Whitehead AS, Gallagher P, Mills JL et al. A genetic defect in 5,10 methylenetetrahydrofolate reductase in neural tube defects. Q. J. Med. 1995 ;88:763-766.
56. Steegers-Theunissen RPM, Boers GHJ, Trijbels FJM, et al. Maternal hyperhomocysteinemia: a risk factor for neural-tube defects? Metabolism 1994;43:1475-1480.
57. Mills JL, McPartlin JM, Kirke PN, et al. Homocysteine metabolism in pregnancies complicated by neural-tube defects. Lancet 1995;345:149-151.
58. Sohda S, Arinami T, Hamada H, Yamada N, Hamaguchi H, Kubo T. Methylenetetrahyrofolate reductase polymorphism and pre-eclampsia. J Med Genet 1997;34 :525-526.
59. Nelen WLDM, Steegers EAP, Eskes TKAB, Blom HJ. Genetic risk factor for unexplained recurrent early pregnancy loss. Lancet 1997;350 :861.
60. Arinami T, Yamada N, Yamakawa-Kobayashi K, Hamaguchi H, Toru M. Methylenetetrahydrofolate reductase variant and schizophrenia/depression. Am J Med Genet 1997 :74 ;526-528.
61. Loewenstein A, Winder A, Goldstein M, Lazar M, Eldor A. Bilateral retinal vein occlusion associated with 5,10-methylenetetrahydrofolate reductase mutation. Am J Ophthalmol 1997;124 :840-841.
62. Neugebauer S, Baba T, Kurokawa K, Watanabe T. Defective homocysteine metabolism as a risk factor for diabetic retinopathy. Lancet 1997;349;473-474.
63. Weatherall DJ, Clegg JB, Higgs DR, Wood WG. . In : Scriver CR, Beaudet AL, Sly WS, Valle D, editors. The metabolic and molecular bases of inherited disease , 7th edition.,New York : McGraw-Hill, 1995 :3417-3484.
64. Ma J, Stampfer MJ, Giovannucci E et al. Methylenetetrahydrofolate reductase polymorphism, reduced risk of colorectal cancer and dietary interactions. Cancer Res 1997; 57 :1098-1102.
65. Weitkamp LR, Tackels DC, Hunter AGW, Holmes LB, Schwartz CE. Heterozygote advantage of the MTHFR gene in patients with neural tube defect and their relatives. Lancet 1998 :351;1554-1555.

# 17. MOLECULAR BIOLOGY OF METHIONINE SYNTHASE: INTERRELATIONSHIPS WITH HOMO-CYSTEINE AND VASCULAR DISEASE

RUMA BANERJEE

## SUMMARY

Methionine synthase is one of two key enzymes that manages cellular homocysteine and is found in most mammalian tissues. It catalyzes the $B_{12}$-dependent transmethylation of homocysteine using methyltetrahydrofolate as a methyl group donor. The cDNA encoding human methionine synthase has been cloned recently and its sequence has been determined. Catastrophic mutations in methionine synthase are found in the cblG class of patients, and are correlated with severe hyperhomocysteinemia with attendant cardio-vascular diseases. However, polymorphisms have yet to be found that are correlated with the moderate hyperhomocysteinemia. A mouse knock out of the methionine synthase gene confers an embryonic lethal phenotype, indicating that it is an essential gene. The activity of methionine synthase is also dependent on redox proteins that reactivate oxidized enzyme. The components of this redox pathway have been described recently to be a cytochrome $P_{450}$-like methionine synthase reductase and soluble cytochrome $b_5$. Mutations in methionine synthase reductase have been identified in the cblE class of patients and are correlated with severe hyperhomocysteinemia.

K. Robinson (ed.), Homocysteine and Vascular Disease, 291-311.

292     *Ruma Banerjee*

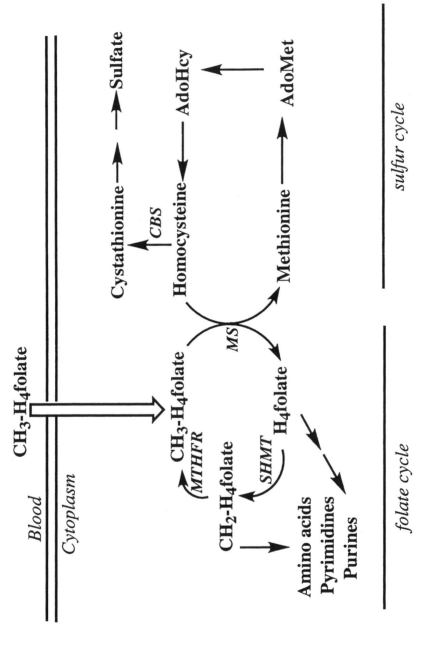

*Figure 1. Position of methionine synthase in folate and sulfur metabolic cycles. MS, SHMT, MTHFR and CBS represent methionine synthase, serine hydroxymethyltransferase, methylenetetrahydrofolate reductase and cystathionine β-synthase respectively. AdoMet and AdoHcy are S-adenosylmethionine and S-adenosylhomocysteine respectively.*

## INTRODUCTION AND HISTORICAL BACKGROUND

Methionine synthase catalyzes a transmethylation reaction at an important metabolic crossroads in mammalian cells (Figure 1). It is poised at the portals of folate traffic and demethylates incoming methyltetrahydrofolic acid ($CH_3$-$H_4$folate), the circulating form of the vitamin, that is delivered to cells from the bloodstream. Its action converts $CH_3$-$H_4$folate to $H_4$folate, which is then available for supporting vital cellular functions including DNA and amino acid biosyntheses. The enzyme also straddles the sulfur metabolic cycle and salvages homocysteine as methionine. Homocysteine, the subject of this book, is a rogue metabolite, whose elevated levels are correlated with cardiovascular diseases (for a recent review see (1)) and neural tube defects (2).

The activity of methionine synthase is dependent on the cofactor, methylcobalamin (MeCbl), a derivative of vitamin $B_{12}$. Studies from du Vigneaud's laboratory on the nutritional needs of rats grown on a diet lacking methionine, demonstrated the connection between homocysteine and choline in the generation of methionine (3, 4). Utilizing germ-free rats, they demonstrated that the deuterium from $D_2O$ was transferred to the methyl groups of choline justifying the conclusion that the synthesis of biologically labile methyl groups occurred in the tissues rather than in intestinal flora (5). It was later demonstrated that rats on a "labile methyl"-free diet grew when homocysteine, folic acid and $B_{12}$ were supplied (6). The role of methylcobalamin (MeCbl) in the enzyme was established in 1962 (7). A $B_{12}$-independent form of this enzyme is found in nature in some eubacteria, archaea and in plants (8). In the remainder of the microbial and in the animal kingdoms, the $B_{12}$-dependent form of the enzyme is found. These proteins appear to represent an evolutionarily convergent solution to the same overall chemical problem, since their gene sequences are unrelated (9, 10).

In addition to the $B_{12}$ cofactor, the activity of methionine synthase is dependent on a reductive activation system (Figure 2). This reliance arises from the oxidative sensitivity of the cofactor that leads to the sporadic generation of inactive enzyme. The latter can be rescued back to the catalytic cycle by a reductive methylation system in which electrons are provided by NADPH, and AdoMet serves as a methyl group donor. In *E. coli,* two flavoproteins, flavodoxin and flavodoxin NADPH oxidoreductase, mediate electron transfer between NADPH and methionine synthase (11-13). In mammals, the redox components have recently been identified, and appear to be a $P_{450}$-like reductase, methionine synthase reductase (14), and soluble cytochrome $b_5$ (15).

Functional deficiency of methionine synthase results most commonly either directly from defects in the enzyme itself, or indirectly from failure of the redox proteins or the cobalamin transport proteins that ensure supply of intra

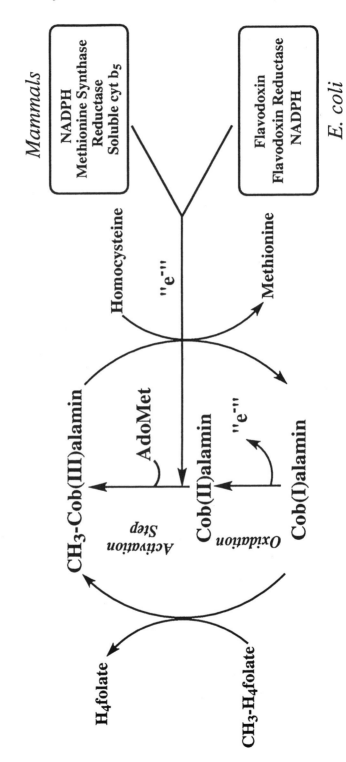

Figure 2. Postulated mechanism for reaction catalyzed by methionine synthase. The pathway for electron transfer for reductive activation of methionine synthase in mammals is not known. Recently identified components of this pathway are indicated.

cellular $B_{12}$ (16, 17). The clinical consequences include homocystinuria (or severe hyperhomocysteinemia), megaloblastic anemia, hypomethioninemia, and neurological disorders with developmental delay and cerebral atrophy (16, 17). In recent years substantial progress has been made in characterizing the mammalian methionine synthase at both the biochemical and molecular genetic levels (for reviews see (18, 19)). The first mutations in its gene that are correlated with severe hyperhomocysteinemia have been described (20, 21), and the association between polymorphisms and mild hyperhomocysteinemia has been examined (22, 23). In this chapter, the recent advances in our understanding of mammalian methionine synthase and its interrelationship with homocysteine, vascular diseases and neural tube defects will be reviewed.


## CHARACTERISTICS OF MAMMALIAN METHIONINE SYNTHASE

### Molecular weight, Kinetic Characteristics and Cofactor Saturation

Methionine synthase is a large monomeric protein with a molecular weight of 140 kDa in humans (24). The bacterial enzyme from *Escherichia coli* is slightly smaller at 136 kDa (25), and is better studied. Its high level of homology to the human protein (55% identity), distributed over most of its length, lends itself to being a good model for the human enzyme. The absorption spectrum of the purified porcine enzyme has maxima at 358, 506 and 536 nm at pH 7.2, characteristic of hydroxocobalamin.

The extent to which methionine synthase exists as holoenzyme has been examined in porcine liver and in human placenta (26). In both tissues, between 90-100% of the protein is present in the holoenzyme form. This issue has also been examined in methionine synthase in bone marrow cells (27). In normal and megaloblastic bone marrows, the percentage of holomethionine synthase is 100 and 13 respectively. Fibroblast cells in culture however, exhibit varying degrees of cofactor saturation of methionine synthase (28). Metal analysis of the purified porcine enzyme by plasma emission spectroscopy has confirmed the presence of one equivalent of cobalt per enzyme active site (24). Like the *E. coli* enzyme (29), porcine methionine synthase also appears to bind stoichiometric zinc (30).


### Enzyme Assays and Kinetics

Under *in vitro* conditions, enzyme activity is monitored in a fixed time radiolabeled assay in which the transfer of the $[^{14}C]$-methyl group from $CH_3$-

H₄folate to methionine is followed (equation 1). The constituents of the reductive activation system that need

$$[^{14}C]\text{-}CH_3\text{-}H_4\text{folate} + \text{Homocysteine} \longrightarrow H_4\text{folate} + [^{14}C]\text{-methionine} \quad [1]$$

to be included in the assay mixture include AdoMet and either (i) dithiothreitol and hydroxocobalamin or (ii) titanium citrate with or without hydroxocobalamin or (iii) NADPH and redox proteins (27). While the first assay with dithiothreitol and hydroxocobalamin is conducted under semianaerobic conditions, the latter two require strict anaerobic conditions (31). A fixed time spectrophotometric assay has been described recently in which the production of H₄folate is determined following its conversion to 5,10,methenyltetrahydrofolate (32). The specific activity of the purified porcine enzyme is 1.6 to 1.7 μmol/min/mg protein at 37ûC, and corresponds to a turnover number of ~250 min⁻¹ (24).

Steady state initial velocity studies are consistent with a sequential mechanism, in which both substrates are bound in a ternary complex with the enzyme for turnover. Product inhibition kinetics indicate that CH₃-H₄folate binding precedes homocysteine, and methionine release precedes H₄folate (24). This is similar to the kinetic pattern observed for the *E. coli* enzyme (33). The $K_m$'s for homocysteine and CH₃-H₄folate are reported to be ~2 μM and 17 μM respectively (24, 34). As with other folate-dependent enzymes, methionine synthase binds polyglutamylated CH₃-H₄folate preferentially. The $K_m$ values for the tri-, penta-, and heptaglutamates are 3-fold lower than that for the monoglutamate substrate. The $V_{max}$ with the penta- to heptaglutamate substrates is 2-fold higher than with the mono- or triglutamate substrates (35). The activity of the rat enzyme has been shown to be stimulated approximately 8- and 12-fold with spermine and spermidine respectively (36). Other polyamines such as putrescine and cadaverine have a weaker effect. Chemical and kinetic details of the reaction mechanism of methionine synthase have been largely elucidated with the bacterial enzyme (recently reviewed in (18, 19, 37)) and will not be discussed here.

## Domain Organization

As mentioned above, the high degree of primary sequence homology between the *E. coli* and human proteins, allows use of the former as a model for the latter. The *E. coli* methionine synthase has a modular organization with apparently discrete domains for binding of substrates and cofactor (Figure 3). Partial proteolysis of methionine synthase results in the generation of an N-terminal homocysteine and CH₃-H₄folate-binding domain, a middle B₁₂-binding domain and a C-terminal AdoMet-binding domain (9, 25). Of these, the structures of the cobalamin- and AdoMet-binding domains have been determined by X-ray crystallography (38, 39). The N-terminal substrate binding domain can be further subdivided. The first 353 residues constitute a homocysteine-binding module (40) in which a catalytically essential zinc activates the thiol substrate (29). Residues extending from 354 to 649 are believed to represent the $CH_3$-$H_4$folate-binding domain since this region is homologous to the methyltransferase from *Clostridium thermoaceticum* that binds the same substrate (41). Residues 650-896 represent the cobalamin-binding domain, and the C-terminal domain extending from residues 897-1227 binds AdoMet. Alternative domain conformations appear to control access of substrates to the cofactor during the catalytic turnover cycle and of AdoMet and redox proteins during the activation reaction (42).

## MOLECULAR CLONING, SEQUENCE ANALYSIS AND CHROMOSOMAL LOCALIZATION OF METHIONINE SYNTHASE

The human cDNA encoding methionine synthase was simultaneously cloned by several groups (21, 43, 44). It contains an open reading frame of 3798 nucleotides encoding a protein of 1265 amino acids with a predicted molecular mass of 140 kDa. The amino acid sequence of the human enzyme is 55% identical with that of the *E. coli* protein, and 64% identical with the predicted *Caenorhabditis elegans* enzyme. The human gene maps to chromosomal location 1q42.3-43 (44). *The E. coli* gene encoding methionine synthase was cloned and overexpressed earlier (9).

The mRNA encoding human methionine synthase has been found in all tissues that were examined including liver, heart, brain, placenta, lung, skeletal, muscle, kidney, pancreas, spleen and thymus. Two predominant mRNA species are observed with sizes corresponding to ~7.5 and 10 kb respectively (43). The shorter cDNA has been sequenced completely (43). The 10 kb band is apparently a preprocessed form of the 7.5 kb message, since it hybridizes to a probe complementary to intron 5 in a Northern blot (44).

## REGULATION OF MAMMALIAN METHIONINE SYNTHASE.

Studies on the regulation of mammalian methionine synthase in HEp-2 cells in culture revealed that supplementation of the medium with $B_{12}$ resulted in a thirty-fold elevation of enzyme activity (45). This was later extended to several other cell lines in which the $B_{12}$-induced activation of methionine synthase ranged from 10- to 30-fold (46). In the initial experiments, methionine and

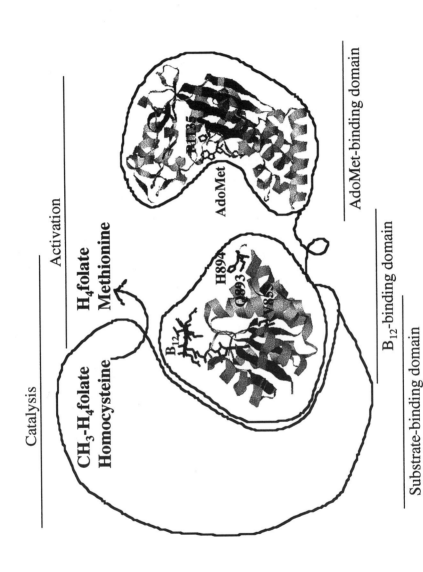

*Figure 3. Modular organization of E. coli methionine synthase showing domain localizations of human mutations and polymorphisms that have been reported to date. Bacterial V855, Q893, H894 and P1135 correspond to human I881, D919, H920 and P1173 respectively. The locations of the bound B₁₂ and AdoMet are indicated.*

choline in the medium were replaced by homocysteine and vitamin $B_{12}$. Homocysteine was however found to have no effect on the activation of methionine synthase, since $B_{12}$ in the presence or absence of homocysteine resulted in the same extent of stimulation (46). The activity of the other $B_{12}$-dependent enzyme, methylmalonyl-CoA mutase, was found to be unchanged upon supplementation of the medium with $B_{12}$ (47).

When methionine in a medium containing $B_{12}$ and folic acid was substituted by homocysteine, methionine synthase activity increased a further 2.5- to 4.0-fold beyond the level induced by $B_{12}$. In animal models, a similar pattern of activation was observed when a deficient diet was supplemented with $B_{12}$ in chicken (48) and rat (49). In addition, activity of methionine synthase increased still further when methionine was removed from the $B_{12}$-containing diet.

In the cell culture system, the effect of the protein synthesis inhibitor, puromycin, on methionine synthase activation was studied. Curiously, activation by $B_{12}$ but not by low methionine, was found to be independent of new protein synthesis (50). Based on these results, the effect of $B_{12}$ on methionine synthase activation was ascribed to result from apoenzyme to holoenzyme conversion. However, since $B_{12}$ relies on a high affinity and efficient transport system for entry into cells, the possibility exists that the kinetics of $B_{12}$ transport surpassed that of puromycin's, accounting for the observed results.

The availability of antibodies to the human methionine synthase, as well as its cDNA sequence, have allowed a reexamination of the mechanism of $B_{12}$ activation by Western and Northern blot analyses (51). These results clearly reveal that induction of enzyme activity is not due to the conversion of preexisting apomethionine synthase to holoenzyme. Western blot analysis shows a clear correspondence between the fold increase in methionine synthase activity and the increase in the methionine synthase protein levels, indicating that new protein is synthesized. Finally, Northern analysis indicates that the level of methionine synthase mRNA remains unchanged during the same period that an increase in activity is measured. While the mechanism of $B_{12}$ activation of methionine synthase is still unknown, both apo- to holoenzyme conversion and transcriptional regulation can now be ruled out. The $B_{12}$-dependent increase in methionine synthase activity may have important implications for the debate on food fortification and homocysteine-lowering intervention studies.

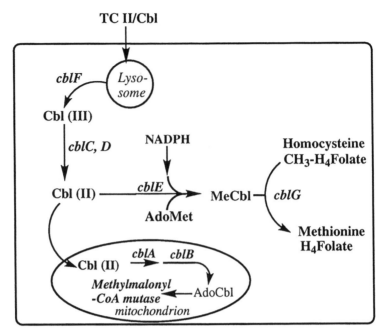

*Figure 4. Intracellular cobalamin metabolism. The various genetic complementation groups, designated* cbl *A-F, that result in impaired intracellular cobalamin metabolism are indicated. Of these,* cblE *and* cblG *result in isolated functional deficiency of methionine synthase. Mutations in methionine synthase and methionine synthase reductase are correlated with the* cblE *and* cblG *conditions respectively. Mitochondrial cobalamin metabolism leads to deoxyadenosylcobalamin, the cofactor for methylmalonyl-CoA mutase. Cbl(III), Cbl(II), Cbl(I), refer to cobalamin in the $3^+$, $2^+$ and $1^+$ oxidation states respectively.*

## METHIONINE SYNTHASE MUTATIONS CORRELATED WITH HYPERHOMOCYSTEINEMIA

Intracellular cobalamin metabolism is complex and compartmentalized (Figure 4). A number of defects have been identified in this pathway based on the genetic complementation between the groups (17). These metabolic steps lead ultimately to the two cofactor forms: MeCbl and deoxyadenosylcobalamin that are required by methionine synthase and methylmalonyl-CoA mutase respectively. Steps that lead to impaired MeCbl synthesis include *cbl*C, D, E, F and G. Of these, only *cbl*G and *cbl*E lead to an isolated functional deficiency of methionine synthase. The others affect the activity of both cobalamin-dependent enzymes.

*Table I. Polymorphisms and mutations identified in methionine synthase*

| Cell line | Mutation | Phenoytype | Reference |
|-----------|----------|------------|-----------|
| *cbl*G WG1892 | 2640DATC | DIle881, single amino acid deletion in $B_{12}$-binding domain | 20,21 |
| | 3517C→T | P1173L, mutation in AdoMet-binding domain | |
| *cbl*G WG1505 | 3517C→T | P1173L, mutation in AdoMet-binding domain | 28 |
| *cbl*G WG2290 | 2758C→G | H920D mutation in $B_{12}$-binding domain | 21 |
| *cbl*G WG1655 | 3378insA | frameshift with premature termination | 56 |
| | mid IVS-6 G→A substitution | generation of cryptic 3'acceptor splice site leading to premature termination | |
| *cbl*G WG1670 and *cbl*G WG1671* | 2112DTC | frameshift with premature termination | 56 |
| | -166IVS-3 A→G | generation of cryptic 3'acceptor splice site leading to premature termination | |
| | 2756 A→G | D919G mutation in $B_{12}$-binding domain | 21, 44, 22 |
| | 2053A→T | K685K, silent polymorphism | 22 |
| | 2127A→G | E709E, silent polymorphism | 22 |
| | 3144A→G | A1048A, silent polymorphism | 22 |

*These cell lines were from siblings*

Catastrophic lesions in methionine synthase leading to severe hyperhomocysteinemia had been suspected based on the genetic and biochemical characterization of *cbl*G patient cell lines (52-54). Two subsets of *cbl*G cell lines were originally described in which the concentration of bound [$^{57}$Co]-cobalamin was either comparable to controls or was virtually undetectable (55). The two groups could also be readily distinguished by their activities in the *in vitro* assays using artificial reductants. Whereas methionine synthase activity in the group with normal levels of bound $B_{12}$ was indistinguishable from that in control fibroblast cell lines, it was drastically reduced in the group with low $B_{12}$ (referred to as the variants). Availability of the human methionine synthase cDNA sequence has allowed molecular characterization of the genetic defects in a number of *cbl*G cell lines and these are summarized in Figure 3 and Table I.

Northern analysis of *cbl*G cell lines has revealed an interesting pattern that corresponds to the enzyme activity levels associated with the two subsets. The *cbl*G variants, 79/96, WG1670, WG1655 and WG1671 show trace levels of the two transcripts that are observed only upon prolonged exposure or by phosphorimager analysis (20, 56). In the other subgroup, the methionine synthase mRNA levels are comparable to those of controls (20). Four mutations have been described in the variant subgroup, all of which are expected to be functionally null since premature termination is predicted to result from the existing deletion or insertion mutations (56). These results however contradict the biochemical studies on at least two of these cell lines, WG1670 and WG1671, in which methionine synthase activity was measurable, albeit very low (28). They also contradict the results from knockout experiments (discussed below) that indicate that methionine synthase is an essential gene in mice. However, one allele in each of these cell lines carries mutations that are expected to unmask cryptic splice sites leading to functionally null phenotypes. Thus, the possibility that normal splicing occurs at low frequency in these cell lines giving rise to very low levels of wild type enzyme needs to be examined.

The biochemical phenotype associated with the *cbl*G nonvariant patients is interesting. The activity of methionine synthase in fibroblast cell extracts is similar to that of control cells when artificial reductants, *viz*. titanium citrate or dithiothreitol/hydroxocobalamin are employed . In contrast, marked differences between the patient and control cell lines are observed when NADPH and the redox proteins present in the cell extract are employed for reductive activation (20, 28). These data indicated that the defects in the *cbl*G nonvariants that were examined, specifically impaired reductive activation rather than catalytic turnover, and led to the prediction that mutations were likely to be localized in the $B_{12}$- or AdoMet-binding domains. This prediction was borne out by mutation detection analysis. All mutations detected so far cluster in two domains, the cobalamin-binding domain and the C-terminal AdoMet-binding domains (Figure 3).

## POLYMORPHISMS IN METHIONINE SYNTHASE

Since two apparently unrelated pathologies, premature vascular diseases (reviewed in (1)), and neural tube defects (2) are both associated with moderately elevated homocysteine levels, the coding sequence of the human methionine synthase gene has been analyzed for associated polymorphisms that may confer risk. To this end, the methionine synthase cDNA from eight patients with mild hyperhomocysteinemia were analyzed by direct sequencing (22). Four of the patients had neural tube defects and four had pregnancies complicated by severe spiral arterial disease. The latter causes infarction of the placenta resulting in either a stillborn or a severely growth-retarded child, resulting predominantly from spiral artery occlusion.

Four polymorphisms, of which three are silent, were detected (Table I). The silent mutations were 2053A→T, 2127 A→G, 3144A→G. Neither the possible correlation of these silent mutations with altered homocysteine levels nor their evaluation as markers in linkage disequilibrium with a possible pathogenic mutation has been reported. The fourth mutation, 2756A→G causes a coding sequence change, D919G, and had been observed previously (21, 44). The frequency of the AA, AG and GG genotypes in the control Dutch population is 0.71, 0.26 and 0.3 respectively. There is no indication that this polymorphism *per se* is a risk factor for either neural tube defects or spiral arterial disease. Likewise, no differences were observed in the mean homocysteine levels and the genotype. No significant association between the D919G genotype and the occurrence of neural tube defects was found in a British population, or between the maternal allele and neural tube defects (23). These studies, although limited in scope, suggest that a common polymorphism in the methionine synthase protein that is correlated with susceptibility to mild hyperhomocysteinemia is unlikely. However, only half of the cDNA constitutes the open reading frame for methionine synthase, with much of the rest representing a 3' untranslated sequence. The existence of polymorphisms in this region that may affect the stability of the message and therefore of methionine synthase levels remains to be examined.

## METHIONINE SYNTHASE REDUCTASE MUTATIONS CORRELATED WITH HYPERHOMOCYSTEINEMIA

The oxidative sensitivity of methionine synthase renders it dependent on a reductive methylation system for reactivation (Figure 2). The components of the reductive activation system in *E. coli* are well characterized (11-13), the mammalian components have been revealed by very recent studies using genetic (14) and biochemical approaches (15). Biochemical studies on *cbl*E cell lines had provided strong evidence that the lesion in this group is associated with the reductive activation system. Moreover, both biochemical and genetic complementation was demonstrated between *cbl*E and *cbl*G cell lines indicating that the defective loci were distinct (28, 57, 58). Since it had been demonstrated that *cbl*G's carry mutations in methionine synthase (20, 21, 28), it was reasonable to conclude that *cbl*E's carried mutations in the redox protein(s).

In *E. coli*, two flavoproteins, flavodoxin oxidoreductase and flavodoxin, transfer reducing equivalents from NADPH to methionine synthase (Figure 2, 11-13). AdoMet serves as the methyl group donor in both bacterial and mammalian enzymes. Based on the homology between the cofactor binding domains of the bacterial flavodoxin (FMN) and flavodoxin reductase (FAD, NADPH) on the one hand and the mammalian $P_{450}$ reductase (FMN, FAD, NADPH) on the other, Gravel and coworkers hypothesized that the human homolog may be a cytochrome $P_{450}$ reductase-like protein (14). Using consensus sequences to the predicted FMN, FAD, and NADPH binding sites, they cloned a cDNA corresponding to soluble cytochrome $P_{450}$ reductase. The gene maps to chromosomal location 5p15.2-15.3. The deduced protein contains 698 amino acids with a predicted molecular mass of 77,000, and is 38% identical to the human microsomal cytochrome $P_{450}$ reductase. Several mutations have been described in the methionine synthase gene in *cbl*E cell lines, providing strong evidence that the gene product is involved in reductive activation of methionine synthase (14, 59).

The biochemical approach to characterization of the reductive activation components has led to a similar but not identical solution (15). Reconstitution of methionine synthase activity in crude liver homogenates fractionated by batch chromatography indicated the involvement of two protein components (28). Using a reconstitution assay, one of the two components was purified to homogeneity, and corresponds to soluble cytochrome $b_5$. The other component is microsomal, and the involvement of cytochrome $b_5$ and NADPH in the assay, suggested its identity as cytochrome $P_{450}$ reductase. Purified cytochrome $P_{450}$ reductase and soluble cytochrome $b_5$ each supports methionine synthase activity in the presence of NADPH and the other component in a saturable manner.

Soluble cytochrome $b_5$ is a small hemeprotein with a molecular mass of 10,977 daltons. The only function previously ascribed to soluble cytochrome $b_5$ is in methemoglobin reduction in erythrocytes (60). The membrane associated form functions both in fatty acid desaturation (61) and in $P_{450}$-dependent monooxygenation reactions (62). The soluble and membrane associated forms are both encoded by the same gene, but differ in the presence of a 24 bp insertion in the cDNA encoding the soluble form. The insertion contains an inframe stop codon and leads to the translation of a 98 residue long polypeptide (63). The membrane associated form has an additional C-terminal membrane anchor.

Soluble cytochrome $b_5$ thus represents an additional target in which polymorphisms and or mutations may be associated with hyperhomocysteinemia. However, the small size of the gene, and the even smaller size of the insert (24 bp) that distinguishes the soluble from the membrane associated form, suggests that viable mutations in soluble cytochome $b_5$ may be very rare. It is interesting to note in this regard, that of the various patients with methemoglobinemia, only one has been described with lesions in cytochrome $b_5$ (64). Mutations in the portion of the gene that is common to the soluble and membrane associated forms would be expected to have pleiotropic and probably severe consequences, due to the importance of the membrane cytochrome $b_5$ in multiple metabolic pathways.

Based on the data presently available, it is difficult to evaluate whether methionine synthase reductase activates methionine synthase directly. If it does, then it would represent an alternative route to the cytochrome $b_5$- cytochrome $P_{450}$ reductase pathway uncovered by the biochemical reconstitution studies (Figure 5). In this context, it is interesting to note that a third complementation group distinct from *cbl*G and *cbl*E, has been reported recently that displays an isolated functional deficiency of methionine synthase (65). Alternatively, reduction of methionine synthase by methionine synthase reductase may be dependent on the presence of soluble cytochrome $b_5$. The connection between cytochrome $b_5$ and the $P_{450}$-like methionine synthase reductase will have to await expression and biochemical characterization of the latter.


MOUSE MODEL FOR METHIONINE SYNTHASE DEFICIENCY

The importance of homocysteine and folate in vascular disease and in neural tube defects has spurred the development of a mouse model for methionine synthase deficiency. Using gene-targeting technology in embryonic stem cells, the methionine synthase gene has been knocked out (66). Heterozygous matings produced wild type (+/+), heterozygous (+/-) and homozygous (-/-) knockouts in a 1:2:0 ratio, indicating that the homozygotes are nonviable. Examination of 12.5 day old embryos of heterozygous crosses reveals that approximately a quarter of them are reabsorbed compared with 4% in wild-type crosses. This demonstrates that the (+/+) embryos implant successfully but succumb before 12.5 days. The heterozygous mice are apparently indistinguishable from the wild-type litter mates and do not exhibit any reduction in fecundity. The homocysteine levels in the heterozygotes is

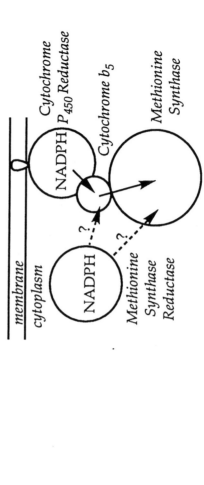

Figure 5. Comparison of reductive activation components of methionine synthase in E. coli and in mammals. Alternative pathways are suggested by the present state of knowledge on the mammalian reductive activation system as discussed in the text. The pathway of electron flow in mammals is presently unknown.

comparable to that of controls (Barry Shane, personal communication). Methionine synthase activity in the livers of heterozygotes is ~65% of the (+/+) controls. As expected, there is no difference in the levels of cystathionine β-synthase or methylmalonyl-CoA mutase activities in the (+/-) versus (+/+) mice.

## CONCLUSIONS

The past few years have witnessed an explosion of new information on the molecular genetic and biochemical characterization of mammalian methionine synthase as well as in the elucidation of details of the reaction mechanism of the bacterial enzyme. The structures of two of the three major regions comprising the bacterial methionine synthase have provided the first glimpse of pieces of this protein, and are also invaluable for modeling and understanding the human enzyme (38, 39). The cloning and sequencing of the human gene encoding methionine synthase (21, 43, 44) have permitted identification of the first mutations in this gene that are correlated with severe hyperhomocysteinemia (20, 21, 28). The methionine synthase knock out model has revealed the indispensability of the gene in mice, and studies are in progress to characterize the cause and timing of the embryonic lethality observed in the homozygous (-/-) mice (66). The mammalian physiological activation system that is required for returning the oxidized enzyme to the catalytic cycle is being revealed by genetic and biochemical studies (14, 15). A $P_{450}$-like oxidoreductase and soluble cyotochrome $b_5$ have been described as components of the mammalian activation system. In addition, numerous mutations in the $P_{450}$-like protein, methionine synthase reductase, have been described thus establishing the cause of the genetic defect in *cbl*E cell lines (14). These developments have opened the doors to evaluation of whether or not polymorphisms in methionine synthase itself or in the auxiliary redox proteins are correlated with mild hyperhomocysteinemia. Early results indicate that the D919G polymorphism in methionine synthase that has a relatively high prevalence, is not correlated with either vascular diseases or neural tube defects (22, 23). However, a full evaluation of whether or not polymorphisms in methionine synthase are associated with susceptibility to disease must await additional characterization of the long cDNA encoding methionine synthase, as well as of the more recently described methionine synthase reductase and soluble cytochrome $b_5$.

*Acknowledgements. This work was supported by grants from the National Institutes of Health (DK45776 and HL58984).*

# REFERENCES

1.  Refsum H, Ueland PM, Nygard O, Vollset SE. Homocysteine and cardiovascular disease. Annu. Rev. Medicine 1998;49:31-62.

2.  Mills JL, McPartlin JM, Kirke PN, Lee YJ, Conle MR, Weir DG. Homocysteine metabolism in pregnancies complicated by neural tube defects. Lancet 1995;345:149-151.

3.  du Vigneaud V, Chandler JP, Moyer AW, Keppel DM. The effect of choline on the ability of homocysteine to replace methionine in the diet. J. Biol. Chem. 1939;131:57-76.

4.  Moyer AW, du Vigneaud V. The structural specificiy of choline and betaine in transmethylation. J. Biol. Chem. 1942;143:373-382.

5.  du Vigneaud V, Ressler C, Rachele JR. The biological synthesis of "labile methyl groups". Science 1950;122:267-271.

6.  Bennett MA. Utilization of homocysteine for growth in presence of vitamin $B_{12}$ and folic acid. J. Biol. Chem. 1950;187:751-756.

7.  Guest JR, Friedman S, Woods DD, Smith EL. A methyl analog of cobamide coenzyme in relation to methionine synthesis by bacteria. Nature 1962;195:340-342.

8.  Whitfield CD, Steers EJJ, Weissbach H. Purification and properties of 5-methyltetrahydropteroyltriglutamate-homocysteine transmethylase. J. Biol. Chem. 1970;245:390-401.

9.  Banerjee RV, Johnston NL, Sobeski JK, Datta P, Matthews RG. Cloning and sequence analysis of the *Escherichia coli* metH gene encoding cobalamin-dependent methionine synthase and isolation of a tryptic fragment containing the cobalamin-binding domain. J. Biol. Chem. 1989;264:13888-13895.

10. Gonzalez JC, Banerjee RV, Huang S, Sumner JS, Matthews RG. Comparison of Cobalamin-Independent and Cobalamin-Dependent Methionine Synthases from Escherichia coli: Two solutions to the Same Chemical Problem. Biochem. 1992;31:6045-6056.

11. Fujii K, Huennekens FM. Activation of methionine synthase by a reduced triphosphopyridine nucleotide-dependent flavoprotein system. J. Biol. Chem. 1974;249:6745-6753.

12. Fujii K, Galivan JH, Huennekens FM. Activation of methionine synthase: Further characterization of the flavoprotein system. Arch. Biochem. Biophys. 1977; 178:662-670.

13. Fujii K, Huennekens FM. in Biochemical aspects of nutrition. (Yagi K, ed.) pp. 173-183 Japan Scientific Societies, Tokyo.

14. Leclerc D, Wilson A, Dumas R, et al. Cloning and mapping of a cDNA for methionine synthase reductase, a flavoprotein defective in patients with homocystinuria. Proc. Natl. Acad. Sci. USA 1998;95:3059-3064.

15. Chen Z, Banerjee R. Purification of soluble cytochrome $b_5$ as a component of the reductive activation system of porcine methionine synthase. J. Biol. Chem. 1998;273:26248-26255.

16. Fenton WA, Rosenberg LE. in *The metabolic and molecular bases of inherited disease.* 1995. (Scriver CR, Beaudet AL, Sly WS, Valle D, eds.) pp 3111-3128 McGraw-Hill, New York

17. Shevell MI, Rosenblatt DS. The neurology of cobalamin. Can. J. of Neurol. Sci. 1992;19:472-486.

18. Banerjee R. The yin-yang of cobalamin biochemistry. Chemistry and Biology 1997;4:175-186.

19. Ludwig ML, Matthews RG. Structure-based perspectives on $B_{12}$-dependent enzymes. Annu. Rev. Biochem. 1997;66:269-313.

20. Gulati SG, Baker P, Fowler B, et al. Mutations in human methionine synthase in cblG patients. Hum. Molec. Genet. 1996;5:1859-1866.

21. Leclerc D, Campeau E, Goyette P, et al. Human methionine synthase: cDNA cloning and identification of mutations in patients of the cblG complementation group of folate/cobalamin disorders. Hum. Molec. Genet. 1996;5:1867-1874.

22. van der Put NMJ, van der Molen EF, Kluijtmans LAG, et al. Sequence analysis of the coding region of human methionine synthase: Relevance to hyperhomocysteinemia in neural-tube defects and vascular disease. Q. J. Med 1997;90:511-517.

23. Morrison K, Edwards YH, Lynch SA. Methionine synthase and neural tube defects. J. Med. Genet 1997;34:958.

24. Chen Z, Crippen K, Gulati S, Banerjee R. Purification and kinetic characterization of methionine synthase from pig liver. J. Biol. Chem. 1994;269:27193-27197.

25. Drummond J, Huang S, Blumenthal RM, Matthews RG. Assignment of enzymatic function to specific protein regions of cobalamin-dependent methionine synthase from *Escherichia coli*. Biochemistry 1993;32:9290-9295.

26. Chen Z, Chakraborty S, Banerjee R. Demonstration that the mammalian methionine synthases are predominantly cobalamin-loaded. J. Biol. Chem. 1995;270:19246-19249.

27. Taylor RT, Weissbach H. $N^5$-Methyltetrahydrofolate-Homocysteine Transmethylase. J. Biol. Chem. 1967;242:1502-1516.

28. Gulati S, Brody LC, Rosenblatt DS, Banerjee R. Defects in auxiliary redox proteins lead to functional methionine synthase deficiency. J. Biol. Chem. 1997;272:19171-19175.

29. Goulding CW, Matthews RG. Cobalamin-dependent methionine synthase from Escherichia coli: Involvement of zinc in homocysteine activation. Biochemistry 1997;36:15749-15757.

30. Chen Z. Ph.D. Thesis, University of Nebraska, Lincoln 1998.

31. Banerjee R, Gulati S, Chen Z. Methionine synthase from pig liver. Methods Enzymol. 1997;281:189-196.

32. Drummond JT, Jarrett J, Gonzalez JC, Huang S, Matthews RG. Characterization of Nonradioactive Assays for Cobalamin-Dependent and Cobalamin-Independent Methionine Synthase Enzymes. Anal. Biochem. 1995;228:323-329.

33. Banerjee R, Frasca V, Ballou DP, Matthews RG. Participation of cob(I)alamin in the reaction catalyzed by methionine synthase from *Escherichia coli:* A steady-state and rapid reaction kinetic analysis. Biochemistry 1990;29:11101-11109.

34. Yamada K, Tobimatsu T, Kawata T, Wada M, Maekawa A, Toraya T. Purification and some properties of cobalamin-dependent methionine synthase from rat liver. J. Nutr. Sci. Vitaminol. 1997;43:177-186.

35. Coward JK, Chello PL, Cashmore AR, Parameswaran KN, DeAngelis LM, Bertino JR. 5-Methyl-5,6,7,8-tetrahydropteroyl Oligo-γ-L-glutamates: Synthesis and Kinetic Studies with Methionine Synthetase from Bovine Brain. Biochem. 1975;14(7):1548-1552.

36. Kenyon SH, Nicolaou A, Ast T, Gibbons WA. Stimulation in vitro of vitamin $B_{12}$-dependent methionine synthase by polyamines. Biochem. J. 1996;316:661-665.

37. Matthews RG, Goulding CW. Enzyme-catalyzed methyl transfers to thiols: the role of zinc. Curr. Op. Chem. Biol. 1997;1:332-339.

38. Drennan CL, Huang S, Drummond JT, Matthews R, Ludwig ML. How a protein binds $B_{12}$: A 3A X-ray structure of $B_{12}$-binding domains of methionine synthase. Science 1994;266:1669-1674.

39. Dixon MM, Huang S, Matthews RG, Ludwig ML. The activation domain of cobalamin-dependent methionine synthase: A novel fold for AdoMet binding. Structure 1996;4:1263-1275.

40. Goulding CW, Postigo D, Matthews RG. Cobalamin-dependent methionine synhtase is a modular protein with distinct regions for binding homocysteine, methyltetrahydrofolate, cobalamin and adenosylmethionine. Biochemistry 1997;36:8082-8091.

41. Roberts DL, Zhao S, Doukov T, Ragsdale SW. The reductive acetyl coenzyme A pathway: sequence and heterologous expression of active methyltetrahydrofolate:corrinoid/iron-sulfur protein methyltransferase from *Clostridium thermoaceticum*. J. Bacteriol. 1994;176:6127-6130.

42. Jarrett JT, Huang S, Matthews RG. Methionine Synthase exists in two distinct conformations that differ in the reactivity towards methyltetrahydrofolate, adenosylmethionine and flavodoxin. Biochemistry 1998;37:5372-5382.

43. Li YN, Gulati S, Baker PJ, Brody LC, Banerjee R, Kruger WD. Cloning, mapping and RNA analysis of the human methionine synthase gene. Hum. Molec. Genetics 1996;5:1851-1858.

44. Chen LH, Liu M-L, Hwang H-Y, Chen L-S, Korenberg J, Shane B. Human methionine synthase. cDNA cloning, gene localization and expression. J. Biol. Chem. 1997;272:3628-3634.

45. Mangum JH, North JA. Vitamin $B_{12}$-dependent methionine biosynthesis in HEp-2 cells. Biochem. Biophys. Res. Commun. 1968;32:105-110.

46. Mangum JH, Murray BK, North JA. Vitamin $B_{12}$ dependent methionine biosynthesis in cultured mammalian cells. Biochemistry 1969;8:3496-3499.

47. Kerwar SS, Spears C, Brian M, Weissbach H. Studies on vitamin $B_{12}$ metabolism in HeLa cells. Arch. Biochem. Biophys. 1971;142:231-237.

48. Dickerman HW, Redfield BG, Bieri JG, Weissback H. The role of vitamin $B_{12}$ in methionine biosynthesis in avian liver. J. Biol.Chem. 1964;239:2888-2895.

49. Finkelstein JD, Kyle WE, Harris BJ. Methionine metabolism in mammals. Regulation of homocysteine methyltransferase in rat tissue. Arch. Biochem. Biophys. 1971;146:84-92.

50. Kamely D, Littlefield JW, Erbe RW. Regulation of 5-methyltetrahydrofolate:homocysteine methyltransferase activity by methionine, vitamin $B_{12}$, and folate in cultured baby hamster kidney cells. Proc. Nat. Acad. Sci. USA 1973;70:2585-2589.

51. Gulati S, Brody L, Banerjee R. Regulation of mammalian methionine synthase by $B_{12}$. BBRC 1999;259:436-442.

52. Watkins D, Rosenblatt DS. Genetic heterogeneity among patients with methylcobalamin deficiency. J. Clin. Invest. 1988;81:1690-1694.

53. Watkins D, Rosenblatt DS. Functional methionine synthase deficiency (cblE and cblG): clinical and biochemical heterogeneity. Amer. J. Med. Genetics 1989;34:427-434.

54. Hall C, Lindenbaum RH, Arenson E, Begley J, Chu R. The nature of the defect in cobalamin G mutation. Clin. Inves. Med . 1989;12:262-269.

55. Sillaots SL, Hall CA, Hurteloup V, Rosenblatt DS. Heterogeneity in cblG: Differential Retention of Cobalamin on Methionine Synthase. Biochem. Med. Metabolic Biol. 1992;47:242-249.

56. Wilson A, Leclerc D, Saberi F, et al. Functionally null mutations in patients with the cblG variant form of methionine synthase deficiency. Am. J. Hum. Genet. 1998;63:409-414.

57. Schuh W, Rosenblatt DS, Cooper BA, et al. Homocystinuria and megaloblastic anemia responsive to vitamin $B_{12}$ therapy. An inborn error of metabolism due to a single defect in cobalamin metabolism. N. Engl. J. Med. 1984;310:686-690.

58. Rosenblatt DS, Cooper BA, Pottier A, Lue-Shing H, Matiaszuk N, Grauer K. Altered Vitamin $B_{12}$ Metabolism in Fibroblasts from Patients with Megaloblastic Anemia and Homocystinuria due to a New Defect in Methionine Biosynthesis. J. Clin. Invest. 1984;74:2149-2156.

59. Wilson A, Leclerc D, Rosenblatt DS, Gravel RA. Identification of eleven novel mutations in patients with cblE form of methionine synthase deficiency. submitted for publication 1998.

60. Hultquist D, Passon P. Catalysis of methaemoglobin reduction by erythrocyte cytochrome $b_5$ and cytochrome $b_5$ reductase. Nature New Biol. 1971;229:252-254.

61. Enoch H, Strittmatter P. Cytochrome $b_5$ reduction by NADPH cytochrome $P_{450}$ reductase. J. Biol. Chem. 1979;254:8976-8981.

62. Pompon D, Coon M. On the mechanism of action of cytochrome P-450 oxidation and reduction of the ferrous dioxygen complex of liver microsomal cytochrome P-450 by cytochrome b5. J. Biol. Chem. 1984;259:15377-15385.

63. VanderMark PK, Steggles AW. The isolation and characterization of the soluble membrane-bound porcine cytochrome $b_5$ cDNAs. Biochem. Biophys. Res. Comm. 1997;240:80-83.

64. Jaffe ER, Hultquist DE. Cytochrome $b_5$ reductase deficiency and enzymopenic hereditary methemoglobinemia. New York: McGraw-Hill Press, 1989. (Scriver CR, Beauder AL, Sly WS, Valle D, eds. The Metabolic Basis of Inherited Disease;

65. Fowler B, Suormala T, Gunther M, Till J, Wraith JE. A new patient with functional methionine synthase deficiency: Evidence for a third complementation class. J. Inher. Dis. 1997;20:21.

66. Swanson DA, Baker P, Liu ML, et al. A methionine synthase knock-out mouse. Am. J. Hum. Genet. 1998;63:A275.

# 18. MOLECULAR BIOLOGY OF CYSTATHIONINE β–SYNTHASE: INTERRELATIONSHIPS WITH HOMOCYSTEINE, PYRIDOXINE, AND VASCULAR DISEASE

WARREN D. KRUGER AND BRIAN FOWLER

SUMMARY

Cystathionine β-synthase (CBS) catalyzes the condensation of homocysteine with serine to form cystathionine, an irreversible step in the biosynthesis of cysteine. This reaction plays a key role in the determination of plasma homocysteine levels. Individuals lacking CBS activity (classical CBS deficiency or homocystinuria) have extremely elevated plasma homocysteine levels and have severe arteriosclerosis at relatively young ages. These findings led to the initial interest in homocysteine as a risk factor for vascular disease. In this chapter we will examine various aspects of CBS and CBS deficiency. We will review CBS enzymology, regulation, and the relationship between CBS and pyridoxine. In addition, we will discuss the molecular genetics of CBS deficiency and how mutations in CBS affect plasma homocysteine in the heterozygous and homozygous state. Finally, we will discuss the potential of drugs targeted at CBS to control plasma homocysteine levels.

*K. Robinson (ed.), Homocysteine and Vascular Disease, 313-333.*
© 2000 *Kluwer Academic Publishers. Printed in the Netherlands.*

## HOMOCYSTINURIA AND CBS DEFICIENCY

The association of a distinct clinical phenotype with the excretion of increased amounts of homocystine was first recognized in 1962 [1,2]. Surveys of patients with mental retardation and dislocated lenses led to the diagnosis of several cases, some of whom had been categorized as cases of Marfan's syndrome on the basis of physical features [3]. As further cases were discovered a clinical phenotype of a progressive multi-organ disorder affecting the ocular, nervous, skeletal and cardiovascular systems emerged and came to represent so called classical homocystinuria. In these patients, disturbed methionine metabolism was characterized by increased levels of methionine, homocystine and cysteine-homocysteine disulfide and low levels of cystine in plasma and urine [4].

The underlying specific enzyme defect, lack of CBS activity, was demonstrated by Mudd et al. first in liver and subsequently in brain, cultured skin fibroblasts, and phytohaemaglutinin-stimulated lymphocytes [5-8]. As more patients were detected a wide spectrum of clinical variation and severity of symptoms became evident. The spectrum of clinical presentation ranged from single system involvement, usually of lens dislocation with mild or absent involvement of other systems, to full multi-system involvement [9-11]. Other organs affected are the hair, skin and liver and several anecdotal reports of additional clinical signs such as pancreatitis, dystonia with parkinsonian features and pneumothorax have appeared [12]. Clinical signs usually appear after the second year, although the age of onset can vary considerably from as early as four weeks [13], to late adulthood [14].

## PYRIDOXINE RESPONSIVENESS

An important indication of genetic heterogeneity was the discovery, first reported by Barber and Spaeth [15], that approximately half of all patients show a clear reduction of plasma and urine methionine and homocystine values on treatment with pharmacological doses of pyridoxine (vitamin $B_6$), the vitamin precursor of pyridoxal 5'-phosphate (PLP) [16]. A large study done in the 1980s examining over 600 patients clearly establishes that the pyridoxine responsive form of the disease is associated with milder disease [17] with later age of onset of symptoms and reduced overall morbidity.

The mechanism underlying pyridoxine responsive homocystinuria is still not clear. Because PLP is a co-factor for CBS, one possible explanation for pyridoxine responsiveness would be that mutant forms of the enzyme could simply have a lower affinity for PLP. Several studies have examined this hypothesis and results are mixed. In some early studies, the addition of PLP to crude liver and cultured fibroblast homogenates resulted in either slight or significant increases in the activity of CBS in some responsive patients, but no stimulation of residual activity in others [18-19]. Detailed studies of PLP binding kinetics showed that some non-responsive patients with detectable residual CBS in fibroblast extracts have an extremely high affinity constant for PLP [20-21]. In such patients tissue levels of the coenzyme reached on pyridoxine treatment would be insufficient to stimulate the enzyme explaining the lack of *in vivo* response in spite of the presence of appreciable residual enzyme activity *in vitro*. In a study of cell lines from 68 responsive patients, our lab (B.F.) found that stimulation of *in vitro* CBS activity by PLP was higher than the normal level in 47 out of 62 cell lines from responsive patients. Taken together, these data suggest that decreased affinity for pyridoxine may be the explanation of some but not all *in vivo* $B_6$ responsiveness.

Another predictor of pyridoxine responsiveness is simply the presence of residual enzyme activity in extracts derived from responders. Based on fibroblast extract measurements in 35 patients, Uhlendorf et al. [22] concluded that *in vivo* pyridoxine responsiveness is associated with the retention of small amounts of residual CBS activity *in vitro*. Studies from a large series of patients in our lab [23 and unpublished data] with carefully defined *in vivo* response to pyridoxine found 26 of 34 non-responsive patients with no detectable residual CBS activity and 62 of 68 responsive patients with measurable activity in cultured fibroblasts (B. Fowler, unpublished data). Thus like *in vitro* stimulation by PLP, there is not a 100% concordance between residual activity and *in vivo* pyridoxine responsiveness.

Treatment with pyridoxine and, in partially and unresponsive patients, other homocysteine lowering treatments such as dietary methionine restriction or betaine administration clearly alters the course of the disease but long term outcome remains unclear [24]. To date the levels of total homocysteine achieved even in the best treated patients is above 50 μmol/L, well above levels associated with premature vascular disease. If a mild increase of homocysteine proves indeed to be a causative agent for vascular disease, homocysteine lowering treatment will need to be even more vigorously applied than to date [25].

In spite of these advances, sufficiently early diagnosis and introduction of adequate treatment to correct the consequences of this severe disorder remains a challenge to workers in this field. Considerable delay often occurs between the appearance of clinical abnormalities and diagnosis [14] and even newborn screening does not detect all cases due to inadequacy of existing methods to detect milder metabolic abnormalities particularly in pyridoxine responsive cases [26].

## HYPERHOMOCYSTEINEMIA

In the literal sense homocystinuria and hyperhomocysteinemia are both defined as the urinary excretion of the disulfide homocystine and the elevation of homocysteine in blood. In fact homocystinuria has come to be synonymous with the severe homozygous genetic deficiency, of one of the three key enzymes of homocysteine metabolism, namely CBS, methylenete-trahydrofolate reductase (MTHFR) and methionine synthase (MS), usually associated with a characteristic clinical phenotype [13]. A caveat is that the finding of elevated homocystine in urine is not consistent in patients with milder forms of the enzyme deficiencies [4].

Conversely hyperhomocysteinemia refers to an increased concentration of homocysteine, free or bound to cysteine residues both free and protein-bound, in blood due to any reason. This can include the homocystinurias, as well as a wide range of acquired causes, including folate and vitamin $B_{12}$ deficiency [27] and various other reasons as summarized in Chapter 5 of this volume.

## CBS AND HOMOCYSTEINE METABOLISM

CBS lies at the branch point of remethylation of homocysteine and its breakdown by transsulfuration. Its action irreversibly commits homocysteine to catabolism, and thus it plays a pivotal role in the fate of homocysteine specifically and in the control of methionine metabolism in general. The control of methionine metabolism is complex due to the need to satisfy the organism's requirements for protein synthesis, for S-adenosylmethionine (Adomet) dependent transmethylation reactions, for polyamine synthesis, for the formation of cystathionine, cysteine and various related metabolites and for the catabolism of choline. Also levels of homocysteine itself, which plays an essential role in folate and methionine metabolism but is highly toxic in excess, must be finely modulated. Much of our knowledge on regulation has been gained from an extensive series of studies by Finkelstein mainly performed in animals [28]. An important, as yet largely unanswered question is how much of this information can be directly transferred to the human situation [29].

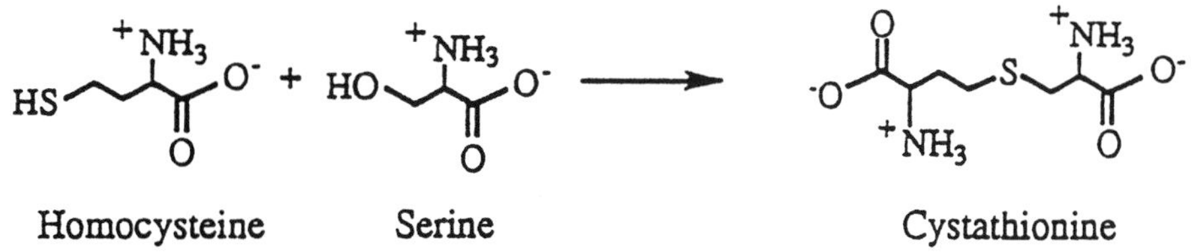

*Figure 1. Reaction catalyzed by CBS.*

CBS is regulated in two general ways. First, the intrinsic kinetic and allosteric properties of the enzyme allow immediate response to metabolite changes [28]. Second, changes in the level of CBS itself, as well as the enzymes of remethylation, can occur in response to a number of factors. These include protein or methionine content of the diet, hormones or age [29,30]. Enzymes of remethylation decrease while those of transsulfuration increase with increasing age in rats, changes which are also seen with increased dietary content of methionine [31,32]. In studies in humans the conversion of homocysteine to cystathionine was much lower on a methionine restricted than on a normal diet [33]. Thus a high methionine intake seems to favor transsulfuration at the expense of recycling of homocysteine through the remethylation pathway.

## CBS REACTION AND REGULATION

Human CBS (EC 4.2.1.22) catalyzes the condensation of homocysteine with serine to form cystathionine and one molecule of water (Figure 1). This reaction was first described by Selim and Greenberg in 1959 in extracts from rat liver [34]. These investigators were also the first to note the importance of PLP in the reaction. CBS enzyme activity is present at high levels in the mammalian liver, kidney and pancreas, and is present at lower levels in most other tissues [6]. In 1964 Mudd and colleagues demonstrated the presence of the enzyme in human liver, and showed that in patients with clinical homocystinuria this activity was absent [5]. Over the next thirty years, much more has become known about the enzyme due to advances in biochemical purification and the cloning of the cDNA for both the human and rat enzyme.

The human and rat CBS cDNAs are predicted to encode a molecule to 63 Kd, which is in good agreement with that observed during denaturing PAGE electrophoresis [35,36]. The enzyme is cytosolic and the predominant form appears to be a tetramer. Historically, there has been some confusion as to

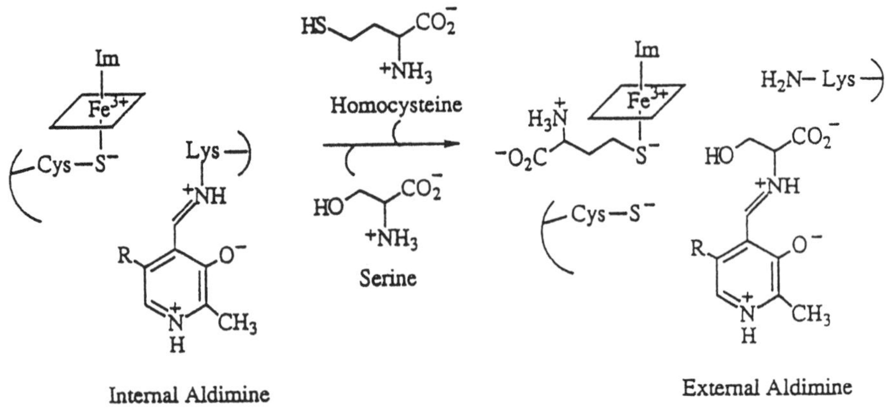

*Figure 2: Model for function of co-factors in CBS reaction. The left side of the reaction arrow shows the heme being bound to CBS by a cysteine and histidine (Im) residues. Another residue in CBS, lysine 119, binds PLP to form an internal Aldimine. When the enzyme binds serine and homocysteine (right of arrow) the homocysteine displaces the internal cysteine in heme binding, while lysine is displaced by serine to bind PLP. This then allows the condensation reaction to take place. Taken from [44] with permission.*

whether the tetramer or a dimer was the active species, and what was the actual size of the monomer. This confusion arose because the enzyme tended to be proteolyzed during purification from the liver [37]. The proteolyzed form runs at about 48Kd and was active as a dimer, while the full length form is a 63Kd protein and is active as a tetramer. Interestingly, the proteolyzed form appears to have about thirty-fold higher specific activity than the full length form. Recent studies suggest that the proteolyzed form is probably missing the C-terminal portion of the protein. Deletion of the C-terminal 145 amino acids results in the recombinant human protein being ten-fold more active *in vitro* [38,39]. Thus the C-terminal portion of CBS appears to be regulatory in nature.

The predicted CBS protein shares significant sequence similarity to several enzymes including prokaryotic cysteine synthase, threonine deaminase, and the β-chain of tryptophan synthase. The region of similarity between all three of these enzymes lies between amino acids 80 to 305 on the protein backbone. This similarity in primary amino acid sequence is also reflected in at least some conservation in tertiary structure as antibodies raized against human CBS strongly cross-react with yeast threonine deaminase [38]. All three of the above mentioned enzymes, like CBS, utilize PLP and catalyze the transformation of serine. Thus the conserved region probably encompasses the key catalytic regions of CBS, at least with regard to PLP and serine. Based on the similarity with the PLP crystal structure of tryptophan synthase [40], it is thought that CBS binds PLP at lysine 119.

A key role in the biochemistry of CBS is played by pyridoxal 5'-phosphate (PLP). The hypothesized role of PLP in the reaction mechanism is to bind serine and help make it more reactive (see [41] for review). The PLP moiety is thought to be bound to the ε-amino group of lysine 119 by a Schiff-base linkage. When serine is bound, this linkage shifts from the lysine to the serine α-amino group. Thus, the aldehyde group of PLP attacks the amine group of serine to produce an aldimine intermediate. The pyridoxal ring can act to stabilize electrons, and this allows the β-carbon of serine to be attacked by the sulfur atom of homocysteine. After the reaction is completed the PLP is transferred back to lysine again. Thus, the co-factor is transiently released by CBS during the actual enzyme chemistry.

Recently, it has been found that CBS also binds heme [42]. In fact the first described mammalian CBS cDNA sequence was initially identified in a search for rat proteins which bound heme [43]. Recombinant human CBS enzyme isolated from bacteria shows a linear relationship between increasing heme-content and activity [42]. This suggests that heme is required for enzyme activity. CBS also appears to bind heme and pyridoxine together in a equimolar ratio, and heme may be required for pyridoxine binding. The role of heme in CBS chemistry is uncertain because other pyridoxine-dependent enzymes such as tryptophan synthase and threonine deaminase are not thought to bind heme. One possible model (See Figure 2) is that the ferric iron in the heme acts to coordinate and activate the homocysteine thiol with its interaction with pyridoxine bound serine [44]. There are two attractive features of this model: First, the model provides an explanation for the absence of heme in other PLP dependent enzymes because the role of heme is specific to the chemistry of homocysteine and not serine. Second, the model provides a mechanism for the activation of the thiol *in lieu* of an active site zinc that is employed by other homocysteine-utilizing enzymes.

Stoichiometry studies suggest that one molecule of heme and one molecule of pyridoxine bind per dimer in the purified enzyme [44]. This relationship suggests that the reaction chemistry is taking place at the dimer interface. This result is somewhat surprising because in tryptophan synthase it is clear that each monomer binds a single PLP molecule. One possible explanation is that in purified preparations of CBS only one-half of the tetramers are actually active and binding PLP and heme. However, similar stoichiometry results have been observed in two different laboratories, in multiple enzyme preparations [42,44].

The activity of CBS is regulated by the presence of Adomet and by the redox state of the heme. Adomet stimulates CBS activity by significantly lowering the $K_m$ of CBS for homocysteine [45]. This results in a two to four fold increase in activity under most *in vitro* reaction conditions. More recently it has been observed that CBS activity can also be influenced *in vitro* by modification of redox conditions [44]. Specifically, under reducing conditions induced by titanium citrate or dithionite, the enzyme exhibits 1.7 fold lower levels of activity. This decrease in activity appears to be due to alteration of the redox state of the iron molecule in the heme of CBS because reducing agents which do not effect iron bound heme do not effect enzyme activity. This redox regulation may be biologically important because glutathione, a downstream product dependent on the CBS reaction, is the major intracellular regulator of redox potential.

## MOLECULAR GENETICS OF CBS DEFICIENCY

The *CBS* gene consists of 19 exons spread over a region of about 30 Kb on chromosome 21q22.3 [46]. There appear to be three transcripts generated for the gene with alternative usage of different exon 1 [47]. The major two transcripts encode for identical proteins and differ only in the use of different exons in the upstream UTR. Another transcript which would produce a N-terminally deleted protein is also produced, but this appears to be a minor transcript. The transcript expression pattern is similar to protein expression, i.e. high expression in the liver and kidney and reduced but detectable expression in most other tissues.

Since the isolation of the cDNA, much effort has revolved around characterizing mutations in the *CBS* gene present in patients with homocystinuria. To date, over 49 alterations in the CBS gene have been described in the literature (see Tab. 1) [35,38,48-63]. Greater than 90% percent of these alterations are predicted to cause missense changes in the protein. There are also two mutations, $G_{1356+1}A$ and $A_{1224-2}C$, in key intronic splicing sites which are predicted to cause in-frame deletions within the CBS protein due to exon skipping. The paucity of nonsense or truncating mutations in CBS deficient patients is surprising. One possible explanation is that a complete null allele of human *CBS* has viability problems. Interestingly, mice homozygous for a *in vitro* generated null allele of CBS show a very high rate of neo-natal lethality [64].

So far, the identified *CBS* mutations are located throughout the coding exons with most of them occurring or affecting exons 3-10. Interestingly only a few mutations have been observed in exons 11-15, which contain sequences which appear to be dispensable for CBS enzyme function [38,39]. The actual mechanism by which a particular CBS missense mutation affects enzyme function is generally not known, although some alleles appear to be associated

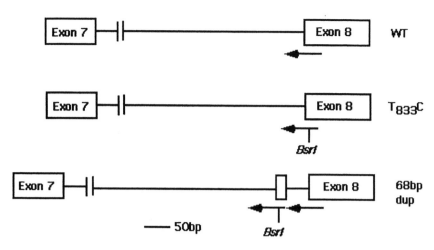

*Figure 3: Relationship between T833C and 68bp duplication allele. The region of CBS containing exon7, intron 7, and exon 8 is presented. The exons are represented by the boxes, while the intron is shown by the line. The large arrow indicates 68bp region that is duplicated in the 68bp duplication. The T833C mutation creates a new BsrI restriction site within this same region. It should be noted that the portion of exon 8 which is duplicated in the 68bp duplication allele is skipped over by the splicing machinery and is not processed into the mature mRNA.*

with pyridoxine responsive homocystinuria, while others do not (see below). It should be noted, however, that not all patients with identical CBS alleles have identical clinical phenotypes. In one report, very different clinical phenotypes were observed in three siblings with identical genotypes [27].

Most of the CBS alleles described to date have only been identified in a single patient, or in a few patients from the same geographic or ethnic population. However, a few of the alleles appear more frequently and deserve special mention. The G307S mutation has been observed to be very frequent in Irish pyridoxine non-responsive homocystinurics. Seventy percent of the mutations identified in Irish patients contain G307S [65]. Interestingly the rate of homocystinuria in Ireland is the highest in the world (about 1:50,000 births), and it is probably due to expansion of this allele. Although this allele has been observed in patients from other countries (USA, Norway, Australia) the frequency is much lower than in Ireland [55,58,59]. Interestingly in Italy, where one would expect little genetic admixture with Ireland, this allele has not been observed [57].

Another commonly observed mutation is the I278T allele. This alteration has been observed in populations throughout the world including Italy, Norway, Czechoslovakia, France, Australia and the United States [55,57,59,63]. It is commonly associated with pyridoxine responsive homocystinuria. This allele is probably derived by intragenic crossing over in chromosomes which contain the so-called 68bp duplication (see Figure 3) [66]. This duplication is found at a frequency of between 5-15% in various populations. The duplication contains a single base pair change which is identical to the I278T alteration. The duplication is benign because the first copy of the duplication is ignored by the splicing machinery. However, a intragenic recombination event which leaves behind the "mutant" copy and eliminates the wild type copy would give the I278T alteration.

At least two other pyridoxine-responsive alleles have been identified. The A114V allele is observed frequently in responders from Italy [57], while the R266K allele is responsible for the majority of pyridoxine responsive patients in Norway [55]. Homozygotes for the R266K mutation are actually "hyper" responsive; upon pyridoxine treatment their plasma tHcy levels are entirely normal. This allele has also been shown to be pyridoxine responsive when expressed in yeast cells.

Because the vast majority of alterations observed in CBS patients are of the missense variety it is difficulty to know whether a particular allele is a disease causing mutation or a benign polymorphism. To address this issue two different functional assays for human CBS have been developed. In the assay developed by Kozich and Kraus the human CBS cDNA containing the mutation to be tested is cloned and expressed in *E. Coli*, and then extracts derived from the bacteria are tested for CBS activity [56]. In the assay developed by Kruger and Cox the human cDNA is tested for function by its ability to complement the cysteine auxotrophy present in a yeast strain which is deleted for its endogenous CBS gene (*CYS4*) [54]. Both systems have been used effectively to characterize mutant *CBS* alleles.

## HETEROZYGOSITY FOR CBS AND VASCULAR DISEASE

The discovery of the association between premature vascular disease in adults and a disorder of homocysteine metabolism of a similar degree to that seen in obligate heterozygotes for CBS deficiency prompted the very important question - do heterozygotes also show vascular abnormalities?. This is significant because although homozygotes are rare, heterozygotes may represent up to 0.5% of the Caucasian population. In a questionnaire based study Mudd et al. [67] found no evidence of a higher frequency of strokes or heart attacks in relatives of CBS deficiency in 203 families. Possible limitations of the study were discussed in subsequent correspondence in the same journal [68,69]. Clarke et al. [70] reported no significant differences between 25 patients and controls using ultrasound measurements of neck arteries suggesting no increased vascular disease in obligate heterozygotes. In contrast, a further ultrasound study revealed slightly lower mean values of ankle/arm systolic pressure in 14 heterozygotes compared with age matched controls as well as the finding of arterial wall changes, 8 of 26 arteries of heterozygotes vs. 2 of 99 control arteries [71]. A later study based on ultrasound measurements of brachial artery diameters at rest, during reactive hyperemia and after nitroglycerin induced vasodilatation, revealed no impairment of flow mediated dilation or nitroglycerin responses in 14 obligate heterozygotes of 33-49 years of age [72]. Furthermore, de Valk et al. found no evidence of premature arteriosclerosis and reported no significant differences in ankle-brachial index or intima-media thickness in 23 heterozygotes aged between 18 and 50 years [73]. These authors pointed out the difficulty in design and interpretation of such studies due to incomparable ages, much lower numbers and the unpredictability of compounding genetic and environmental factors in obligate heterozygotes compared with hyperhomocysteinemic subjects.

Summarizing, studies so far have generally not found evidence of a higher incidence of premature vascular disease in obligate heterozygotes for CBS deficiency. A final answer to this question requires further studies with larger numbers and full consideration of compounding factors.


ENZYME STUDIES IN OBLIGATE HETEROZYGOTES

A number of studies have examined whether CBS heterozygotes have decreased CBS activity [22,70,74-81]. Most of these studies have measured enzyme activity in patient fibroblast extracts, although in two studies liver biopsies were used [82,83]. In almost all of these studies there was some overlap in values between the controls and obligate heterozygotes. In six studies in which the mean values in heterozygotes could be ascertained, CBS activity ranged from 20--41% of the mean control value with an average in all studies of 25%. This suggests a dominant negative effect in heterozygotes.

These studies taken together indicate a clear difference between group values but there is considerable overlap. Studies in cultured fibroblasts suffer from a number of difficulties. Tissue culture is time consuming and conditions can vary considerably. The collection of sufficient heterozygous subjects is tedious so that studies take place over a long period of time if sufficient numbers are to be included and thus exaggerating variations due to culture conditions. Also, the more controls that are included, the wider the distribution of values and the greater the likelihood of including heterozygotes in the control group.

Finally it must be noted that very low activities have been found in some obligate heterozygotes whilst some homocystinuric patients have appreciable residual activity. These reservations must be borne in mind when enzyme assay in fibroblasts is performed for diagnostic purposes [4].

## METABOLIC MEASUREMENTS: POST-METHIONINE LOADING

Because CBS has a higher $K_m$ for homocysteine than MS, it has been speculated that heterozygosity for CBS may be more easily detected under conditions of excess homocysteine. To produce such conditions, subjects are fed a large oral dose of methionine and then plasma homocysteine levels are determined at a pre-selected time after ingestion.

Early studies on the nature of the disorder based on methionine loading observed no consistent differences in metabolite levels, including sulfur amino acids in plasma [84-88] and sulfate excretion [89], between the very small numbers of heterozygotes investigated and control subjects. Sardharwalla et al. [90] first reported evidence for mildly disturbed metabolism of homocysteine in obligate heterozygotes in a detailed study of sulfur-containing amino acids in plasma and urine after a load of 100 mg of methionine per kg body weight. Features of the study were plasma measurements at 5 time points within the 12 hour post-load period and the use of a specific detection method for sulfur amino acids in urine. Small but clearly measurable amounts of homocystine and cysteine-homocysteine disulfide in plasma and urine all helped to distinguish the 12 heterozygous subjects from controls. A number of subsequent studies (reviewed by McGill [91]) confirmed differences on a group basis although a varying degree of overlap was found particularly in studies where only a single time point was measured. It must be noted that early studies measured free amino acids whereas later ones determined total homocysteine. For example, Murphy-Chutorian et al. [92] found free homocystine values, measured 6 hours post load, above the 95th centile of controls in 7 of 8 obligate heterozygotes. Boers et al. [78] measured the "peak total homocysteine" calculated from homocystine and cysteine-homocysteine values measured at 6 post load time points and were able to discriminate 18 of 20 heterozygotes but only if the menopausal status was considered. Brattstrom et al. [93] reported discrimination of only 12 out of 20 obligate heterozygotes by measuring total homocysteine in a single four hour post load sample.

Thus not only the exact metabolite measured but also the number and time of post load samples seem to play a role in the effectiveness of such tests. With regard to the time of post load increases of homocysteine we (B.F.) found maximum post load total homocysteine levels to vary widely in control subjects ranging from 2--12 hours, with a mean value of 7.2 hours [94]. Furthermore McGill et al. [91] pointed out that the inability of metabolic changes to consistently distinguish heterozygotes reflects complex properties of homeostasis of the pool size of a compound such as homocysteine which has more than one metabolic route.

## FASTING LEVELS

Although methionine loading can identify some heterozygous individuals, it is not a widely used procedure as it is cumbersome. A number of studies have measured fasting levels of total homocysteine, made possible by the introduction of more sensitive methods, but discrimination between obligate heterozygotes is considerably poorer than after methionine loading. For example, Sartorio et al. [77] found overlap with controls in 3 out of 9 heterozygotes when protein bound homocysteine was measured, while other studies found overlap of total homocysteine in 5 out of 10 [81] and 16 out of 20 [93] heterozygous subjects.

Recently Boddie et al. [95] claimed good discrimination between controls and the seven heterozygotes studied by measuring fasting total homocysteine/cysteine and homocysteine/folate ratios. This approach needs to be evaluated in much larger numbers to allow final assessment of its value as a practical test. This is reminiscent of the findings of Sardharwalla and Fowler [90] who reported homocysteine-cysteine disulfide to cystine, homocysteine to cystine, and homocysteic acid to cysteic acid ratios in urine of heterozygotes.

Brattström et al. [93] reported a significant negative correlation between fasting total homocysteine, folic acid, and $B_{12}$ and also that pyridoxine administration reduced post methionine homocysteine levels but not fasting levels. Thus fasting total homocysteine probably reflects disturbed remethylation of homocysteine whereas post methionine levels are possibly related to CBS activity.

Recent information relating metabolite levels to mutations showed post methionine load total homocysteine levels within the control range in 4 subjects heterozygous for the I278T allele (associated with $B_6$ responsive homocystinuria) [81,96] and in one carrying the G307S allele [97] although Sperandeo et al. [96] reported only one post-load measurement. This indicates variability of phenotypic expression in heterozygotes.

The large degree of overlap between obligate heterozygotes and controls, especially with the more simplified tests used in studying vascular disease patients, prevents definitive identification of heterozygosity in an individual. This has important implications for studies of vascular disease patients since it cannot be certain whether such studies underestimate or overestimate "abnormal" methionine metabolism within these patients.

## CBS AND MILD HYPERHOMOCYSTEINEMIA

Several reports have appeared associating low levels of CBS activity in patient fibroblasts with increased risk of vascular disease. In two studies patient fibroblast CBS activities were shown to be decreased in vascular disease patients who also showed increased post methionine load homocysteine values [70,98], to a similar extent as those in obligate heterozygotes for CBS deficiency. Subsequently Dudman et al. [99] described a group of 15 subjects with vascular disease and post load hyperhomocysteinemia with mean CBS activity of 48% of control values. Nordstrom and Kjellstrom [79] also found low fibroblast activities of this enzyme in vascular disease patients but these could not be interpreted as abnormal due to the low values found in older controls.

Molecular genetic studies have failed to identify a mutation in the structural domain of the CBS gene as a cause of hyperhomocysteinemia in these patients. Kozich et al. [100] analyzed 7 of the 8 possible individual alleles from four such patients in a bacterial expression system and found that normal catalytic activity was encoded. In addition, sequence analysis of cDNA from both alleles in cells of one patient showed no evidence of a mutation. Nevertheless decreased amounts of normally active enzyme molecules were shown to be present in the patient cultures thereby explaining the decreased specific activity of CBS. Two studies reported no increased prevalence of a CBS mutation known to be common in homozygous homocystinuric patients in the particular population in vascular disease patients with mild hyperhomocysteinemia. Thus the I278T mutation was absent in 60 vascular disease patients in Holland and the G307S mutation was not detected in 100 Irish patients [101].

Therefore, mild hyperhomocysteinemia seems not to be caused by heterozygosity for CBS. However decreased CBS activity due to some other possibly subtle change affecting expression of the enzyme remains to be excluded. Also mutations in the promoter or control region of the gene have not been excluded.

## CBS AS A PHARMACOLOGIC TARGET

Given the key role of CBS in the regulation of homocysteine metabolism, some thought must be given to its potential as a target for drugs which could be used to lower plasma homocysteine levels, and thus reduce one's risk for vascular disease. Until recently, CBS seemed to be a poor target, since most drugs work by inhibiting the function of specific proteins and not enhancing their function. However, the recent discovery that the C-terminal quarter of CBS acts as a negative regulatory domain suggests that this domain of CBS may be a reasonable pharmacologic target [38]. Conceivably, drugs could be developed which interact with the C-terminal domain in such a way as to stimulate CBS activity, and thus lower plasma homocysteine levels. As more structural and functional data on CBS are accumulated the feasibility of this strategy for lowering plasma homocysteine levels will become clearer.

*Acknowledgments. B. Fowler acknowledges the support of the Swiss National Science Foundation (Grant No. 32-45988.95). W. Kruger acknowledges support of the National Institutes of Health (Grant No. HL57288). Special thanks to Rose Sonlin for secretarial support.*

## REFERENCES

1.  Carson NAJ, Neill DW. Metabolic abnormalities detected in a survey of mentally backward individuals in Northern Ireland. Arch Dis Childh 1962;37:505-13.
2.  Gerritsen T, Vaughn JG, Waisman HA. The identification of homocystine in the urine. Biochem Biophys Res Commun 1962;9:493-96.
3.  Schimke NR, McKusick VA, Huang Th, Pollack AD. Homocystinuria. A study of 20 families with 38 affected members. JAMA 1965;193:711-19.
4.  Fowler B, Jakobs C. Post- and prenatal diagnostic methods for the homocystinurias. Eur J Pediat 1998;157:S88-93.
5.  Mudd SH, Finkelstein JD, Irreverre F, Laster L. Homocystinuria: an enzymatic defect. Science 1964;143:1443-45.
6.  Mudd S, Finkelstein J, Irreverre F, Laster L. Transsulfuration in mammals: microassays and tissue distributions of three enzymes of the pathway. J Biol Chem 1965;240:4382-92.
7.  Uhlendorf BW, Mudd SH. Cystathionine synthase in tissue culture derived from human skin: enzyme defect in human fibroblasts. Science 1968;160:1007-09.
8.  Goldstein JL, Cambell B, Gartler S. Cystathionine synthase activity in human lymphocytes: induction by phytohemaglutinin. J Clin Invest 1972;51:1034-37.

9. McKusick VA, Hall JG, Char F. The clinical and genetic characteristics of homocystinuria. In: Carson NAJ, Raine DN, editors. Inherited disorders of sulfur metabolism. London: Churchill Livingstone Ltd, 1971: 179-203.

10. Wicken B, Turner G. Homocystinuria in New South Wales. Arch Dis Childh 1978;53:242-45.

11. Boers GHJ, Polder TW, Cruysberg JRM, et al. Homocystinuria versus Marfan's syndrome: the therapeutic relevance of the differential diagnosis. Neth J Med 1984;27:206-12.

12. de Franchis R, Sperandeo MP, Sebastio G, Andria G. Clinical aspects of cystathionine β-synthase deficiency: how wide is the spectrum? Eur J Pediat 1998;157 Suppl:S67-70.

13. Mudd SH, Levy HL, Skovby F. Disorders of transsulfuration. In: Scriver CR, Beaudet AL, Sly WS, Valle D, editors. The metabolic and molecular basis of inherited disease. 7th ed. New York: McGraw-Hill Book Co, 1995: 1279-327.

14. Cruysberg JRM, Boers GHJ, Trijbels JMF, Deutman AF. Delay in diagnosis of homocystinuria: retrospective study of consecutive patients. Br Med J 1996;313:1037-40.

15. Barber GW, Spaeth GL. The successful treatment of homocystinuria with pyridoxine. J Pediatr 1969;75:463-78.

16. Fowler B. Recent advances in the mechanism of pyridoxine-responsive disorders. J Inher Metab Dis 1985;8(Suppl. 1):76-83.

17. Mudd SH, Skovby F, Levy HL, et al. The natural history of homocystinuria due to cystathionine β-synthase deficiency. Am J Hum Genet 1985;37:1-31.

18. Gaull GE, Rassin DK, Sturman JA. Enzymatic and metabolic studies of homocystinuria: effects of pyridoxine. Neuropaediatrie 1969;1:199-226.

19. Mudd SH, Edwards WA, Loeb PM, Brown MS, Laster L. Homocystinuria due to cystathionine synthase deficiency. The effect of pyridoxine. J Clin Invest 1970;49:1762-73.

20. Lipson MH, Kraus J, Rosenberg LE. Affinity of cystathionine β-synthase for pyridoxal 5′-phosphate in cultured cells. J Clin Invest 1980;66:188-93.

21. Lipson MH, Kraus J, Solomon L.R, Rosenberg LE. Depletion of cultured human fibroblasts of pyridoxal 5′-phosphate: effect on activities of aspartate aminotransferase, alanine aminotransferase, and cystathionine β-synthase. Arch Biochem Biophys 1980;204:486-93.

22. Uhlendorf BW, Conerly EB, Mudd SH. Homocystinuria: studies in tissue culture. Pediat Res 1973;7:645-58.

23. Fowler B, Kraus J, Packman S, Rosenberg LE. Homocystinuria: evidence for three distinct classes of cystathionine β-synthase mutants in cultured fibroblasts. J Clin Invest 1978;61:645-53.

24. Walter JH, Wraith JE, White FJ, Bridge C, Till J. Strategies for the treatment of cystathionine β-synthase deficiency: the experience of the Willink Biochemical Genetics Unit over the past 30 years. Eur J Pediat 1998;157 Suppl:S71-S76.

25. Wilcken DEL, Wilcken B. The natural history of vascular disease in homocystinuria and the effects of treatment. J Inher Metab Dis 1997;20: 295-300.

26. Naughten ER, Yap S, Mayne PD. Newborn screening for homocystinuria: Irish and world experience. Eur J Pediat 1998;157 Suppl:S84-87.

27. Stabler SP, Marcell PD, Podell ER, Allen RH, Savage DG, Lindenbaum J. Elevation of total homocysteine in the serum of patients with cobalamin or folate deficiency detected by capillary gas chromatography-mass spectrometry. J Clin Invest 1988;81:466-74.

28. Finkelstein JD. Methionine metabolism in mammals. J Nutr Biochem 1990;1:228-37.

29. Löhrer FMT, Schwab R, Angst CP, Haefeli WE, Fowler B. Influence of S-adenosylmethionine administration on S-adenosylhomocysteine, homocysteine and 5-methyltetrahydrofolate in healthy humans. J Pharmacol Exper Therapeut 1997;292:845-50.

30. Finkelstein JD. Control of sulfur metabolism. In: Oldfield JE, Muth OH, editors. Sulfur in nutrition. Westport, CT: Avi Press, 1970: 46-60.

31. Finkelstein JD. Regulation of methionine metabolism in mammals. In: Usdin E, Borchardt RT, Creveling CR, editors. Transmethylation. New York: Elsevier/North-Holland, 1979: 49-58.

32. Finkelstein JD, Martin JJ. Methionine metabolism in mammals. Adaptation to methionine excess. J Biol Chem 1986;261:1582-87.

33. Finkelstein JD, Mudd SH. Transsulfuration in mammals. The methionine sparing effect of cystine. J Biol Chem 1967;242:873-80.

34. Selim AS, Greenberg DM. An enzyme that synthesizes cystathionine and deaminates L-serine. J Biol Chem 1959;234:1474-80.

35. Kraus JP, Le K, Swaroop M, et al. Human cystathionine β-synthase cDNA: sequence, alternative splicing and expression in cultured cells. Hum Mol Genet 1993;2(10):1633-38.

36. Skovby F, Kraus JP, Rosenberg LE. Homocystinuria: biogenesis of cystathionine β-synthase subunits in cultured fibroblasts and in an in vitro translation system programmed with fibroblast messenger RNA. Am J Hum Genet 1984;36(2):452-59.

37. Skovby F, Kraus JP, Rosenberg LE. Biosynthesis and proteolytic activation of cystathionine β-synthase in rat liver. J Biol Chem 1984;259(1):588-93.

38. Shan X, Kruger WD. Correction of disease-causing CBS mutations in yeast. Nat Genet 1998;19:91-3.

39. Kery V, Poneleit L, Kraus JP. Trypsin cleavage of human cystathionine β-synthase into an evolutionarily conserved active core: structural and functional consequences. Arch Biochem Biophys 1998;355(2):222-32.

40. Isupov MN, Antson AA, Dodson EJ, et al. Crystal structure of tryptophanase. J Mol Biol 1998;276(3):603-23.

41. Zubay G. Biochemistry. Reading, MA: Addison-Wesley Publishing, Inc, 1989:202-07.

42. Kery V, Bukovska G, Kraus JP. Transsulfuration depends on heme in addition to pyridoxal 5′-phosphate. Cystathionine β-synthase is a heme protein. J Biol Chem 1994;269(41):25283-88.

43. Ishihara S, Morohashi K, Sadano H, Kawabata S, Gotoh O, Omura T. Molecular cloning and sequence analysis of cDNA coding for rat liver hemoprotein H-450. J Biochem 1990;108(6):899-902.

44. Taoka S, Ohja S, Shan X, Kruger WD, Banerjee R. Evidence of heme-mediated redox regulation of human cystathionine β-synthase activity. J Biol Chem 1998 (in press).

45. Roper MD, Kraus JP. Rat cystathionine β-synthase: expression of four alternatively spliced isoforms in transfected cultured cells. Arch Biochem Biophys 1992;298(2):514-21.

46. Chasse JF, Paly E, Paris D, et al. Genomic organization of the human cystathionine β-synthase gene: evidence for various cDNAs. Biochem Biophys Res Commun 1995;211(3):826-32.

47. Chasse JF, Paul V, Escanez R, Kamoun P, London J. Human cystathionine β-synthase: gene organization and expression of different 5′ alternative splicing. Mamm Genome 1997;8(12):917-21.

48. de Franchis R, Kozich V, McInnes RR, Kraus JP. Identical genotypes in siblings with different homocystinuric phenotypes: identification of three mutations in cystathionine β-synthase using an improved bacterial expression system. Hum Mol Genet 1994;3(7):1103-08.

49. Sebastio G, Sperandeo, M.P., Panico, M., de Franchis, R., Kraus, J.P., Andria, G. The molecular basis of homocystinuria due to cystathionine β-synthase deficiency in Italian families, and report of four novel mutations. Am J Hum Genet 1995;56:1324-33.

50. Kozich V, de Franchis R, Kraus JP. Molecular defect in a patient with pyridoxine-responsive homocystinuria. Hum Mol Genet 1993;2(6):815-16.

51. Kluijtmans L. Molecular genetic analysis in hyperhomocysteinemia. Nijmegen: University of Nijmegen, 1998: 190.

52. Marble M, Geraghty MT, de Franchis R, Kraus JP, Valle D. Characterization of a cystathionine β-synthase allele with three mutations in cis in a patient with B₆ nonresponsive homocystinuria. Hum Mol Genet 1994;3(10):1883-86.

53. Shih VE, Fringer JM, Mandell R, et al. A missense mutation (I278T) in the cystathionine β-synthase gene prevalent in pyridoxine-responsive homocystinuria and associated with mild clinical phenotype. Am J Hum Genet 1995;57(1):34-9.

54. Kruger WD, Cox DR. A yeast assay for functional detection of mutations in the human cystathionine β-synthase gene. Hum Mol Genet 1995;4(7):1155-61.

55. Kim CE, Gallagher PM, Guttormsen AB, et al. Functional modeling of vitamin responsiveness in yeast: a common pyridoxine-responsive cystathionine β-synthase mutation in homocystinuria. Hum Mol Genet 1997;6(13):2213-21.

56. Kozich V, Kraus JP. Screening for mutations by expressing patient cDNA segments in E. coli: homocystinuria due to cystathionine β-synthase deficiency. Hum Mutat 1992;1(2):113-23.

57. Sperandeo MP, Panico M, Pepe A, et al. Molecular analysis of patients affected by homocystinuria due to cystathionine β-synthase deficiency: Report of a new mutation in exon 8 and a deletion in intron 11. J Inherit Metab Dis 1995;18(2):211-14.

58. Hu FL, Gu Z, Kozich V, Kraus JP, Ramesh V, Shih VE. Molecular basis of cystathionine β-synthase deficiency in pyridoxine responsive and nonresponsive homocystinuria. Hum Mol Genet 1993;2(11):1857-60.

59. Dawson PA, Cox AJ, Emmerson BT, Dudman NP, Kraus JP, Gordon RB. Characterisation of five missense mutations in the cystathionine β-synthase gene from three patients with B₆-nonresponsive homocystinuria. Eur J Hum Genet 1997;5(1):15-21.

60. Kraus JP. Komrower Lecture. Molecular basis of phenotype expression in homocystinuria. J Inherit Metab Dis 1994;17(4):383-90.

61. Aral B, Coude M, London J, et al. Two novel mutations (K384E and L539S) in the C-terminal moiety of the cystathionine β-synthase protein in two French pyridoxine-responsive homocystinuria patients. Hum Mutat 1997;9(1):81-2.

62. Tsai MY, Wong PW, Garg U, Hanson NQ, Schwichtenberg K. Identification of a splice site mutation in the cystathionine β-synthase gene resulting in variable and novel splicing defects of pre-mRNA. Biochem Mol Med 1997;61(1):9-15.

63. Kozich V, Janosik M, Sokolova J, et al. Analysis of CBS alleles in Czech and Slovak patients with homocystinuria: report on three novel mutations E176K, W409X and 1223 + 37 del99. J Inherit Metab Dis 1997;20(3):363-66.

64. Watanabe M, Osada J, Aratani Y, et al. Mice deficient in cystathionine β-synthase: animal models for mild and severe homocyst(e)inemia. Proc Natl Acad Sci USA 1995;92(5):1585-89.

65. Gallagher PM, Ward P, Tan S, et al. High frequency of cystathionine β-synthase mutation g307s in Irish homocystinuria patients. Hum Mutat 1995;6:177-80.

66. Tsai MY, Bignell MK, Schwichtenberg KA, Hanson NQ. High prevalence of a mutation in the cystathionine β-synthase gene. Am J Hum Genet 1996;59(6):1262-67.

67. Mudd SH, Havlik R, Levy HL, McKusick VA, Feinleib M. A study of cardiovascular risk in heterozygotes for homocystinuria. Am J Hum Genet 1981;33:883-93.

68. Swift M, Morrell D. Cardiovascular risk in homocystinuria family members. Am J Hum Genet. 1982;34:1016-18.

69. Mudd SH, Havlik R, Levy HL, McKusick VA, Feinleib M. Cardiovascular risk in heterozygotes for homocystinuria. Am J Hum Genet. 1982;34:1018-21.

70. Clarke R, Daly L, Robinson K, Naughten E, Cahalane S, Fowler B, Graham I. Hyper-homocysteinemia: an independent risk factor for vascular disease. N Engl J Med 1991; 324:1149-55.

71. Rubba P, Faccenda F, Pauciullo P, et al. Early signs of vascular disease in homocystinuria - a noninvasive study by ultrasound methods in eight families with cystathionine-β-synthase deficiency. Metabolism 1990;39:1191-95.

72. Celermajer DS, Sorensen K, Ryalls M, et al. Impaired endothelial function occurs in the systemic arteries of children with homozygous homocystinuria but not in their heterozygous parents. J Am Coll Cardiol 1993;22:854-58.

73. Devalk H W, Vaneeden MKG, Banga JD, et al. Evaluation of the presence of premature atherosclerosis in adults with heterozygosity for cystathionine-β-synthase deficiency. Stroke 1996;27:1134-36.

74. Fleisher LD, Tallan HH, Beratis NG, Hirschhorn K, Gaull GE. Cystathionine synthase deficiency: heterozygote detection using cultured skin fibroblasts. Biochem Biophys Res Comm 1973 55:38-45.

75. Bittles AH, Carson NAJ. Tissue culture techniques as an aid to prenatal diagnosis and genetic counseling in homocystinuria. J Med Genet 1973;10:120-21.

76. Bittles AH, Carson NAJ. Homocystinuria: studies on cystathionine β-synthase, S-adenosylmethionine synthetase and cystathionase activities in skin fibroblasts. J Inher Metab Dis 1981;4:3-6.

77. Sartorio R, Carrozzo R, Corbo L, Andria G. Protein-bound plasma homocyst(e)ine and identification of heterozygotes for cystathionine-synthase deficiency. J Inher Metab Dis 1986;9:25-9.

78. Boers GHJ, Fowler B, Smals AGH, et al. Improved identification of heterozygotes for homocystinuria due to cystathionine β-synthase deficiency by the combination of methionine loading and enzyme determination in cultured fibroblasts. Hum Genet 1985;69:164-69.

79. Nordstrom M, Kjellstrom T. Age dependency of cystathionine β-synthase activity in human fibroblasts in homocyst(e)inemia and atherosclerotic vascular disease. Atherosclerosis 1992;94:213-21.

80. Steegers-Theunissen RP, Boers GH, Trijbels FJ, et al. Maternal hyperhomocysteinemia: a risk factor for neural-tube defects? Metabolism 1994;43:1475-80.

81. Tsai MY, Garg U, Key NS, Hanson NQ, Suh A, Schwichtenberg K. Molecular and biochemical approaches in the identification of heterozygotes for homocystinuria. Atherosclerosis 1996;122:69-77.

82. Laster L, Spaeth GL, Mudd SH, Finklestein JD. Homocystinuria due to cystathionine synthase deficiency. Combined clinical staff conference at the National Institutes of Health. Annals Int Med 1965;63:1117-42.

83. Gaull G, Sturman JA, Schaffner F. Homocystinuria due to cystathionine synthase deficiency: enzymatic and ultrastructural studies. J Pediat 1974;84:381-90.

84. White HH, Araki S, Thompson HL, Rowland LP, Cowen D. Homocystinuria. Trans Am Neurol Assoc 1964;89:24-7.

85. Brenton DP, Cusworth DC, Gaull GE. Homocystinuria: metabolic studies of 3 patients. J Pediatr 1965;67:58.

86. Kennedy C, Shih VE, Rowland LP. Homocystinuria: a report in two siblings. Pediatrics 1965;36:736-41.

87. Dunn HG, Perry TL, Dolman CL. Homocystinuria, a recently discovered cause of mental defect and cerebrovascular thrombosis. Neurology 1966;16:407-20.

88. Chase HP, Goodman SI, O'Brian D. Treatment of homocystinuria. Arch Dis Childh 1967;42:514-20.

89. Laster L, Mudd SH, Finkelstein JD, Irreverre F. Homocystinuria due to cystathionine synthase deficiency; the metabolism of L-methionine. J Clin Invest 1965;44:1708-19.

90. Sardharwalla IB, Fowler B, Robins AJ, Komrower GM Detection of heterozygotes for homocystinuria. Study of sulfur-containing amino acids in plasma and urine after L-methionine loading. Arch Dis Childh 1974;49:553-59

91. McGill JJ, Mettler G, Rosenblatt DS, Scriver CR. Detection of heterozygotes for recessive alleles. Homocyst(e)inemia: paradigm of pitfalls in phenotypes. Am J Med Genet 1990;36:45-52.

92. Murphy-Chutorian DR, Wexman MP, Grieco AJ, et al. Methionine intolerance: a possible risk factor for coronary artery disease. J Am Coll Cardiol 1985;6:725-30.

93. Brattstrom L, Israelsson B, Norrving B, et al. Impaired homocysteine metabolism in early onset cerebral and peripheral occlusive arterial disease. Effects of pyridoxine and folic acid treatment. Atherosclerosis 1990;81:51-60.

94. Löhrer FMT, Angst CP, Brown G, Frick G, Haefeli WE, Fowler B. The effect of methionine loading on 5-methyltetrahydrofolate, S-adenosylmethionine and S-adenosylhomocysteine in plasma of healthy humans. Clin Sci 1996;91:79-86.

95. Boddie AM, Steen MT, Sullivan KM, et al. Cystathionine-β-synthase deficiency: detection of heterozygotes by the ratios of homocysteine to cysteine and folate Metabolism 1998;47:207-11.

96. Sperandeo MP, Candito M, Sebastio G, et al. Homocysteine response to methionine challenge in four obligate heterozygotes for homocystinuria and relationship with cystathionine β-synthase mutations. J Inher Met Dis 1996;19:351-56.

97. Dawson PA, Kraus JP, Cochran DAE, Dudman NPB, Emmerson BT, Gordon RB. Variable hyperhomocysteinemia phenotype in heterozygotes for the Gly307Ser mutation in cystathionine β-synthase. Austral New Zealand J Med 1996;26:180-85.

98. Boers GHJ, Smals AGH, Trijbels FJM, Fowler B, Bakkeren AJM, Schoonderwaldt HC, Kleijer, WJ Kloppenborg PWC. Heterozygosity for homocystinuria in premature peripheral and cerebral occlusive arterial disease. N Engl J Med 1985;313:709-15.

99. Dudman NPB, Wilcken DEL, Wang J, Lynch JF, Macey D Lundberg P. Disordered methionine homocysteine metabolism in premature vascular disease - its occurrence cofactor therapy and enzymology. Arterio Thromb 1993;13:1253-60.

100. Kozich V, Kraus E, de Franchis R, Fowler B, Boers GHJ, Graham I, Kraus JP. Hyperhomocysteinemia in premature arterial disease: examination of cystathionine β-synthase alleles at the molecular level. Hum Mol Genet 1995;4:623-29.

101. Kluijtmans LAJ, van den Heuvel LPWJ, Boers GHJ, et al. Molecular genetic analysis in mild hyperhomocysteinemia: a common mutation in the methylenetetrahydrofolate reductase gene is a genetic risk factor for cardiovascular disease. Am J Hum Genet 1996;58:35-41.

# 19. HOMOCYSTEINE AND CHOLESTEROL: BASIC AND CLINICAL INTERACTIONS

HENK J. BLOM

## SUMMARY

Homocysteine in its reduced form is a two-edged sword. On the one hand its oxidation to disulfides can produce reactive oxygen species. On the other hand its free thiol function can scavenge reactive oxygen species. The use of un-physiologic forms and amounts of homocysteine blur most in vitro and animal studies on the pathobiochemical mechanism of hyperhomocysteinemia. Cholesterol itself has few atherogenic properties and requires oxidative modification to expose its cytotoxicity. If hyperhomocysteinemia leads to increased production of reactive oxygen species *in vivo*, homocysteine may interact with cholesterol cytotoxicity by oxidative modification of LDL.

There is virtually no evidence of increased lipid peroxidation in patients with mild or severe hyperhomocysteinemia. In these patients hyper-homocysteinemia may even lead to an increased anti-oxidant capacity. Also no strong interaction between homocysteine and cholesterol is observed in case/control studies. The relation between hyperhomocysteinemia and choles-terol as risk factors for cardiovascular disease is no more than additive in pa-tients with vascular disease. No synergistic interactions were observed. Evi-dence is accumulating that homocysteine inhibits endothelial dependent vaso-dilation. Hyperhomocysteinemia seems to affect the acute atherothrombotic process, in contrast to hypercholesterolemia where long exposure will eventu-ally lead to lipid accumulation in the vascular wall resulting in arterial ob-struction. In conclusion, in humans hyperhomocysteinemia does not seem to

*K. Robinson (ed.), Homocysteine and Vascular Disease, 335-348.*
© 2000 *Kluwer Academic Publishers. Printed in the Netherlands.*

cause increased lipid peroxidation. It even may be that increased homocysteine concentrations may protect lipids against peroxidation.


## INTRODUCTION

The story of hyperhomocysteinemia as a common risk factor for arterial and venous occlusive disease arises from the observations that patients with the rare inborn error of metabolism cystathionine β-synthase (CBS) deficiency suffer from a very high risk of arteriosclerosis and thrombosis (1). Further observations showed that patients with defects of homocysteine remethylation also have a very high risk of obstruction of the arterial or venous system (2). These findings show that, irrespective of its cause, severe elevations of homocysteine are toxic for the vascular system.

More than 20 years ago Wilcken and Wilcken (3) were the first to investigate whether mild elevations of homocysteine are also related to an increased risk for coronary artery disease (CAD). More than 80 studies of different retrospective and prospective design have lead to the acceptance of mild hyperhomocysteinemia as a common risk factor for arterial as well as venous occlusive disease (4).

In the field of hyperhomocysteinemia two main questions are yet unanswered:

A.  Will homocysteine lowering therapy reduce the risk of vascular and venous obstruction in patients with mild hyperhomocysteinemia?

B.  Via which mechanism(s) does homocysteine affects the vascular system?

A. Again studies on patients with inborn errors of homocysteine metabolism revealed what we may expect from homocysteine lowering therapy. Administration of vitamin $B_6$ singly or in combination with folic acid and betaine to patients with CBS deficiency not only strongly reduces their homocysteine concentrations but also significantly reduces their risk of arterial and venous disease (1,5). In mild hyperhomocysteinemia the use of these B-vitamins will decrease plasma homocysteine by about 30%, but whether this will also reduce the risk of vascular disease in patients with mild hyperhomocysteinemia is yet unanswered. Intervention studies are currently initiated or executed (6).

B. Although many studies on possible pathogenic properties of homocysteine have been performed (4,7), there is yet no satisfying mechanism available. Two reasons can explain this lack of success: 1. the use of physiologically irrelevant forms of homocysteine, like D-homocysteine 2. in many studies an extremely high concentration of homocysteine in its reduced form is used (8). In biochemistry it is well known that the use of β-mercapto-ethanol or dithio

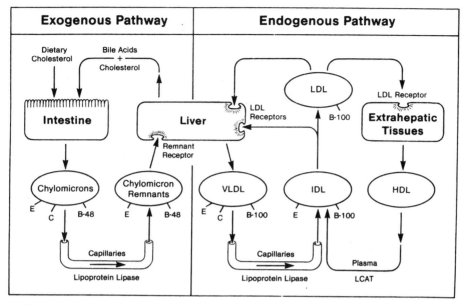

*Figure 1. Exogenous and endogenous cholesterol metabolism. HDL denotes high-density lipoprotein, LDL low-density lipoprotein, IDL intermediate-density lipoprotein, VLDL very-low-density lipoprotein, LCAT lecithin:cholesterol acyltransferase.*

threitol (DDT) effects the function of most proteins by converting disulfide bounds to free sulfhydryl groups. This effect will also be achieved if homocysteine is applied in millimolar concentrations. It should be kept in mind that in plasma only about 1% of the total homocysteine is present as reduced homocysteine (9-15). This means that in mild hyperhomocysteinemia with a total homocysteine concentration of about 20 μmol/L, only about 0.2 μmol/L is present as free reduced homocysteine.

CHOLESTEROL

In the body cholesterol is transported by different lipoproteins (Fig. 1). About 70% of total cholesterol in blood is contained in low density lipoproteins (LDL) particles, which transports cholesterol from the liver to different tissues in the body. The LDL concentration of blood is mediated by LDL-receptors (16) and occurs mainly by the liver. High density lipoproteins (HDL) contain about 20% of blood total cholesterol and transport cholesterol from the tissues back to the liver (reverse cholesterol transport). In the liver cholesterol can be degraded or excreted in the gut (as bile acids) or incorporated again into LDL.

338     *Henk J. Blom*

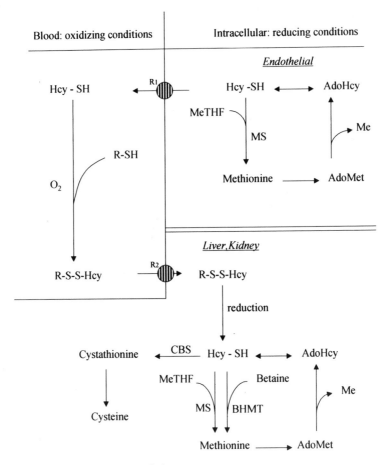

*Figure 2. Homocysteine metabolism.*

LDL is considered the atherogenic component of total cholesterol, whereas HDL cholesterol is inversely associated with coronary heart disease. A total cholesterol determination is much simpler than the measurement of all the different cholesterol containing lipoproteins. Therefore, in large epidemiological studies total cholesterol is measured as an indication of LDL levels because of the strong correlation between LDL cholesterol and total cholesterol concentrations.

Cholesterol itself has few atherogenic properties. Only after oxidative modification does cholesterol become cytotoxic. After depletion of all the antioxidants present in LDL, the lipid peroxidation process of LDL starts with the peroxidation of poly-unsaturated fatty acids in LDL lipids, which is followed by their degradation to a complex variety of products as conjugated dienes and aldehydes (17,18). Thus, the anti-oxidant content as well as the poly-unsaturated fatty acid composition and concentration of LDL play an important role in determining the susceptibility of LDL to oxidative modification. This oxidative modification is not likely to occur in the circulation because of the high anti-oxidant content. It is assumed that the oxidative modification takes place primarily in the intima, in micro domains, which are devoid of well equipped anti-oxidant mechanisms. Oxidized LDL is taken up by the macrophages via specific scavenger receptors, which do not recognize native LDL and are not under control of intracellular cholesterol (19-21). This uncontrolled uptake of excess modified lipoprotein lipids leads to accumulation in the macrophages, which eventually will result in conversion to foam cells. In the arterial wall this will give rise to the formation of fatty streaks, the early stage of the atherosclerotic lesion. Continuation of this process can result in arterial obstruction.


## HOMOCYSTEINE

### Metabolism

For understanding the role of homocysteine in the aetiology of arterial and venous disease an insight into homocysteine metabolism and transport is required. This is extensively reviewed in Chapter 3. In the liver all homocysteine metabolizing enzymes are present. On the one hand homocysteine can be irreversibly degraded to cystathionine by CBS, which requires for adequate function pyridoxal-5-phosphate (PLP), an active form of vitamin $B_6$. Cystathionine can further be converted to cysteine by cystathionase. On the other hand the homocysteine moiety can be salvaged by remethylation to methionine by either methionine synthase (MS) or betaine-homocysteine-methyltransferase (BHMT). Methionine synthase is a complex enzyme, which in addition to 5-methyltetrahydrofolate (MeTHF) for methyl donation, also requires cobalamin for methyltransport and S-adenosylmethionine (AdoMet) for activation (22). MeTHF is formed out of methylene-THF by MTHFR.

The product of homocysteine remethylation is methionine, which is required for protein synthesis. An unique property of methionine is its activation to AdoMet by methionine adenosyl transferase (MAT) and ATP. AdoMet donates its methyl group in over 100 different reactions such as methylation of DNA, proteins and phospholipids. The product S-adenosyl-homocysteine (AdoHcy) is hydrolyzed to adenosine and homocysteine.

Outside the liver and kidney homocysteine metabolism is fully dependent on the folate and cobalamin dependent remethylation or on homocysteine export out of the cell, because BHMT is virtually not present. Although CBS is measurable in most tissues, its peripheral activity seems to be too low to contribute to homocysteine metabolism (23,24). Concerning the vascular endothelial cells, this means that as soon as capacity of the folic acid dependent homocysteine remethylation is exceeded homocysteine will be exported into the blood.

## Homocysteine export and consequences

Homocysteine export has gained relatively little attention (24-27), although it may regulate homocysteine concentrations in the cell within strict limits. In the cell glutathione, cysteine and homocysteine are present in their reduced form. Due to the high oxygen content, homocysteine in the blood is oxidized to a disulfide with different thiol containing compounds: itself, cysteine or proteins. Homocysteine can also perform a disulfide exchange reaction with any other disulfide. Consequently, in blood only a minimal amount of about 1% of the total concentration of homocysteine is present as reduced homocysteine (11-15). So, as soon as homocysteine is exported to the blood it will oxidize to a disulfide with itself, cysteine and plasma proteins (Fig. 2). As a consequence, plasma homocysteine present in disulfides cannot directly be imported to the endothelial cells by the homocysteine exporting carrier. The oxidized forms of homocysteine present in plasma probably need to be taken up by the cell via another mechanism, before homocysteine can be liberated from its disulfide bonds by reduction and become available for conversion by the different homocysteine converting enzymes. During the filtering of blood in the kidney most homocysteine binding compounds except proteins will pass through the kidney cells, where homocysteine can be liberated by reduction of the disulfides. This may explain why proper kidney function is extremely important for maintaining normal homocysteine concentrations in plasma, although in man there is little net extraction of homocysteine by the kidney (see chapter 15).

## Experiments with non-physiologic concentrations of homocysteine.

As indicated above only about 1% of total plasma homocysteine is present as reduced homocysteine, thus with a free sulfhydryl function. As a consequence in cardiovascular patients with hyperhomocysteinemia of about 20 μmol/L, only 0.2 μmol/L of their homocysteine is present as reduced homocysteine. Performing in vitro or in vivo experiments with reduced homocysteine in the mmol range (like most studies) is 10,000 times out of the physiological range and therefore of no clinical relevance. In biochemistry it is well known that compounds with a free sulfhydryl function like β-mercapto-ethanol or dithiothreitol in millimolar concentrations influences protein functions. In this light it is not surprising that the homocysteine literature is replete with studies on effects of homocysteine on all kinds of different proteins. Millimolar concentrations of reduced homocysteine should not be applied in pathobiochemical studies. This chapter on homocysteine and cholesterol is limited to those studies using homocysteine in physiologic forms and concentrations.

## CHOLESTEROL AND HOMOCYSTEINE

### Basic interactions

Cholesterol and homocysteine metabolism are not linked according to current knowledge, but both compounds may share (parts) of their pathogenic mechanisms. As described above oxidative modification of LDL is believed to constitute the link between increased cholesterol concentrations and arteriosclerosis. Oxidation of amino acids or peptides with a free thiol moiety such as homocysteine, cysteine and glutathione, can result in generation of reactive oxygen species, such as superoxide, hydrogen peroxide and the hydroxyl radical (28-30). Thiol oxidation is facilitated in the presence of trace amounts of $Fe^{3+}$ or $Cu^{2+}$, in a Fenton-type reaction with ensuing radical production. If an increased export of homocysteine to plasma will lead to an increased generation of reactive oxygen species, a synergistic interaction between homocysteine and cholesterol can be expected. Rats, who were made hyperhomocysteinemic by a folate deficient diet, showed increased plasma lipid peroxidation products (31). On the other hand amino acids or peptides with a free thiol function like glutathione and N-acetylcysteine are well known for their radical scavenging properties. Indeed, Halvorsen et al. (57) observed that normal plasma concentrations of homocysteine have no significant effects on the lipid peroxidation of LDL, whereas moderately elevated and high concentrations of homocysteine even protected LDL against in vitro oxidative modification. However, when copper was used to initiate oxidation low concentrations of homocysteine of 6 and 25 µmol/L caused a small but significant generation of lipid peroxides. The pro-oxidant effects of homocysteine on copper or iron catalyzed LDL oxidation in cell free systems is also reported by others (29,32).

Young et al (33) induced very severe hyperhomocysteinemia (about 500 µmol/L) in pigs by inhibition of methionine synthase with $N_2O$. These pigs had a small but significant increase of malondialdehyde, a marker of lipid peroxidation, in their heart tissue. Their coronary arteries revealed no histologic abnormalities. Rabbits fed a methionine rich diet for 6-9 months had elevated thiobarbituric acid reactive substances (TBARS) in their aorta (34). Whether these animal studies can be extrapolated to humans in not clear.

## Clinical interactions

So far in vitro and animal investigations have not lead to a satisfying pathobiochemical mechanism of hyperhomocysteinemia. In part this can be explained because many studies applied homocysteine in forms and/or concentrations of no physiologic relevance (see above). For the moment it seems that the pathophysiology of homocysteine and its interaction with cholesterol can best be evaluated in patients with hyperhomocysteinemia.

A possible link between hyperhomocysteinemia and lipid accumulation in the vascular wall is indicated by some studies. Selhub et al (35) observed a strong relation between homocysteine concentrations and the carotid-arteriostenosis in elderly. Tonstad et al (36) reported on total homocysteine as an independent predictor of carotid intimal-medial in hyperlipidemics. Furthermore, homocysteine correlates with cholesterol levels (4) indicating that interactions between homocysteine and cholesterol may be possible.

Lipid peroxidation in hyperhomocysteinemia is investigated in different studies of different design. Patients with severe hyperhomocysteinemia due to CBS deficiency may serve as an extreme model to study a possible relation between lipid peroxidation and hyperhomocysteinemia. Four studies of different design of three different research groups found no evidence of increased radical formation in patients with severe hyperhomocysteinemia. We investigated *in vitro* LDL oxidation (oxidation resistance, maximal oxidation rate, extent of oxidation, time needed for maximal diene production), LDL vitamin E content and fatty acid composition, and TBARS (thiobarbituric acid reactive substances) in 10 patients (30) and measured fluorescent lipid peroxidation in 8 patients (37) with severe hyperhomocysteinemia due to CBS deficiency, and no indication of increased lipid peroxidation was found. The TBARS concentration was even lower in patients with severe hyperhomocysteinemia than in controls indicating that homocysteine may rather scavenge than generate radicals. Dudman et al (38) reported reduced levels of high-density lipoprotein cholesterylester hydroperoxides, and an elevated ubiquinol-10/ubiquinone-10 ratio in CBS deficient patients, again indicating a decreased rather than an increased lipid peroxidation in severe hyperhomocysteinemia. More recently, Cordoba-Poras (39) investigated the presence of oxidized LDL and the susceptibility of LDL to oxidative modification in 6 CBS deficient patients and 6 controls. Again no indication of increased lipid peroxidation was obtained.

Hladovec et al. (40) described increased circulating endothelial cells in patients with peripheral arterial occlusive disease after a load of 0.1 g L-methionine/kg bodyweight which is known to cause increased plasma homo-cysteine concentrations. A dose of 0.05 g L-methionine did not lead to an in-crease of circulating endothelial cells, indicating an existence of a threshold for homocysteine to produce endothelial lesions. Studies in animals lead to com-parable observations. Whether mild hyperhomocysteinemia is related to in-creased radical formation is discussed below. Clarke et al (41) examined obli-gated heterozygous for CBS deficiency, who have mild hyperhomocysteinemia in particularly after methionine loading. Free radical formation was measured by neutrophil chemiluminescence and the cellular anti-oxidant capacity was examined by measuring the activities of superoxide dismutase, glutathione peroxidase and their co-factors (selenium, copper), vitamin E and vitamin A. No differences between heterozygotes and controls were found. Fonseca et al (42) studied the effect of homocysteine on TBARS in a methionine loading test in non-insulin-dependent diabetes mellitus. As expected TBARS were elevated in diabetics. The additional presence of hyperhomocysteinemia was not associ-ated to a further increase of TBARS. In 66 patients with vascular disease the total anti-oxidant capacity was studied by Currie et al (43). Hyperhomocyste-inemia was found in 29% of the patients and their anti-oxidant capacity was increased.

Taken together, all studies performed in patients with mild or severe hyper-homocysteinemia showed no evidence of increased lipid peroxidation. Three studies (30,38,43) even provided evidence of increased anti-oxidant capacity or decreased lipid peroxidation in hyperhomocysteinemia.

If hyperhomocysteinemia is not causing increased lipid peroxidation, a syn-ergistic interaction between elevated homocysteine and cholesterol seems less likely. The relationship between elevated homocysteine and cholesterol, and also smoking and high blood pressure, was systematically studied in the Euro-pean Concerted Action Project (44). The risk attributed to elevated homocys-teine was independent and of equal strength as of the conventional risk factors for cardiovascular disease. Intriguing synergistic (more than multiplicative) interactions were observed between hyperhomocysteinemia and blood pressure and smoking, in particular in women. However, the interaction between hyper-homocysteinemia and cholesterol was about additive, which is in line with the data described above that hyperhomocysteinemia does not lead to oxidative modification of LDL.


## HOMOCYSTEINE AND NITRIC OXIDE (NO)

Evidence is emerging that the atherogeneity of homocysteine is mediated via its interaction with endothelium-dependent vascular relaxation. *In vitro* low concentrations of homocysteine of 10 µmol/L can inhibit relaxation of rabbit aorta rings induced by NO (45). In normal human coronary artery rings the disulfide homocystine in concentrations of 10-20 µmol/L induced endothelium modulated vasoconstriction (46). Cynomolgus monkeys, who were made hyperhomocysteinemic by a diet high in methionine, low in folate and free of choline, showed a marked resistance of endothelium-dependent vasodilation (47). Healthy humans with mild hyperhomocysteinemia have impaired endothelium-dependent vasodilation, which was reported by three independent studies (48-50), although Hanratti et al (51) found no change in endothelial function after methionine supplementation in 16 healthy volunteers. Children with severe hyperhomocysteinemia due to CBS deficiency also demonstrated abnormal endothelium-dependent vasodilation, although their parents who may have mild hyperhomocysteinemia due to heterozygosity for CBS deficiency had normal endothelial function (52). Verhaar et al (53) infused MeTHF in the forearm of patients with familial hypercholesterolenemia, which restored their endothelium-dependent vasodilation. In controls MeTHF had no effect on endothelial function.

These data provide a new and compelling physiologic mechanism how elevated homocysteine levels in blood may be related to arterial obstruction. A high plasma homocysteine concentration may participate in the acute cardiovascular event, rather than generating radicals and concomitant lipid accumulation in the vascular wall. In line with this hypothesis are the recent observations that mild hyperhomocysteinemia is a risk factor for vascular disease in children (54,55) and the high mortality of patients with coronary artery disease and mild hyperhomocysteinemia (56).

*Acknowledgement.Support was obtained by grant (D97.021) of the Dutch Heart Foundation. The author gratefully acknowledges Anita Kerkhof-van Loon for expert assistance in preparation of this manuscript.*

## REFERENCES

1.   Mudd SH, Skovby F, Levy HL, Pettigrew KD, Wilcken B, Pyeritz RE, Andria G, Boers GH, Bromberg IL, Cerone R, et al. The natural history of homocystinuria due to cystathionine beta-synthase deficiency. Am J Hum Genet 1985;37:1-31.
2.   McCully KS. Vascular Pathology of homocysteinemia: implications for the pathogenesis of arteriosclerosis. Am J Pathol 1969;56:111-128.
3.   Wilcken DEL, Wilcken B. The pathogenesis of coronary artery disease. A possible role for methionine metabolism. J Clin Invest 1976;57:1079-1082.

4. Refsum H, Ueland PM, Nygard O, Vollset SE. Homocysteine and cardiovascular disease. Annu Rev Medicine 1998;49:31-62.

5. Kluijtmans LA, Boers GH, Verbruggen B, Trijbels FJ, Novakova IR, Blom HJ. Homozygous cystathionine beta-synthase deficiency, combined with factor V Leiden or thermolabile methylenetetrahydrofolate reductase in the risk of venous thrombosis. Blood 1998;91:2015-2018.

6. Willems HPI, Gerrits WBJ, Rozendaal FR, den Heijer M, Blom HJ, Bos GMJ. The VITRO trial: study design. Neth J Med 1998;52:S43(Abstract)

7. Welch GN, Loscalzo J. Homocysteine and atherothrombosis. N Engl J Med 1998;338:1042-1050.

8. Blom HJ, van der Molen EF. Pathobiochemical implications of hyperhomocysteinemia. Fibrinolysis 1994;8:86-87.

9. Ueland PM, Refsum H, Stabler SP, Malinow MR, Andersson A, Allen RH. Total homocysteine in plasma or serum: methods and clinical applications. Clin Chem 1993;39:1764-1779.

10. Ueland PM. Homocysteine species as components of plasma redox thiol status [editorial; comment]. Clin Chem 1995;41:340-342.

11. Andersson A, Lindgren A, Hultberg B. Effect of thiol oxidation and thiol export from erythrocytes on determination of redox status of homocysteine and other thiols in plasma from healthy subjects and patients with cerebral infarction [see comments]. Clin Chem 1995;41:361-366.

12. Hultberg B, Andersson A, Arnadottir M. Reduced, free and total fractions of homocysteine and other thiol compounds in plasma from patients with renal failure. Nephron 1995;70:62-67.

13. Mansoor MA, Guttormsen AB, Fiskerstrand T, Refsum H, Ueland PM, Svardal AM. Redox status and protein binding of plasma aminothiols during the transient hyperhomocysteinemia that follows homocysteine administration. Clin Chem 1993;39:980-985.

14. Ueland PM, Mansoor MA, Guttormsen AB, Muller F, Aukrust P, Refsum H, Svardal AM. Reduced, oxidized and protein-bound forms of homocysteine and other aminothiols in plasma comprise the redox thiol status--a possible element of the extracellular antioxidant defense system. J Nutr 1996;126:1281S-4S.

15. Svardal A, Refsum H, Ueland PM. Determination of in vivo protein binding of homocysteine and its relation to free homocysteine in the liver and other tissues of the rat. J Biol Chem 1986;261:3156-3163.

16. Brown MS, Goldstein JL. A receptor-mediated pathway for cholesterol homeostasis. Science 1986;232:34-47.

17. Esterbauer H, Juergens G, Quehenberger O, Koller E. Autoxidation of human low density lipoprotein: loss of polyunsaturated fatty acids and vitamin E and generation of aldehydes. J Lipid Res 1987;28:495-509.

18. Esterbauer H, Dieber-Rotheneder M, Waeg G, Striegl G, Juergens G. Biochemical, structural and functional properties of oxidized low-density lipoprotein. Chem Res Toxicol 1990;3:77-92.

19. Goldstein JL, Anderson RGW, Brown MS. Degradation of cationized low density lipoprotein and regulation of cholesterol metabolism in homozygous familial hypercholesterolemia fibroblasts. Proc Natl Acad Sci USA 1976;73:3178-3182.

20. Goldstein JL, Ho YK., Basu SK, Brown MS. Binding site on macrophages that mediates uptake and degradation of acetylated low density lipoprotein, producing massive cholesterol deposition. Proc Natl Acad Sci USA 1979;76:333-337.

21. Brown MS, Basu SK, Falck JR, Ho YK, Goldstein JL. The scavenger cell pathway for lipoprotein degradation: Specificity of the binding site that mediates the uptake of negatively-charged LDL by macrophages. J Supramol Struct 1980;13:67-81.

22. Banerjee RV, Matthews RG. Cobalamin-dependent methionine synthase. FASEB J 1990;4:1450-1459.

23. Finkelstein JD. The metabolism of homocysteine: pathways and regulation. Eur J Pediatr 1998;157 Suppl 2:S40-4.

24. Vandermolen EF, Hiipakka MJ, Vanlithzanders H, Boers GHJ, Vandenheuvel LPWJ, Monnens LAH, Blom HJ. Homocysteine metabolism in endothelial cells of a patient homozygous for cystathionine beta-synthase (CS) deficiency. Thromb Haemost 1997;78:827-833.

25. Christensen B, Refsum H, Vintermyr O, Ueland PM. Homocysteine export from cells cultured in the presence of physiological or superfluous levels of methionine: methionine loading of non-transformed, transformed, proliferating, and quiescent cells in culture. J Cell Physiol 1991;146:52-62.

26. Christensen B, Refsum H, Garras A, Ueland PM. Homocysteine remethylation during nitrous oxide exposure of cells cultured in media containing various concentrations of folates. J Pharmacol Exp Ther 1992;261:1096-1105.

27. Refsum H, Guttormsen AB, Fiskerstrand T, Ueland PM. Hyperhomocysteinemia in terms of steady-state kinetics. Eur J Pediatr 1998;157 Suppl 2:S45-9.

28. Starkebaum G, Harlan JM. Endothelial cell injury due to copper-catalyzed hydrogen peroxide generation from homocysteine. J Clin Invest 1986;77:1370-1376.

29. Heinecke JW, Kawamura M, Suzuki L, Chait A. Oxidation of low density lipoprotein by thiols: superoxide-dependent and -independent mechanisms. J Lipid Res 1993;34:2051-2061.

30. Blom HJ, Kleinveld HA, Boers GH, Demacker PN, Hak Lemmers HL, te Poele Pothoff MT, Trijbels JM. Lipid peroxidation and susceptibility of low-density lipoprotein to in vitro oxidation in hyperhomocysteinemia. Eur J Clin Invest 1995;25:149-154.

31. Durand P, Prost M, Blanche D. Pro-thrombotic effects of a folic acid deficient diet in rat platelets and macrophages related to elevated homocysteine and decreased n-3 polyunsaturated fatty acids. Atherosclerosis 1996;121:231-243.

32. Hirano K, Ogihara T, Miki M, Yasuda H, Tamai H, Kawamura N, Mino M. Homocysteine induces iron-catalyzed lipid peroxidation of low-density lipoprotein that is prevented by alpha-tocopherol. Free Radic Res 1994;21:267-276.

33. Roge Canales M, Rodrigo Gonzalo de Liria C, Prats Vinas LJ, Vaquero Perez M, Ribes Rubio A, Rodes Monegal M, Pintos Morell G. [Neonatal hemolytic-uremic syndrome associated with methylmalonic aciduria and homocystinuria] Sindrome hemolitico-uremico neonatal asociado a aciduria metilmalonica y homocistinuria. An Esp Pediatr 1996;45:97-98.

34. Toborek M, Kopieczna Grzebieniak E, Drozdz M, Wieczorek M. Increased lipid peroxidation as a mechanism of methionine-induced atherosclerosis in rabbits. Atherosclerosis 1995;115:217-224.

35. Selhub J, Jacques PF, Bostom AG, D'Agostino RB, Wilson PW, Belanger AJ, O'Leary DH, Wolf PA, Schaefer EJ, Rosenberg IH. Association between plasma homocysteine concentrations and extracranial carotid-artery stenosis [see comments]. N Engl J Med 1995;332:286-291.

36. Tonstad S, Joakimsen O, Stensland Bugge E, Leren TP, Ose L, Russell D, Bonaa KH. Risk factors related to carotid intima-media thickness and plaque in children with familial hypercholesterolemia and control subjects. Arterioscler Thromb Vasc Biol 1996;16:984-991.

37. Blom HJ, Engelen DP, Boers GH, Stadhouders AM, Sengers RC, de Abreu R, TePoele Pothoff MT, Trijbels JM. Lipid peroxidation in homocysteinemia. J Inherit Metab Dis 1992;15:419-422.

38. Dudman NP, Wilcken DE, Stocker R. Circulating lipid hydroperoxide levels in human hyperhomocysteinemia. Relevance to development of arteriosclerosis. Arterioscler Thromb 1993;13:512-516.

39. CordobaPorras A, SanchezQuesada JL, GonzalezSastre F, OrdonezLlanos J, BlancoVaca F. Susceptibility of plasma low- and high-density lipoproteins to oxidation in patients with severe hyperhomocysteinemia. J Mol Med 1996;74:771-776.

40. Hladovec J, Sommerova Z, Pisarikova A. Homocysteine and endothelial damage after methionine load. Thrombosis Research 1997;88:361-364.

41. Clarke R, Naughten E, Cahalane S, Sullivan KO, Mathias P, McCall T, Graham I. The role of free radicals as mediators of endothelial cell injury in hyperhomocysteinemia. Ir J Med Sci 1992;161:561-564.

42. Fonseca VA, Stone A, Munshi M, Baliga BS, Aljada A, Thusu K, Fink L, Dandona P. Oxidative stress in diabetic macrovascular disease: does homocysteine play a role? South Med J 1997;90:903-906.

43. Currie IC, Wilson YG, Scott J, Day A, Stansbie D, Baird RN, Lamont PM, Tennant WG. Homocysteine: an independent risk factor for the failure of vascular intervention. Br J Surg 1996;83:1238-1241.

44. Graham IM, Daly LE, Refsum HM, Robinson K, Brattstrom LE, Ueland PM, Palmareis RJ, Boers GHJ, Sheahan RG, Israelsson B, Uiterwaal CS, Meleady R, Mcmaster D, Verhoef P, Witteman J, Rubba P, Bellet H, Wautrecht JC, Devalk HW, Luis ACS, Parrotroulaud FM, Tan KS, Higgins I, Garcon D, Medrano MJ, Candito M, Evans AE, Andria G. Plasma homocysteine as a risk factor for vascular disease: The European concerted action project. JAMA 1997;277:1775-1781.

45. Jia L, Liu XJ, Furchgott RF. Blockade off nitric oxide-induced relaxation of rabbit aorta by cysteine and homocysteine. Acta Pharmacol Sin 1997;18:11-20.

46. Tyagi SC, Smiley LM, Mujumdar VS, Clonts B, Parker JL. Reduction-oxidation (Redox) and vascular tissue level of homocyst(e)ine in human coronary atherosclerotic lesions and role in extracellular matrix remodeling and vascular tone. Mol Cell Biochem 1998;181:107-116.

47. Lentz SR, Sobey CG, Piegors DJ, Bhopatkar MY, Faraci FM, Malinow MR, Heistad DD. Vascular dysfunction in monkeys with diet-induced hyperhomocyst(e)inemia [see comments]. J Clin Invest 1996;98:24-29.

48. Tawakol A, Omland T, Gerhard M, Wu JT, Creager MA. Hyperhomocyst(e)inemia is associated with impaired endothelium-dependent vasodilation in humans. Circulation 1997;95:1119-1121.

49. Woo KS, Chook P, Lolin YI, Cheung ASP, Chan LT, Sun YY, Sanderson JE, Metreweli C, Celermajer DS. Hyperhomocyst(e)inemia is a risk factor for arterial endothelial dysfunction in humans. Circulation 1997;96:2542-2544.

50. Chambers JC, Mcgregor A, Jeanmarie J, Kooner JS. Acute hyperhomocysteinemia and endothelial dysfunction. Lancet 1998;351:36-37.

51. Hanratti CG, McAuley DF, McGurk C, Young IS, Johnston GD. Homocysteine and endothelial vascular function [letter]. Lancet 1998;351:1288-1289.

52. Celermajer DS, Sorensen K, Ryalls M, Robinson J, Thomas O, Leonard JV, Deanfield JE. Impaired endothelial function occurs in the systemic arteries of children with homozygous homocystinuria but not in their heterozygous parents. J Am Coll Cardiol 1993;22:854-858.

53. Verhaar MC, Wever RMF, Kastelein JJP, Vandam T, Koomans HA, Rabelink TJ. 5-methyltetrahydrofolate, the active form of folic acid, restores endothelial function in familial hypercholesterolemia. Circulation 1998;97:237-241.

54. Van Beynum IM, Smeitink JAM, den Heijer M, Te Poele Pothoff MTWB, Blom HJ. Hyperhomocysteinemia: a risk factor for ischaemic stroke in children. Circulation 1999;99:2070-2072.

55. Vilaseca MA, Moyano D, Artuch R, Ferrer I, Pineda M, Cardo E, Campistol J, Pavia C, Camacho JA. Selective screening for hyperhomocysteinemia in pediatric patients. Clin Chem 1998;44:662-664.

56. Nygard O, Nordrehaug JE, Refsum H, Ueland PM, Farstad M, Vollset SE. Plasma homocysteine levels and mortality in patients with coronary artery disease. N Engl J Med 1997;337:230-236.

57. Halvorsen B, Brude I, Drevon CA, Nysom J, Ose L, Christiansen EN, nenseter MS. Effect of homocysteine in copper-ion catalized, azo componend initiated, and mononuclear cell-mediated oscidative modification of low density liroprotein. J Cipid Res 1996;37:1591-1600.

# 20. HOMOCYSTEINE AND COAGULATION FACTORS: BASIC INTERACTIONS AND CLINICAL STUDIES

RALPH GREEN

## SUMMARY

Hyperhomocysteinemia of genetic, nutritional or metabolic origin is associated with an increased predisposition to thromboembolism. Several mechanisms have been put forward to explain the basis for this association. This review examines evidence from animal and cell culture experiments upon which hypotheses concerning the proposed mechanisms are based. Disruption of endothelial cell function is likely to be the central mechanism responsible for perturbation of coagulant or anticoagulant pathways that results in thromboembolism associated with increased homocysteine levels. Evidence from experimental studies on endothelial cells implicate homocysteine as having effects on: (i) factor V, its modulator, protein C, or thrombomodulin, the docking site required by thrombin for activation of protein C; (ii) antithrombin III binding to heparan sulfate; (iii) tissue plasminogen activator binding to endothelial cells through its annexin II attachment site; (iv) von Willebrand factor processing and secretion; (v) tissue factor expression and; (vi) the affinity of Lp(a) for plasmin-modified fibrin. Modifications of platelet activation, aggregation and survival by homocysteine have also been described. Additionally, clinical evidence is presented for and against the notion that the coexistence of hyperhomocysteinemia with other prothrombotic conditions, such as lupus erythematosus and factor V Leiden, increases the risk of thromboembolism. While there is a preponderance of evidence that

K. Robinson (ed.), Homocysteine and Vascular Disease, 349-370.
© 2000 Kluwer Academic Publishers. Printed in the Netherlands.

hyperhomocysteinemia is a risk factor for thromboembolism, it is still not certain whether raised levels of homocysteine are causative or incidental in the association.


INTRODUCTION

Raised levels of homocysteine in the blood (hyperhomocysteinemia), whether the consequence of genetic or acquired conditions, have been linked to increased risk of atherothrombosis, resulting in occlusive vascular disease. The biochemical pathways involved in homocysteine metabolism, as well as the varied features of classical homocystinuria and severe hyperhomocysteinemia associated with inborn errors of metabolism, are detailed elsewhere in this volume. An outline of the homocysteine metabolic pathways is shown in Chapter 3. In homocystinuria, an inborn metabolic disorder associated with several skeletal, connective tissue, ocular, neurological and occlusive vascular complications, the vascular complications are serious and protean, and constitute the major cause of morbidity and mortality among affected individuals. Autopsy of patients with homocystinuria often discloses multiple thrombi and emboli contained within large and small arteries and veins, which frequently show pathological change [1]. Changes in the arterial wall consist of intimal thickening which may be concentric or patchy. The media is also involved, with increased deposition of collagen between split muscle fibers as well as disruption of the internal elastic lamina [2]. The association of vascular pathological changes and thrombotic complications with homocystinuria indicates a profound disruption of normal endothelial cell function and blood coagulation. Because of the conspicuous and intriguing occurrence of vascular and thrombotic complications with homocystinuria, a potential role for homocysteine in the induction of both atherosclerosis and thrombosis in the population at large has received increasing attention.

Various mechanisms have been proposed to explain the pathogenesis of vascular damage and predisposition to thrombosis that are associated with hyperhomocysteinemia. These include thiol reactivity with free protein cysteinyl residues on endothelial cell surfaces, adhesion molecules, platelets, or clotting factor agonists and their inhibitors, and free radical generation during disulfide bond formation. Free radicals are believed to be injurious to blood vessels and are held responsible for atherogenesis [3]. These theories are extensively reviewed in Chapter 21. Homocysteine can also undergo autocyclization to form homocysteine thiolactone in a mechanism involved in error-correction during amino acid selection for protein synthesis. Jakubowski [4] has proposed that the activated carboxyl group of homocysteine thiolactone can cause post-translational modification of proteins through acylation of their lysine epsilon amino groups. Additionally, homocysteine has been linked to several biochemical mechanisms that result in perturbed regulation of apoptotic programmed cell death and replication [5, 6], and apoptotic vascular endothelial cells manifest procoagulant properties [7]. Finally, there is a possible role for S-adenosylhomocysteine (SAH), the immediate metabolic precursor of homocysteine, in the pathogenesis of vascular occlusive disease, a topic which has received little attention [8]. Intracellular concentrations of SAH are considerably higher than those of homocysteine, and the compound is a powerful inhibitor of S-adenosylmethionine-dependent methyltransferases. Consequently, a variety of biological reactions that require methylation may become impaired, including gene activation and repression, transcription factor expression, membrane biosynthesis and repair, induction of cellular differentiation and catecholamine production, all of which could affect endothelial cell, platelet and coagulation factor production or function. For example, Kokame and associates [9] have reported up-regulation of expression of a number of genes in cultured human umbilical vein endothelial cells exposed to 1–10 mM homocysteine. Several of the above mechanisms have been implicated in the pathogenesis of thrombosis associated with raized levels of homocysteine. They will be considered in relation to the effect that these interactions might have on the various molecular and cellular components involved in the maintenance of normal blood fluidity or the promotion of blood coagulation.

## PROPOSED MECHANISMS OF HOMOCYSTEINE THROMBOGENICITY

Disruption of the normal functioning of endothelial cells, considered central protagonists in antithrombotic homeostasis, can result in multiple perturbations of the regulatory components involved in blood coagulation. The normal vascular endothelium generates several compounds that are important in the maintenance of vessel patency and blood fluidity. These include prostacyclin, which inhibits platelet and monocyte activation; the vasodilator, nitric oxide; and ecto-adenosine diphosphatase which inhibits platelet aggregation by degrading ADP. In addition, vascular endothelial cells also express at least two key surface anticoagulant molecules, thrombomodulin, the molecular mooring site required by thrombin for activation of protein C, and heparin-like molecules capable of serving as cofactors for antithrombin III. Additionally, endothelial cells maintain fibrinolysis by secreting tissue plasminogen activator. Finally, certain procoagulant functions are also vested in endothelial cells, notably the production of von Willebrand factor, which promotes adhesion and shear stress-induced aggregation of platelets. Endothelial injury can therefore lead to thrombosis through synergistic mechanisms involving the negation of anticoagulant mediators and the promotion of procoagulant factors [10]. A compelling example of the global disruption of endothelial cell-mediated homeostasis is seen in experimentally induced vascular endothelial apoptosis which activates a profusion of procoagulant mediators while at the same time suppressing a number of anticoagulant membrane components [7]. Homocysteine may, indeed, have such a global effect through induction of endothelial cell death, as has been demonstrated in experimental hyperhomocysteinemia [5], as well as in cultured pulmonary artery endothelial cells [6].

A major criticism of many experimental studies designed to elucidate the mechanisms of homocysteine-mediated vascular damage, is that the dose of homocysteine used far exceeds that seen in most clinical settings associated with cardiovascular disease, including homocystinuria. It should also be pointed out that despite the mounting body of compelling epidemiological evidence linking hyperhomocysteinemia with vascular disease, no clear cause and effect relationship has been demonstrated. It remains possible that rather than a causal relationship, the raized homocysteine level seen in association with vascular occlusion represents a marker of some other underlying biochemical mechanism, such as a derangement in the vitamin-dependent pathways necessary for homocysteine metabolism. Thus, folate or vitamin $B_6$ deficiency might be the ultimate causative factors in vessel wall damage or thrombosis [11].

The integrity and normal function of the vascular endothelium are critical factors in the prevention of intravascular thrombosis and several endothelium-dependent mechanisms have been identified which mitigate the thrombotic process. Disruption or disease of the vascular endothelium is therefore frequently a cogent initiating event in thrombogenesis, or may contribute to a thrombotic diathesis [12]. Indeed, endothelial damage or changes in the vessel wall are directly responsible for thrombus formation in patients with raized plasma levels of homocysteine. It is probable, at least as far as arterial thrombosis is concerned, that vascular endothelial damage always precedes thrombosis. Putative mechanisms for vascular damage and atherogenesis, outlined below, are extensively reviewed in Chapter 19 and 21. It would be intellectually preferable to explain the vascular occlusive phenomena that occur in hyperhomocysteinemia through a single integrated hypothesis. It is, however, possible that the several complications and pathological processes that have been reported either clinically or experimentally and that lead to interdiction of vascular patency or integrity, may arise through different mechanisms.

# EXPERIMENTAL STUDIES

Information concerning the association of hyperhomocysteinemia with thrombosis has come from several sources. Generally, these consist of clinical case or epidemiological studies in which plasma homocysteine is analyzed as a risk factor for thrombosis and experimental studies in which the direct effects of homocysteine on coagulation factors are examined in various *in vitro* or animal model systems. While individual studies have often focused on specific components of the complex cascade of factors that lead to thrombosis, there is a myriad of interactions among and between various steps involved in the regulation of this process. Disruption of one step may have downstream or upstream feedback effects on other steps in the pathway. Consequently, the observations made and conclusions drawn from these reports may not be so much competing as complementary.

Several experimental studies designed to examine the effect of homocysteine on prothrombotic and antithrombotic pathways have been carried out. These have either been *in vitro* studies generally involving the use of cultured arterial and venous endothelial cells, or have been conducted in experimental animals. Since the optical enantiomer of homocysteine used is not always specified in the studies described in this review, concentrations are stated without reference to whether they refer to the biologically active L-form, or to a racemic mixture of D- and L-homocysteine. The potential twofold difference in biological activity is small in relation to the wide range of concentrations used in these various experiments, and the reader is therefore referred to the original source for details. In the studies here reviewed, one or more appropriate controls were always included in the *in vitro* experiments. Such controls include similar concentrations of one or more other naturally occurring reduced thiols (e.g. cysteine), oxidized thiols (including homocystine, the oxidized homocysteine dimer) and in some experiments synthetic reducing thiols (e.g. β-mercaptoethanol). In some experiments, the metabolic precursor (methionine) and product (S-adenosylhomocysteine) for the reversible SAH-hydrolase reaction (see Chapter 3) were also included. Space limitations in a review of this nature preclude presentation of full details of these control experiments.

## Effects on Cultured Vascular Endothelial Cells

Experiments with bovine aortic endothelial cells (BAEC), human aortic endothelial cells (HAEC) and human umbilical vein endothelial cells (HUVEC), have focused on impairment of endothelial cell resistance to thrombosis and the stimulation of procoagulant activities by homocysteine. In the response-to-injury hypothesis of atherogenesis, Ross and coworkers [3] proposed that injury to the endothelium was the initiating event in the development of atherosclerosis. Endothelial cells mediate numerous cytokine and growth factor responses that undoubtedly play important roles in atherogenesis [3]. During the 1980's, *in vitro* studies were carried out to assess the effect of homocysteine on cultured endothelial cells. Extremely high concentrations of homocysteine or homocysteine thiolactone (1-10 mM), exceeding the levels encountered even under the most severe pathological conditions, were used in these studies. Wall et al. [13] found that 0.1 to 10 mM homocysteine thiolactone caused release and detachment of HUVEC in a cytotoxicity assay. Catalase, but not superoxide dismutase, protected against cytotoxicity suggesting that hydrogen peroxide production from thiol autooxidation might be involved. In a study using HUVEC from normal and obligate heterozygotes for cystathionine β-synthase deficiency, De Groot et al. [14] observed that the cells from heterozygotes — assumed to contain 50% of cystathionine β-synthase enzyme activity — were more sensitive to 10 mM homocystine and methionine in a cytotoxicity assay. HUVECS from both normals and cystathionine β-synthase heterozygotes were equally sensitive to 10 mM homocysteine. Starkebaum and Harlan [15] reported that BAEC were lysed by an hydrogen peroxide-generating system consisting of 0.5-1.0 mM homocysteine in the presence of cupric ions or ceruloplasmin. Studies by Dudman et al. [16], however, cast serious doubt on the significance of *in vivo* desquamation [17, 18, 19] or *in vitro* detachment [13, 19] of endothelial cells as an indicator of homocysteine-induced cell injury. They pointed out that the levels of homocysteine in these studies were excessive and that higher concentrations of cysteine, not known to be atherogenic, were equally effective in causing desquamation or detachment.

Other investigators have focused on the possible effect of homocysteine on several of the components involved in blood coagulation or the maintenance of antithrombotic homeostasis. Rodgers and Kane [20] found increased activation rather than synthesis of factor V by BAEC and HUVEC treated with 0.5-10 mM homocysteine. They further demonstrated that this was caused by non-thrombin-mediated proteolytic conversion of factor V to Va. Methionine and cysteine also activated factor V, but to a far lesser extent. In a subsequent study using the same cell lines, Rodgers and Conn [21] reported that protein C activation was reduced by as much as one-third with homocysteine concentrations as low as 0.6 to 1.25 mM and by as much as 90% with homocysteine concentrations of 7.5-10 mM. Lentz and Sadler [22] found that 5 mM homocysteine increased thrombomodulin mRNA and protein synthesis in HUVEC and CV-1(18A) cells without affecting viability. Thrombomodulin was not expressed on the surface of these cells, however, suggesting that homocysteine interfered with the secretory process by partially blocking glycosylation and sulfation of the protein. The authors also reported that homocysteine and other thiols irreversibly inactivated protein C and thrombomodulin, but not thrombin. Confirming these findings, Hayashi et al. [23], using HUVEC cells, found that 10 mM homocysteine inactivated the cofactor activity of thrombomodulin, despite a twofold to threefold increase in thrombomodulin mRNA. Although these are perhaps the most interesting and provocative of all the experimental studies to date, their significance is open to question in view of the relatively high levels of homocysteine used. Animal experiments and human studies on the thrombomodulin and protein C activation pathway will be discussed below.

Apart from the thrombomodulin-mediated protein C activation mechanism, which has received the most attention, there have been a few other studies on the possible role of homocysteine in causing perturbations of other antithrombotic pathways. Nishinaga and associates [24] examined another endothelial anticoagulant mechanism, the interaction of heparin-like glycosaminoglycans with antithrombin III. Using cultured porcine aortic endothelial cells, these workers found that homocysteine reduced the amount of antithrombin III bound to the endothelial cell surface. This effect was observed with homocysteine concentrations as low as 0.1 mM, but reached a maximum (30% of control) at 1.0 mM homocysteine. Interesting as these findings are, considering that an effect was demonstrated at much lower concentrations than in other *in vitro* studies, they were not specific for homocysteine. Cysteine and β-mercaptoethanol, but not methionine, caused similar effects on antithrombin III binding. The authors speculate that the homocysteine effect on expression of anticoagulant heparan sulfate is mediated by sulfhydryl generation of peroxides, since the homocysteine effect was augmented by copper and was prevented by catalase, but not superoxide dismutase. Hajjar [25] reported that 1-5 mM homocysteine blocked tissue plasminogen activator (t-PA), but not plasminogen, binding to human endothelial cells in a time- and dose-dependent fashion. Interestingly the blockade appeared to be specific. L-cysteine did not block t-PA binding but did reverse homocysteine-associated reduction in t-PA binding. This implies that thiol displacement may be involved in the mode of interaction of homocysteine with critical proteins in the procoagulant and anticoagulant cascades. In later studies, Hajjar et al. [26, 27] identified that the inhibition of t-PA binding to endothelial cells by homocysteine was mediated through an interaction of the amino acid with annexin II, the phospholipid binding protein that serves as the docking site for t-PA. Lentz and Sadler [28] reported that 1.0 mM homocysteine significantly inhibits endoplasmic reticulum-dependent processing and secretion of von Willebrand factor by HUVEC cells. Finally, with respect to procoagulant modification of endothelial cells by homocysteine, Fryer et al. [29] demonstrated that 0.1-0.6 mM homocysteine induced an increase in mRNA and expression of tissue factor by cultured human endothelial cells. Although the homocysteine effect was greater than other sulfur-containing amino acids, including cysteine and methionine, the chemical reductants β-mercaptoethanol and dithiothreitol were more potent than homocysteine.

Nitric oxide, or endothelium-derived relaxing factor, has potent vasodilatory and antiplatelet effects. Murphy et al. [30] reported that extracellular cysteine diminished nitric oxide production in cultured porcine aortic endothelial cells. Stamler et al. [31] found that exposure to homocysteine of BAEC, stimulated to secrete nitric oxide, resulted in its conversion to S-nitroso-homocysteine, which also has potent vasodilatory and antiplatelet effects. They speculated that nitrosothiol formation detoxifies homocysteine by blocking autooxidation and hydrogen peroxide generation as well as homocysteine thiolactone formation. This topic is more extensively discussed in Chapter 21.

### Homocysteine-modified plasma proteins

A substantial portion of homocysteine in the serum of homocystinuric patients and normal individuals is protein-bound [32] and individuals who may be mildly hyperhomocysteinemic (e.g., heterozygotes for CBS deficiency) are reported to have higher levels of protein-bound homocysteine [32, 33]. It is possible that excessive homocysteine entering the circulation might, by participating in disulfide bond exchange reactions, alter plasma proteins. After an oral methionine load, protein-bound homocysteine increased dramatically over a six to eight hour period while protein-bound cysteine and cysteinylglycine decreased rapidly during the first hour [34]. Most evidence indicates that albumin carries homocysteine in circulation [35], but other plasma proteins that may interact with homocysteine *in vivo* have not been identified. Harpel et al. [36] have reported that concentrations of homocysteine as low as 8 μM dramatically increased the affinity of Lp(a) for plasmin-modified fibrin surfaces. These results suggest that homocysteine-modified Lp(a) may compete with plasminogen for binding sites on fibrin-coated surfaces thereby creating a more thrombogenic environment.

### Animal and Human Experiments

Harker et al. [17, 18] carried out studies in baboons given long-term infusions of homocysteine thiolactone which resulted in a plasma level of about 200 μmol/L homocystine over a five day period (protein-bound homocysteine was not measured). When baboons were continuously infused with L-homocysteine over a three-month period, plasma levels of 100 to 200 µmol/L homocystine were obtained [17]. Endothelial desquamation followed by shortened platelet survival was observed. There was a marked reduction in the formation of homocysteine-induced patchy intimal lesions when dipyridamole or sulfinpyrazone was administered suggesting that platelets played a role in lesion development [19]. Harker's [18] group also reported shortened platelet survival in cystathionine β-synthase deficient patients and concluded that high levels of homocysteine were directly toxic to the endothelial cells, resulting in their exfoliation with secondary effects on platelets. Uhlemann et al. [37] were not able to reproduce these studies, however, when they studied six patients with cystathionine β-synthase deficiency including two of the four patients studied by Harker et al. [18].

While the levels of total plasma homocysteine achieved in Harker's baboon studies [17-19] probably exceeded those usually found in homocystinuric patients, and cannot therefore be extrapolated to the clinical setting, these studies focused attention on the vascular endothelium and endothelial-platelet interactions as the potential target site of homocysteine-induced injury.

## Effect on platelets

Earlier studies on the possible effect of homocysteine on platelet aggregation and survival have been equivocal, or were carried out using extremely high concentrations of homocysteine, far beyond what would be encountered even in homocystinuria [17, 18, 37, 38]. Graeber and associates [39] examined the effect of 1 mM homocysteine on platelet arachidonic acid metabolism *in vitro* and found that both homocysteine and its oxidized disulfide homocystine caused an increase in thromboxane $A_2$, a platelet proaggregatory substance. Production by human umbilical artery rings of vascular prostacyclin, an inhibitor of platelet aggregation, was not affected [39]. Wang et al. [40] concluded that in the presence of human serum (20%), homocysteine had no specific effect on prostacyclin production by cultured human endothelial cells. Studying HUVECs, they demonstrated no effect of homocysteine, cysteine or homocystine at concentrations of 100 mmol/L. At concentrations above 1 mmol/L, however, substantial inhibition was observed for both homocysteine and cysteine [40]. Furthermore, these investigators also found no difference in the production of prostacyclin by cells cultured in medium containing sera from patients with homocystinuria. Panganamala et al. [41] reported that while concentrations of homocysteine below 100 mM stimulated prostacyclin synthesis by rat aortas *ex vivo*, higher concentrations (1 and 10 mM) decreased secretion of this potent inhibitor of platelet and macrophage activation. These effects were mirrored by similar low and high concentrations of hydrogen

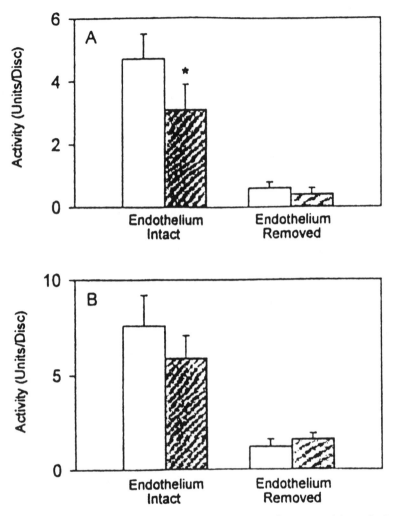

*Figure 1. Thrombomodulin-activated protein C in arteries from normal (open bar) and hyperhomocysteinemic (filled bar) monkeys. Aortic (A) and carotid arteries (B) are shown. Differences for aortic protein C activity were significant (p < 0.05) (Data from Lentz, et al. [43]).*

peroxide, leading the authors to conclude that the homocysteine effects were mediated through peroxide generation. Durand et al. [42], also using a rat model, showed that a methionine load caused a transient fourfold elevation in plasma homocysteine associated with increased platelet aggregation in response to thrombin and ADP, as well as increased thrombin-induced thromboxane synthesis. An increase in basal and LPS-induced tissue factor activity of peritoneal macrophages as well as lipid peroxidation products was also observed. These changes were not amplified in rats fed a folic acid-deficient diet. The authors attributed these changes to the induction of oxidative stress.

Lentz et al. [43] studied vasomotor and coagulation-related changes in a diet-induced hyperhomocysteinemic nonatherosclerotic monkey model. In experimental animals with mean plasma homocysteine of $10.6 \pm 2.6$mM, aortic thrombomodulin anticoagulant activity was reduced by $34 \pm 15\%$ compared with control animals (homocysteine $4.0 \pm 0.2$mM). Whereas the observed difference was statistically significant ($p = 0.03$), the observed difference in carotid artery thrombomodulin activity was not (Fig 1). In a subsequent extension of these studies reported more recently by the same group, additional questions are raized concerning the role of hyperhomocysteinemia in the observed changes in thrombomodulin activity that they had reported earlier. In these experiments, monkeys rendered atherosclerotic through hypercholesterolemia demonstrated a threefold increase in thrombomodulin activity, regardless of whether or not they were hyperhomocysteinemic [44].


## CLINICAL STUDIES

### Thrombotic complications of hyperhomocysteinemia

Mudd, in 1985, [45] comprehensively analyzed the clinical course of 629 patients homozygous for cystathionine β-synthase deficiency and found 42 of 59 deaths that appeared to be related to the genetic disorder were directly attributable to thromboembolism and five more in which it was a contributory factor. Fatal cardiovascular events occurred at a younger age among patients not responsive to pyridoxine than in pyridoxine-responsive patients. The site of vascular occlusion varied, but peripheral venous thrombosis with subsequent pulmonary embolism was relatively common. Of the 629 surveyed, 158 patients had suffered a thromboembolic event following peripheral venous thrombosis. The next most frequent occurrence was cerebral vascular accident. Peripheral arterial thrombosis and myocardial infarction were also noted. Even among untreated patients, thromboembolic events occurred at a younger age among patients subsequently found to be unresponsive to pyridoxine than in those who later responded to large doses of the vitamin. This interesting observation becomes even more intriguing in light of the recent reports that all patients with homocystinuria treated with pyridoxine have a reduced incidence of thrombosis, regardless of whether or not their homocysteine levels responded to pyridoxine [46]. The vitamin may therefore play a more direct

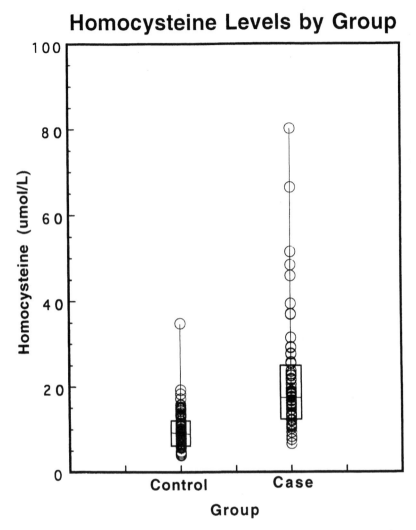

*Figure 2. Distribution of plasma homocysteine levels in patients with otherwise unexplained documented thrombosis and controls (for each group, n = 60). Boxes represent interquartile ranges for homocysteine with median value shown in the center. (Data from Kottke-Marchant, et al. [54]).*

antithrombotic role, as was suggested by Schroeder in 1955 [47] and more recently has been noted in studies on patients with coronary artery disease [48, 49]. Furthermore, though not entirely clear, the implications of the findings of a beneficial effect of pyridoxine in homocystinuric patients, regardless of its apparent effect on homocysteine levels, are intriguing. They raise the possibility that homocysteine, rather than being directly responsible for causing vascular damage and thrombosis, serves merely as a metabolic marker of vitamin deficiency or enzymatic dysfunction [11]. Alternatively, high doses of the vitamin may exert a beneficial effect beyond its role in catalytic concentrations.

There have been a large number of clinical studies that have reported an association of hyperhomocysteinemia of varying degrees with vascular disease (reviewed in other sections of this volume), and both arterial [50] and venous [51] thrombosis. Hyperhomocysteinemia can vary in severity and for convenience may be defined as mild, moderate or severe, on the basis of a total plasma homocysteine concentration that lies within the ranges of 15 to 25 μmol/L, 26 to 50 μmol/L or >50 μmol/L, respectively [52]. Studies in the literature, with some notable exceptions, broadly support the conclusion that hyperhomocysteinemia is an independent risk factor for arterial occlusive disease affecting coronary, cerebral and peripheral vessels, as well as venous thrombosis and pulmonary embolism. In an extensive study on a large group of patients with venous thrombosis reported by den Heijer and associates [53], these workers concluded that both initial and recurrent thrombotic events showed a strong association with the fasting plasma homocysteine concentration. Levels above the 95th percentile for controls conferred an odds ratio of 2.5 (95% CI 1.2-5.2) for the first event and 3.1 (95% CI 1.4-6.8) for recurrence [53]. Curiously, however, the same investigators also noted that risk of venous thrombosis appeared to become evident only in individuals with homocysteine concentrations above a threshold (>22 μmol/L), unlike arterial occlusive disease which generally shows a continuous dose-response relationship [48].

Kottke-Marchant et al. [54], in a study on 183 patients being evaluated for a hypercoagulable state on the basis of documented previous venous or peripheral arterial thrombosis or pulmonary embolism, identified 60 in whom standard risk factors for thromboembolism were absent and a screening profile for thrombophilia was normal. Exclusion risk factors included obesity, cancer, recent surgery or trauma, immobilization, renal failure, pregnancy and known thrombogenic medications. The thrombophilia screen included prothrombin, activated partial thromboplastin and reptilase times, as well as measurements of total fibrinogen, antithrombin III, protein C, protein S, plasminogen and plasminogen activator inhibitor, and tests for the lupus-like anticoagulant. Testing for activated protein C resistance caused by factor V Leiden was not available when the study was carried out. Homocysteine concentrations (Fig 2) were significantly higher than matched healthy controls (21.8 ± 13.8 vs. 11.0 ± 4.7 μmol/L, p = 0.001). Using a 13 μmol/L cut point, the calculated odds ratio for thrombosis was 7.8 (95% CI 3.0-20.2) [54].

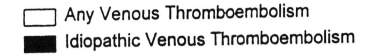

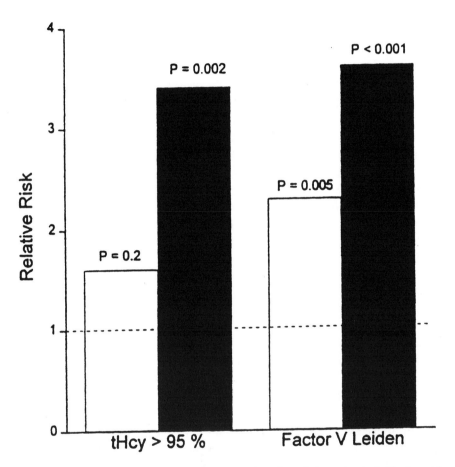

*Figure 3. Relative risk (RR) of venous thromboembolism in individuals with hyperhomocysteinemia or factor V Leiden as isolated risk factors. The RR associated with factor V Leiden is statistically significant for* any *or* idiopathic *thromboembolism. For hyperhomocysteinemia, statistical significance is attained only for idiopathic venous thromboembolism. (Data from Ridker, et al. [62]).*

In addition to collation of data in a number of earlier reviews and meta-analyses [50-52, 55, 56], the clinical association of mild to moderate hyperhomocysteinemia with arterial and venous thrombosis is extensively reviewed in  other chapters contained within this volume, most notably chapters 8, 9, 10, 11 and 13. Though there is substantial evidence that hyperhomocysteinemia con-fers an identifiable increase in the risk of thrombosis, it is not clear what other factors might determine occurrence of a thrombotic event. Of particular interest were the findings of the recent large scale European Concerted Action Project [57]. The authors of this study came to the conclusion that a raized plasma homocysteine was not only an independent risk factor for vascular disease, but also substantially increased the disease probability associated with other risk factors such as smoking and hypertension [57]. A further example of incremental risk of arterial thrombosis resulting from hyperhomocysteinemia has been reported in patients with systemic lupus erythematosus. In 337 such patients in the Hopkins Lupus Cohort Study, risk of stroke and arterial thrombotic events were significantly increased by raized homocysteine concentrations (odds ratio 2.24 and 3.74 respectively) [58]. This was not the case for venous thrombotic events (odds ratio 1.15) [58]. This is in keeping with the concept that whereas there appears to be synergism between conditions that predispose to arterial thrombosis, this does not apply to venous thrombosis which is considered to relate to discrete risk factors [59]. In relation to homocysteine, however, it has recently been suggested that an amplification of risk for occurrence of thrombosis may relate to coexistence of a second prothrombotic condition in addition to hyperhomocysteinemia.

Sporadic case or family reports have appeared in the literature of precocious or unusual thrombotic events occurring in individuals or family members in whom both hyperhomocysteinemia and a second inherited risk factor for thromboembolism were described. For example, Franken et al. [60], described a family in which two family members who co-inherited hyperhomocysteinemia of unspecified type and protein C deficiency developed thrombosis, whereas those with protein C deficiency alone did not. To explain why only about one-third of patients homozygous for homocystinuria develop venous and arterial thromboembolism, Mandel et al. [61] postulated that the coexistence of another thrombophilic disorder might also be necessary for the development of thrombosis. They studied 11 patients with homocystinuria from 7 kindreds with cystathionine β-synthase deficiency, methylenetetrahydrofolate reductase deficiency, the cobalamin C/D defect or selective cobalamin malabsorption. All 6 of the 11 who developed thrombosis had hereditary resistance to activated protein C, a missense mutation (G1691A) in the gene coding for factor V, (factor V Leiden), in which the altered coagulation factor is resistant to inactivation by protein C. Four of the 5 patients without a history of thrombosis did not have factor V Leiden. The only one without thrombosis who did have factor V Leiden had received warfarin therapy since birth.

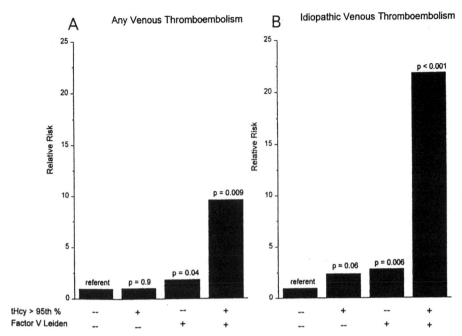

*Figure 4. Relative risk of venous thromboembolism associated with hyperhomocysteinemia or factor V Leiden alone and in combination for* any *and for* idiopathic *thromboembolism. A combination of these risk factors substantially increase the risk. (Data from Ridker, et al. [62]).*

Strong support for these findings were provided by the data of Ridker et al. [62] who, in a prospective cohort study (Physician's Health Study), compared 145 healthy men who subsequently developed venous thromboembolism with 646 men who remained free of any vascular disease during a 10-year period of observation. These investigators assessed the relative risk for venous thromboembolism in individuals with either total plasma homocysteine above the 95th percentile (>17.25 μmol/L) or the factor V Leiden mutation. They found that each condition considered as an isolated risk factor conferred a statistically significant increased relative risk for idiopathic venous thromboembolism. The relative risk (RR) for hyperhomocysteinemia was 3.4 and for factor V Leiden 3.6. (Fig 3). Men with both disorders showed a 20-fold increase in the risk of idiopathic venous thromboembolism (Fig 4). The risk for *any* venous thromboembolic event, including those associated with cancer, recent surgery and trauma, was also analyzed. Factor V Leiden alone (RR = 2.3) or in association with hyperhomocysteinemia (RR = 9.65) conferred a statistically significant risk compared with the referent population. The RR for hyperhomocysteinemia alone did not, however, attain statistical significance in this analysis. The results of this study lend strong endorsement to the proposal that coexistence of an additional risk factor does considerably augment the likelihood of thrombosis in individuals with hyperhomocysteinemia. On the other hand, it should be noted that the finding by Ridker et al [62], of no statistically significant risk for *any* (as opposed to only idiopathic) venous thromboembolic event in association with hyperhomocysteinemia alone, is not fully in agreement with earlier studies. These studies reported an association of hyperhomocysteinemia with venous thromboembolism regardless of the presence of activated protein C resistance [63] or factor V Leiden [51].

Other groups have challenged the notion that concurrent hyperhomocysteinomia and factor V Leiden increases the risk of thrombosis. Quere et al. [64], who studied 15 patients homozygous for cystathionine β-synthase deficiency, found that only two of 5 who had suffered deep vein thrombosis also had factor V Leiden [64]. D'Angelo and associates [65, 66, 67], reporting 307 patients with early-onset or unusual site venous or arterial thrombotic occlusion, did not find a statistically significant difference in concurrence rate of isolated resistance to activated protein C and increased fasting or post-methionine load homocysteine than would be expected in the normal population. In the study reported by den Heijer et al [51], exclusion of subjects with resistance to activated protein C and other established risk factors for thrombosis (deficiencies of protein C, protein S or antithrombin) did not materially affect the risk estimates for raized homocysteine. Kluijtmans et al. [68], studying patients with factor V Leiden found that the prevalence of homozygosity for the thermolabile 5,10-methylenetetrahydrofolate reductase (MTHFR) variant, which is associated with hyperhomocysteinemia, was not different (OR 1.01) between the 471 patients with deep-vein thrombosis and 474 controls. Furthermore, being a factor V Leiden carrier did not modify the risk associated with being homozygous for the MTHFR thermolabile variant. From this, the authors concluded that the homozygous MTHFR mutation is not a genetic risk factor *per se* for deep vein thrombosis, regardless of factor V Leiden genotype. The same group of investigators also screened 24 patients with homocystinuria caused by homozygous cystathionine β-synthase deficiency for factor V Leiden and the C677T mutation in MTHFR [69, 70]. Only one of six patients with thrombosis was a carrier for factor V Leiden, whereas three (50%) were found to be homozygous for the thermolabile MTHFR variant. This compares with a frequency of 10% for homozygosity in the 18 patients without thrombosis as well as the general Dutch population. In contrast to Mandel et al. [61], these authors concluded that factor V Leiden is neither a prerequisite nor a major determinant of thrombotic risk in homocystinuria. On the other hand, they found that compound inheritance of cystathionine β-synthase and MTHFR mutations do constitute a situation of heightened risk for thromboembolism.

At this time, therefore, it must be concluded that while there is clear indication from a number of clinical studies that hyperhomocysteinemia is associated with an increased predisposition to thrombosis, the precise importance of associated risk factors remains in question. There is certainly a preponderance of evidence, concerning hyperhomocysteinemia and factor V Leiden, that supports the concept that prothrombotic mutations in two or more genes create an inherited predisposition to thrombosis [71]. To what extent epigenetic factors influence the expression of inherited risk factors is not known. Occurrence of thrombosis is influenced by several other factors that may mitigate or aggravate risk, and in the case of hyperhomocysteinemia that has a hereditary basis, it is possible that nutritional status may modify the risk burden associated with a particular genotype. For example, adequate folate intake appears to neutralize the tendency to high homocysteine levels in individuals bearing an MTHFR mutation, and may therefore exert a protective effect in vascular disease risk [72, 73]. Also, high doses of pyridoxine are known to ameliorate the risk of vascular complications in homozygotes deficient for cystathionine β-synthase [46]. Little is known about the temporal relationships between elevated levels of homocysteine and thrombosis risk. The duration as well as the degree of hyperhomocysteinemia may play a role in the initiation and progression of the prothrombotic process. It is possible that chronic sustained levels of mild or moderate hyperhomocysteinemia may be more injurious to antithrombotic mechanisms than shorter periods of more marked plasma homocysteine elevations. This could explain why thrombosis has not been noted to occur in association with megaloblastic anemia caused by severe nutritional folate deficiency. The short time to depletion of folate stores, rapid progression to folate deficiency with interdiction of DNA synthesis and development of frank megaloblastic anemia may be too short for the necessary thrombogenic changes to occur [8].

## REFERENCES

1. Mudd SH, Levy HL, Skovby F. Disorders of transulfuration. In: Scriver, CR, Beaudet AL, Sly WS, Valle D, eds. The Metabolic Basis of Inherited Diseases. 6th ed. New York: McGraw-Hill, 1989:693-734.
2. Gibson JB, Carson NAJ, Neill DW. Pathological changes in homocystinuria. J Clin Pathol 1964;17:427-437.
3. Ross R. Mechanisms of disease: Atherosclerosis – an inflammatory disease N Engl J Med 1999;340:115-126.
4. Jakubowski H. Metabolism of homocysteine thiolactone in human cell cultures. Possible mechanism for pathological consequences of elevated homocysteine levels. J Biol Chem 1997;272:1935-1942.

Homocysteine and Coagulation Factors 367

5.  Hladovec J. Experimental homocystinemia, endothelial lesions and thrombosis. Blood Vessels 1979; 16:202-205.
6.  Rounds S, Yee WL, Dawicki DD, et al. Mechanism of extracellular ATP- and adenosine-induced apoptosis of cultured pulmonary artery endothelial cells. Am J Physiol 1998; 275:L379-388.
7.  Bombeli T, Karsan A, Tait JF, Harlan JM. Apoptotic vascular endothelial cells become procoagulant. Blood 1997; 89:2429-2442.
8.  Green R, Miller JW. Folate deficiency beyond megaloblastic anemia: hyperhomocysteinemia and other manifestations of dysfunctional folate status. Semin Hematol. 1999;36:47-64.
9.  Kokame K, Kato H, Miyata T. Homocysteine-respondent genes in vascular endothelial cells identified by differential display analysis. J Biol Chem 1996; 271:29659-29665.
10. Wu KK, Thiagarajan P. Role of endothelium in thrombosis and hemostasis. Annu Rev Med 1996; 47:315-331.
11. Green R. Homocysteine and occlusive vascular disease: culprit or bystander? Prev Cardiol. 1998;1:31-33.
11b Kuller LH, Evans RW. Homocysteine, Vitamins, and cardiovascular disease. Circulation 1998;98:196-199.
12. Nabel EG. Biology of the impaired endothelium. Am J Cardiol 1991; 68:6C-8C.
13. Wall RT, Harlan JM, Harker LA, Striker GE. Homocysteine-induced endothelial cell injury in vitro: a model for the study of vascular injury. Thromb Res 1980; 18:113-121.
14. De Groot PG, Willems C, Boers GH, et al. Endothelial cell dysfunction in homocystinuria. Eur J Clin Invest 1983; 13:405-410.
15. Starkebaum G, Harlan JM. Endothelial cell injury due to copper-catalyzed hydrogen peroxide generation from homocysteine. J Clin Invest 1986; 77:1370-1376.
16. Dudman NPB, Hicks C, Wang J, Wilcken DEL. Human arterial endothelial cell detachment in vitro: its promotion by homocysteine and cysteine. Atherosclerosis 1991; 91:77-83.
17. Harker LA, Ross R, Slichter SJ, Scott RC. Homocystine-induced arteriosclerosis. The role of endothelial cell injury and platelet response in its genesis. J Clin Invest 1976; 58:731-741.
18. Harker LA, Slichter SJ, Scott CR, Ross R. Homocystinemia. Vascular injury and arterial thrombosis. N Engl J Med 1974; 291:537-543.
19. Harker LA, Harlan JM, Ross R. Effect of sulfinpyrazone on homocysteine-induced endothelial injury and arteriosclerosis in baboons. Circ Res 1983; 53:731-739.
20. Rodgers GM, Kane WH. Activation of endogenous factor V by a homocysteine-induced vascular endothelial cell activator. J Clin Invest 1986; 77:1909-1916.
21. Rodgers GM, Conn MT. Homocysteine, an atherogenic stimulus, reduces protein C activation by arterial and venous endothelial cells. Blood 1990; 75:895-901.
22. Lentz SR, Sadler JE. Inhibition of thrombomodulin surface expression and protein C activation by the thrombogenic agent homocysteine. J Clin Invest 1991; 88:1906-1914.
23. Hayashi T, Honda G, Suzuki K. An atherogenic stimulus homocysteine inhibits cofactor activity of thrombomodulin and enhances thrombomodulin expression in human umbilical vein endothelial cells. Blood 1992; 79:2930-2936.

24. Nishinaga M, Ozawa T, Shimada K. Homocysteine, a thrombogenic agent, suppresses anticoagulant heparan sulfate expression in cultured porcine aortic endothelial cells. J Clin Invest 1993; 92:1381-1386.

25. Hajjar KA. Homocysteine-induced modulation of tissue plasminogen activator binding to its endothelial cell membrane receptor. J Clin Invest 1993; 91:2873-2879.

26. Hajjar KA, Mauri L, Jacovina AT, et al. Tissue plasminogen activator binding to the annexin II tail domain. Direct modulation by homocysteine. J Biol Chem 1998; 273:9987-9993.

27. Hajjar KA, Jacovina AT. Modulation of annexin II by homocysteine: implications for atherothrombosis. J Investig Med 1998; 46:364-369.

28. Lentz SR, Sadler JE. Homocysteine inhibits von Willebrand factor processing and secretion by preventing transport from the endoplasmic reticulum. Blood 1993; 81:683-689.

29. Fryer RH, Wilson BD, Gubler DB, Fitzgerald LA, Rodgers GM. Homocysteine, a risk factor for premature vascular disease and thrombosis, induces tissue factor activity in endothelial cells. Arterioscler Thromb 1993; 13:1327-1333.

30. Murphy ME, Piper HM, Watanabe H, Sies H. Nitric oxide production by cultured aortic endothelial cells in response to thiol depletion and replenishment. J Biol Chem 1991; 266:19378-19383.

31. Stamler JS, Osborne JA, Jaraki O, et al. Adverse vascular effects of homocysteine are modulated by endothelium-derived relaxing factor and related oxides of nitrogen. J Clin Invest 1993; 91:308-318.

32. Kang S-S, Wong PWK, Becker N. Protein-bound homocyst(e)ine in normal subjects and in patients with homocystinuria. Pediatr Res 1979;13:1141-1143.

33. Wiley VC, Dudman NPB, Wilcken DEL. Interrelations between plasma free and protein-bound homocysteine and cysteine in homocystinuria. Metabolism 1988;37:191-195.

34. Mansoor MA, Svardal AM, Schneede J, Ueland PM. Dynamic relation between reduced, oxidized, and protein-bound homocysteine and other thiol components in plasma during methionine loading in healthy men. Clin Chem 1992; 38:1316-1321.

35. Refsum H, Helland S, Ueland PM. Radioenzymatic determination of homocysteine in plasma and urine. Clin Chem 1985;31:624-628.

36. Harpel PC, Chang VT, Borth W. Homocysteine and other sulfhydryl compounds enhance the binding of lipoprotein(a) to fibrin: a potential biochemical link between thrombosis, atherogenesis, and sulfhydryl compound metabolism. Proc Natl Acad Sci USA 1992; 89:10193-10197.

37. Uhlemann ER, TenPas JH, Lucky AW, et al. Platelet survival and morphology in homocystinuria due to cystathionine synthase deficiency. N Engl J Med 1976; 295:1283-1286.

38. Hill-Zobel RL, Pyeritz RE, Scheffel U, et al. Kinetics and distribution of [111]Indium-labeled platelets in patients with homocystinuria. N Engl J Med. 1982;307: 781-786.

39. Graeber JE, Slott JH, Ulane RE, Schulman JD, Stuart MJ. Effect of homocysteine and homocystine on platelet and vascular arachidonic acid metabolism. Pediatr. Res. 1982;16:490-493.

40. Wang J, Dudman NPB, Wilcken DEL. Effects of homocysteine and related compounds on prostacyclin production by cultured human vascular endothelial cells. Thromb Haem 1993; 70:1047-1052.

41. Panganamala RV, Karpen CW, Merola AJ. Peroxide mediated effects of homocysteine on arterial prostacyclin synthesis. Prostaglandins Leukot Med 1986; 22:349-356.

42. Durand P, Lussier-Cacan S, Blache D. Acute methionine load-induced hyperhomocysteinemia enhances platelet aggregation, thromboxane biosynthesis, and macrophage-derived tissue factor activity in rats. FASEB J 1997; 11:1157-1168.

43. Lentz SR, Sobey CG, Piegors DJ, et al. Vascular dysfunction in monkeys with diet-induced hyperhomocyst(e)inemia. J Clin Invest 1996; 98:24-29.

44. Lentz SR, Malinow MR, Piegors DJ, et al. Consequences of hyperhomocyst(e)inemia on vascular function in atherosclerotic monkeys. Arterioscler Thromb Vasc Biol 1997;17:2930-2934.

45. Mudd SH, Skovby F, Levy HL, et al. The natural history of homocystinuria due to cystathionine beta-synthase deficiency. Am J Hum Genet 1985; 37:1-31.

46. Wilcken DEL, Wilcken B. The natural history of vascular disease in homocystinuria and the effects of treatment. J Inherit Metab Dis. 1997;20:295-300.

47. Schroeder HA. Is atherosclerosis a conditioned pyridoxal deficiency? J Chron Dis. 1955;2:28-41.

48. Robinson K, Mayer EL, Miller DP, et al. Hyperhomocysteinemia and low pyridoxal phosphate. Common and independent reversible risk factors for coronary artery disease. Circulation. 1995;92:2825-2830.

49. Folsom AR, Nieto FJ, McGovern PG, et al. Prospective study of coronary heart disease incidence in relation to fasting total homocysteine, related genetic polymorphisms, and B vitamins: the atherosclerosis risk in communities (ARIC) study. Circulation. 1998; 98:204-210.

50. Boushey CJ, Beresford SAA, Omenn, GS, Motulsky AG. A quantitative assessment of plasma homocysteine as a risk factor for vascular disease. Probable benefits of increasing folic acid intakes. JAMA. 1995;274:1049-1057.

51. den Heijer M, Koster T, Blom HJ, et al. Hyperhomocysteinemia as a risk factor for deep-vein thrombosis. N Engl J Med 1996; 334:759-762.

52. Green R, Jacobsen DW. Clinical implications of homocysteinemia. In: Bailey L, ed. Folate in Health and Disease. New York, NY, Marcell Dekker, 1994; pp75-122.

53. den Heijer M, Blom HJ, Gerrits WBJ, et al. Is hyperhomocysteinemia a risk factor for recurrent venous thrombosis? Lancet 1995; 345:882-885.

54. Kottke-Marchant K, Green R, Jacobsen DW, et al. High plasma homocysteine: a risk factor for arterial and venous thrombosis in patients with normal coagulation profiles. Clin Appl Thromb/Hemostasis 1997; 3:239-244.

55. Mayer EL, Jacobsen DW, Robinson K. Homocysteine and coronary atherosclerosis. J Am Coll Cardiol 1996; 27:517-527.

56. Refsum H, Ueland PM, Nygård O, Vollset SE. Homocysteine and cardiovascular disease. Annu Rev Med 1998; 49:31-62.

57. Graham IM, Daly LE, Refsum HM, et al. Plasma homocysteine as a risk factor for vascular disease. The European Concerted Action Project. JAMA. 1997;277:1775-1781.

58. Petri M, Roubenoff R, Dallal GE, et al. Plasma homocysteine as a risk factor for atherothrombotic events in systemic lupus erythematosus. Lancet 1996; 348:1120-1124.

59. Phillips MD. Interrelated risk factors for venous thromboembolism. Circulation 1997;95:1749-1751.

60. Franken DG, Vreugdenhil A, Boers GHJ, et al. Familial cerebrovascular accidents due to concomitant hyperhomocysteinemia and protein C deficiency type Numeral 1. Stroke 1993; 24:1599-1600.

61. Mandel H, Brenner B, Berant M, et al. Coexistence of hereditary homocystinuria and factor V Leiden - effect on thrombosis. N Engl J Med 1996; 334:763-768.

62. Ridker PM, Hennekens CH, Selhub J, et al. Interrelation of hyperhomocyst(e)inemia, factor V Leiden, and risk of future venous thromboembolism. Circulation 1997; 95:1777-1782.

63. Falcon CR, Cattaneo M, Panzeri D, Martinelli I, Mannucci PM. High prevalence of hyperhomocyst(e)inemia in patients with juvenile venous thrombosis. Arterioscler Thromb 1994; 14:1080-1083.

64. Quere I, Lamarti H, Chadefaux-Vekemans B. Thrombophilia, homocystinuria,and mutation of the factor V gene. N Engl J Med. 1996;335:289.

65. D'Angelo A, Fermo I, D'Angelo SV. Thrombophilia, homocystinuria, and mutation of the factor V gene. N Engl J Med. 1996;335:289.

66. D'Angelo A, Mazzola G, Crippa L, Fermo I, D'Angelo SV. Hyperhomocysteinemia and venous thromboembolic disease. Haematologica 1997; 82:211-219.

67. Fermo I, D'Angelo SV, Paroni R, et al. Prevalence of moderate hyperhomocysteinemia in patients with early-onset venous and arterial occlusive disease. Ann Intern Med 1995;123:747-753.

68. Kluitjmans LAJ, Boers GHJ, Verbruggen B, et al. Homozygous cystathionine $\beta$-synthase deficiency, combined with factor V Leiden or thermolabile methylenetetrahydrafolate reductase in the risk of venous thrombosis. Blood 1998; 91:2015-2018.

69. Kluitjmans LAJ, den Heijer M, Reitsma PH, et al. Thermolabile methylenetetrahyrofolate reductase and factor V Leiden in the risk of deep-vein thrombosis. Thromb Haemost 1998;79:254-258.

70. Boers GHJ. Hyperhomocysteinemia as a risk factor for arterial and venous disease. A review of evidence and relevance. Thromb Haemost 1997; 78:520-522.

71. Miletich JP. Thrombophilia as a multigenic disorder. Semin Thromb Hemost 1998;24 Suppl 1:13-20.

72. Jacques PF, Bostom AG, Williams RR et al. Relation between folate status, a common mutation in methylenetetrahydrofolate reductase, and plasma homocysteine concentrations. Circulation 1996;93:7-9.

73. Girelli D, Friso S, Trabetti E et al. Methylenetetrahydrofolate reductase $C_{677}T$ mutation, plasma homocysteine, and folate in subjects from Northern Italy with or without angiographically documented severe coronary atherosclerotic disease: evidence for an important genetic-environmental interaction. Blood 1998;91: 4158-4163.

# 21. HOMOCYSTEINE AND ENDOTHELIAL DYSFUNCTION

ROBERT T. EBERHARDT AND JOSEPH LOSCALZO

## SUMMARY

Hyperhomocysteinemia has been linked to the development of atherothrombotic disorders in both experimental and clinical investigations. The precise molecular mechanisms responsible for the pathogenicity of hyperhomocysteinemia remain uncertain; however, endothelial injury and dysfunction are paramount. Production of reactive oxygen species, termed oxidative stress, during the auto-oxidation of homocysteine may incite endothelial injury if it exceeds intrinsic antioxidant protection. Endothelial injury leads to endothelial dysfunction with an impairment of endothelial vasoregulatory action and antithrombotic mechanisms. Central to the vasomotor dysregulation is an impairment of endothelium-dependent vasodilation due to an attenuation of nitric oxide-mediated bioaction. Elevated homocysteine may lead to diminished endothelial nitric oxide production *in vitro*. Furthermore, hyperhomocysteinemia leads to diminished responsiveness to endothelium-dependent agonists *in vivo*. Additionally, homocysteine may lead to disturbances in the antithrombotic activities of the endothelium, thus predisposing to platelet adhesion and thrombus formation. These effects of hyperhomocysteinemia on vascular endothelial function contribute to atherothrombogenesis with a heightened predilection toward clinical thrombosis and atherosclerotic vascular disease. Therapeutic interventions that enhance homocysteine metabolism or attenuate oxidative mechanisms may

*K. Robinson (ed.), Homocysteine and Vascular Disease, 371-387.*
© 2000 *Kluwer Academic Publishers. Printed in the Netherlands.*

improve endothelial function and, thus, limit the development of atherothrombotic disorders.


## INTRODUCTION

In 1969, McCully observed arteriosclerotic (and "pre-atherosclerotic") vascular lesions among children with marked elevation in plasma homocysteine levels due to inborn errors of metabolism, thus implicating homocysteine in the pathogenesis of atherosclerosis [1]. His postmortem findings in these children with hyperhomocysteinemia included focal intimal and medial fibrosis with disruption of the internal elastic lamina in large and medium-sized arteries, and focal proliferation of perivascular connective tissue surrounding small arteries [1]. Since that time, numerous epidemiological data have supported that even moderate elevations of plasma homocysteine concentrations are associated with an increased risk of atherosclerotic vascular disease [2-4]. Furthermore, a defect in homocysteine metabolism was unmasked among individuals with mild elevations in fasting homocysteine concentrations with the development of the methionine challenge test [5]. In fact, even mild hyperhomocysteinemia is a risk factor for the development of systemic atherosclerosis, including coronary, cerebral, and peripheral arterial disease, as well as acute atherothrombotic disorders, including myocardial infarction and stroke [2-5].

Experimental models of hyperhomocysteinemia have produced conflicting results regarding the contribution of homocysteine to the development of atherosclerosis. McCully and Ragsdale observed the development of arteriosclerotic (and "pre-atherosclerotic") lesions in rabbits with hyperhomocysteinemia induced by subcutaneous injection of homocysteine thiolactone for 35 days [6]. These findings were unable to be duplicated by Donahue and colleagues using similar experimental techniques [7]. Conflicting findings were also observed in other animal models, including monkeys and pigs, with hyperhomocysteinemia induced either by infusion of homocysteine (or an oxidative by-product) or a methionine-rich and/or pyridoxine-deficient diet [8-12]. In contrast, Harker and colleagues have consistently demonstrated the development of arteriosclerotic (and pre-atherosclerotic) lesions in baboons with hyperhomocysteinemia induced by infusion of homocysteine [13-15]. The reproducibility of these vascular lesions in hyperhomocysteinemic baboons suggests that a species-dependent response may be playing an important role.

The mechanisms responsible for the contribution of hyperhomocysteinemia to the pathogenesis of vascular disease are incompletely understood. Homocysteine may incite its adverse effects upon the vasculature at several potential sites, including platelets or other circulating blood elements, vascular smooth muscle, and/or vascular endothelium. Since the vascular endothelium plays a dynamic role in providing an antithrombotic milieu and in controlling vascular tone and blood flow, homocysteine may adversely effect endothelial vasomotor regulation and antithrombotic mechanisms by causing endothelial injury and dysfunction. This chapter will focus on the impact of hyperhomocysteinemia on endothelial function, the mechanisms of homocysteine-induced endothelial dysfunction, and the effects of homocysteine-induced endothelial dysfunction on endothelial vasoregulatory and antithrombotic mechanisms.

## ENDOTHELIAL METABOLISM AND INJURY

Homocysteine has been shown to cause endothelial cell injury both *in vitro* and *in vivo*. Harker and colleagues demonstrated frank endothelial injury in baboons with hyperhomocysteinemia induced by an infusion of homocysteine [14]. The surface of large arteries showed patchy desquamation of the endothelium with a loss of surface cells and an increase in circulating endothelial cells [14]. Despite a 25-fold increase in endothelial cell regeneration, the aorta showed patchy endothelial cell desquamation that comprized 10% of the surface area [14]. It was suggested that platelet-rich thrombi might be forming in these areas of endothelial injury owing to exposure of the subendothelial matrix. In addition, homocysteine has been shown to induce cell detachment and [$^{51}$Cr]-release from human endothelial cells in culture [16]. These findings support the possibility that by causing endothelial injury *in vivo*, chronic hyperhomocysteinemia may contribute to the pathogenesis of atherothrombosis.

An understanding of the mechanisms responsible for homocysteine-mediated endothelial injury requires a brief discussion of homocysteine biochemistry and its effects on endothelial metabolism. This is more extensively discussed in Chapter 3. Homocysteine is a sulfur-containing amino acid formed during methionine metabolism. The metabolic fates of homocysteine include remethylation to form methionine or entry into the transulfuration pathway by the action of cystathionine β-synthase (CBS) to form cystathionine. Emphasizing the importance of CBS in homocysteine metabolism are the consequences of genetic deficiencies in CBS. Homozygous CBS deficiency results in the marked elevation in plasma homocysteine levels of homocystinuria, while heterozygous CBS deficiency results in a mild elevation in fasting plasma homocysteine levels and impaired homocysteine handling with a methionine challenge. Deficiencies of any of the essential cofactors in these reactions, including folate, vitamin B$_{12}$, and vitamin B$_6$, will contribute to abnormal homocysteine metabolism. Homocysteine may also undergo auto-oxidation to form homocysteine, and conversion to homocysteine thiolactone, with the generation of hydrogen peroxide [17]. As with other thiols, by-products of homocysteine oxidation include superoxide, hydrogen peroxide, and hydroxyl radical. It is primarily the generation of hydrogen peroxide (and subsequent hydroxyl radical) that is felt to impart the major toxicity of homocysteine, serving as the key source of oxidative stress [18].

There has been reasonable consistency in the experimental evidence supporting the contribution of hydrogen peroxide to the pathogenesis of homocysteine-induced endothelial injury. Starkebaum and Harlan demonstrated spontaneous hydrogen peroxide generation from homocysteine in a copper-dependent manner [19]. Furthermore, this hydrogen peroxide generation resulted in lysis of endothelial cells [19]. The toxic effects of homocysteine on endothelial cells are attenuated by incubation of cell cultures with catalase, strongly suggesting a role for hydrogen peroxide [19]. Additionally, the generation of hydroxyl radical has been implicated to mediate the effects of hydrogen peroxide; this conclusion is based upon the ability of desferrioxamine to attenuate the endothelial toxicity of homocysteine [20]. In contrast, superoxide is felt to play only a minor role in homocysteine toxicity, as benefits similar to those of catalase have not been observed with superoxide dismutase [17].

The generation of hydrogen peroxide during the oxidation of homocysteine may play a major role in the pathogenesis of arterial injury in homocystinuria. Patients with homozygous CBS deficiency have an elevated plasma copper level that may promote the oxidative stress of hyperhomocysteinemia and the spontaneous generation of hydrogen peroxide [21]. In addition, endothelial cells partially deficient in CBS are more susceptible to methionine- and homocysteine-mediated cell injury [22]. When exposed to homocysteine, vascular endothelial cells derived from an obligate CBS heterozygote had higher [$^{51}$Cr]-release and greater platelet adhesion than wild-type cells, thus supporting greater susceptibility to endothelial injury [22].

The cellular effects of hydrogen peroxide generation and increased oxidative stress may lead to cell damage and death. These cellular changes include loss of ATP, DNA damage, activation of poly-ADP ribose polymerase, loss of NAD$^+$, oxidation of glutathione, and lipid peroxidation [23]. In addition, superoxide anion and hydroxyl radical may initiate lipid peroxidation and oxidation of low-density lipoprotein [17]. Blundell and colleagues suggested that the major oxidative threat to endothelial cells is derived from radicals generated intracellularly [24]. The toxicity of homocysteine toward endothelial cells was prevented by free radical scavengers with access to the intracellular compartment, but not those with access only to the extracellular space [24].

Alternative or additional mechanisms through which homocysteine may induce endothelial injury have been entertained. The reactive sulfhydryl group of homocysteine has been implicated in its pathogenicity independent of hydrogen peroxide generation, acting directly on cellular targets. In addition, increased production of homocysteine thiolactone may lead to "homocysteinylation" (thiolation) of cellular and extracellular protein amino groups [25].

Within endothelial cells there are multiple mechanisms that serve to attenuate the toxicity of homocysteine, including glutathione, cellular glutathione peroxidase (GPX), catalase, and nitric oxide (NO) [17]. Glutathione maintains the sulfhydryl groups of cellular proteins and other compounds in their reduced form. GPX catalyzes the reduction of lipid and hydrogen peroxides to their corresponding alcohols. The actions of GPX have also been shown to prevent the oxidative inactivation of NO [26]. The benefit of exogenous catalase in attenuating the toxic effects of homocysteine *in vitro* suggests a similar role of catalase *in vivo*. NO may interact with homocysteine to form S-nitrosohomocysteine, which attenuates its toxicity [27]. S-nitrosohomocysteine does not support the generation of hydrogen peroxide nor undergo conversion to homocysteine thiolactone, while still maintaining the bioactivity of NO as a nitric oxide donor [27]. Thus, endothelial cells possess several mechanisms to counterbalance the detrimental actions of homocysteine. In fact, brief exposure to homocysteine may stimulate endothelial cells to produce NO, thus aiding in its detoxification [28].

With persistent exposure to homocysteine, many of these protective mechanisms are overwhelmed and the damaging effects of homocysteine ensue. The dysfunctional endothelium is unable to sustain NO production, and this depletion of endothelial NO synthetic capacity leaves the endothelium vulnerable to damage [29]. In addition, homocysteine impairs the ability of endothelial cells to detoxify hydrogen peroxide by impairing cellular antioxidant defenses, including a reduction in cellular glutathione and a lower proportion of reduced thiols [30, 31]. Intracellular $NAD^+$ stores are also reduced in response to homocysteine-induced toxicity, and this effect closely correlates with endothelial cell viability [24]. Furthermore, exposure of endothelial cells to homocysteine decreases the expression and activity of the intracellular isoform of GPX [29]. In addition, unlike most endothelial perturbants, homocysteine fails to induce expression of HSP70, which is critical for the survival of a variety of cells exposed to oxidative stress [32]. Thus, homocysteine impairs the cellular mechanisms that attenuate its toxic effects. By causing endothelial injury and alterations in endothelial metabolism, homocysteine may cause endothelial dysfunction with impairment of vasoregulatory and antithrombotic mechanisms (Table 1). Endothelial dysfunction is an established early step in the development and contributes to the pathogenesis of atherosclerosis.

*Table 1. Effects of homocysteine on endothelial cell function*

| Endothelium-generated mediator | Consequence of exposure to homocysteine |
|---|---|
| Nitric oxide NO | Brief exposure increases NO production *in vitro* [28], while prolonged exposure decreases NO production and bioaction both *in vitro* and *in vivo* [29,38] |
| Prostacyclin (PGI₂) | Inconsistent data with both stimulation and inhibition of PGI₂ production reported *in vitro* [34,35] |
| Thrombomodulin (TM) | Decreases TM expression and activation, both *in vitro* and *in vivo* [46,47], resulting in diminished protein C activation [38,46] and greater factor V activity [45] |
| Heparan sulfate | Modulates surface expression of heparan sulfate and, thus, regulates antithrombin III activity *in vitro* [48] |
| Tissue-type plasminogen vator (t-PA) | Selectively reduces binding sites and acti-activity of t-PA *in vitro* [50] |
| ecto-ADPase | Reduces the activity of ecto-ADPase *in vitro* [44] |

## ENDOTHELIAL VASOREGULATORY FUNCTION

The vascular endothelium plays a critical role in the control of vascular tone and regulation of blood flow. The release of NO and other mediators from the endothelium is a key determinant of the vascular response to many physiological stimuli [33]. Hyperhomocysteinemia may lead to a depletion of NO by impairing its production, by generating reactive oxygen species, and by impairing antioxidant defenses [30]. Primarily by altering the bioaction of NO homocysteine may lead to endothelial vasomotor dysfunction. Endothelial dysfunction is characterized by impaired endothelium-dependent vasodilation that may lead to heightened vascular tone, a propensity toward vasospasm, and dysregulation of blood flow. The effects of homocysteine upon endothelial NO release and endothelium-dependent vascular function have

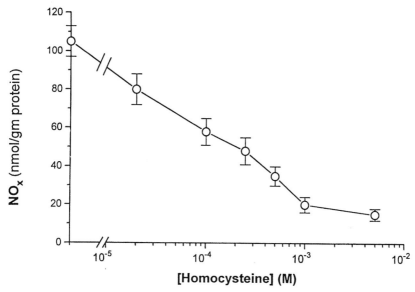

*Figure 1. The effect of homocysteine on endothelial nitric oxide production. Confluent bovine aortic endothelial cells were incubated for 4 hours with media containing the indicated concentrations of homocysteine. The concentration of $NO_x$ within the media was measured using photolysis/chemiluminscence. Each point represents the mean ± S.E.M. of 5 experiments performed in duplicate (p<0.001 by ANOVA). Reproduced with the permission of the American Society for Biochemistry and Molecular Biology from Upchurch et al; J. Biol. Chem 1997;272:17012.*

been studied both *in vitro* and *in vivo*.

## IN VITRO STUDIES

Exposure of cultured endothelial cells to homocysteine may lead to stimulation or impairment of the release and bioaction of NO. The variable reported effects of homocysteine on endothelial NO production are a consequence of the duration and concentration of homocysteine exposure. Stimulation of NO production from endothelial cells transiently exposed to homocysteine leads to increased S-nitrosohomocysteine formation, which was associated with a 78% increase in nitric oxide synthase (NOS) activity and a 58% increase in *Nos3* messenger RNA [28]. These findings support the view that stimulation of NO production by homocysteine may provide a protective, detoxifying mechanism. In contrast, prolonged exposure of endothelial cells to homocysteine results in diminished NO bioaction with an attenuation of the ability of homocysteine-

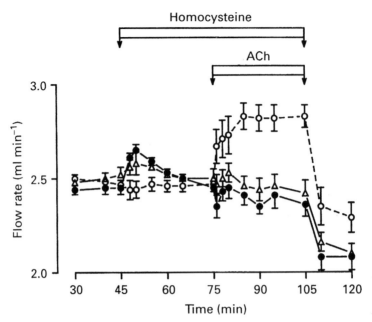

*Figure 2. The effect of homocysteine on acetylcholine (Ach)-induced vasodilation of the rat pancreatic bed. Flow rates in isolated perfused rat pancreas were determined in response to 0.05 μM acetylcholine alone (O), 0.05 μM acetylcholine and 2 mM homocysteine (●), and 0.05 μM acetylcholine and 200 μM homocysteine (Δ). Each point represents the mean ± S.E.M. of 5 experiments. Reproduced with the permission of Stockton Press from Quéré et al; Br. J. Pharmacol. 1997;122:351.*

exposed endothelial cells, stimulated to release NO, to inhibit ADP-induced platelet aggregation [27, 29]. In addition, we found that treatment of bovine aortic endothelial cells with homocysteine leads to a dose-dependent reduction in $NO_x$ production that is independent of NOS activity or *Nos3* gene transcription (Fig. 1) [29]. Thus, it appears that with persistent exposure to homocysteine over time, the endothelium is unable to maintain adequate NO production to detoxify the thiol [30].

In addition to the effect on NO, homocysteine may influence the metabolism and action of other vasoactive mediators. There have been conflicting reports regarding the effect of homocysteine on prostacyclin ($PGI_2$) metabolism. In one study, $PGI_2$ production from isolated rat aortae was inhibited by 1 and 10 mM homocysteine but stimulated by 1 and 100 μM homocysteine [34]. These effects of homocysteine were mimicked by hydrogen peroxide and prevented by incubation with catalase. Similarly, homocysteine inhibited $PGI_2$ production by human endothelial cells cultured in medium containing 20% fetal calf serum [35]. In contrast, in medium containing 20% human serum, free or protein-bound homocysteine had no effect on $PGI_2$ production by human endothelial cells [35]. Thus, the effect of homocysteine on endothelial prostacyclin production remains unclear and still requires further investigation for clarification, especially regarding its effect *in vivo*.


ANIMAL STUDIES

Several experimental models have been utilized to evaluate the effects of hyperhomocysteinemia on vascular endothelial function. These have included hyperhomocysteinemia induced by acute or chronic infusion of homocysteine (or one of its oxidative metabolites), or by a methionine-rich, folate-deficient or a pyridoxine-deficient diet. There are, however, problems with these models, such that they poorly mimic the human disease. Infusion of homocysteine thiolactone may produces changes itself that are not a consequence of homocysteine's effects. In addition, vitamin deficiencies may result in metabolic changes that contribute to vascular dysfunction independent of their effect on homocysteine metabolism. More recently a model of hyperhomocysteinemia was developed by targeted disruption of the cystathionine β-synthase gene [36]. This model may more accurately mimic the human disease and allow for a detailed exploration into the pathogenic mechanisms of hyperhomocysteinemia.

Quéré and colleagues evaluated the effects of an acute infusion of homocysteine on vascular function in the isolated rat pancreatic bed [37]. Infusion of homocysteine at concentrations of 200 μM and 2 mM into the isolated rat pancreatic bed abolished the endothelium-dependent vasodilation induced by acetylcholine, but did not alter adenosine-induced vasodilation (Fig. 2) [37]. The increase in pancreatic flow induced by the acetylcholine infusion was completely suppressed by an acute infusion of homocysteine. In contrast, the increase in pancreatic flow induced by adenosine was not modified by the acute infusion of homocysteine. These effects of homocysteine were not a consequence of direct antimuscarinic actions, as demonstrated by normal contraction of the rat ileum with coincubation of acetylcholine and homocysteine. Thus, an acute infusion of homocysteine may impair the endothelium-dependent vasodilation of a vascular bed *in situ*. This acute model is devoid of the confounding effect of possible alterations in vascular structure, but lacks the long-term effects and utilized higher concentrations of homocysteine than are encountered clinically.

Lentz and colleagues assessed the effect of diet-induced hyperhomocysteinemia in monkeys on endothelium-dependent vascular function [38]. A moderate increase in plasma homocysteine concentrations (from $4.0 \pm 0.2$ μM to $10.6 \pm 2.6$ μM) occurred when monkeys were fed a methionine-rich, folic acid-deficient diet for 4 weeks [38]. The monkeys fed the methionine-rich diet had a diminished vasodilator response to the endothelium-dependent agonists, acetylcholine and ADP, with an attenuation of the increase in hind limb blood flow *in vivo* [38]. There was, however, also a diminished response to the endothelium-independent agent nitroprusside [38]. Similarly, a more dramatic decrease in hind limb blood flow in response to an intraarterial infusion of collagen in these hyperhomocysteinemic monkeys appeared to be a consequence of diminished endothelial responsiveness to platelet-generated ADP rather than heightened platelet aggregation [38]. A similar impairment in vasorelaxation with diminished response to acetylcholine and ADP, and to a lesser extent nitroprusside, was seen *ex vivo* in precontracted carotid arteries from monkeys fed the methionine-rich diet [38]. Thus, long-term exposure to moderate hyperhomocysteinemia, induced by dietary modification, is associated with altered endothelium-dependent and -independent vascular function. Importantly, these alterations in vasodilator response were observed in the absence of structural alterations in the vasculature.

The primary genetic model of hyperhomocysteinemia developed thus far is the cystathionine β-synthase (CBS)-deficient mouse created using "knock out" technology [36]. Homozygous CBS deficient mice have marked hyperhomocysteinemia and manifest growth retardation and diminished survival. Heterozygous CBS-deficient mice have a 2-fold elevation in plasma homocysteine levels with normal growth and survival characteristics [36]. We have recently reported a defect in endothelium-dependent vascular function in both the heterozygous and homozygous CBS-deficient mice [39]. We assessed endothelium-dependent vascular function measuring the relaxation to acetylcholine in precontracted aortic rings using a horizontal myograph and the vasodilator response of mesenteric arterioles during superfusion of methacholine using videomicroscopy. These mice manifest impaired acetylcholine-induced aortic relaxation *in vitro* and paradoxical vasoconstriction of the mesenteric microcirculation with superfusion of methacholine *in vivo* [39]. Thus, both mild and severe hyperhomocysteinemia due to heterozygous and homozygous CBS deficiency, respectively, impairs endothelium-dependent (NO-mediated) vascular function. This model may more accurately mimic the human disease than diet-induced hyperhomocysteinemic models.

## HUMAN INVESTIGATIONS

Human studies evaluating the impact of hyperhomocysteinemia on endothelium-dependent vascular function have included an assessment of the effect of an oral methionine challenge, a comparison of vascular function in

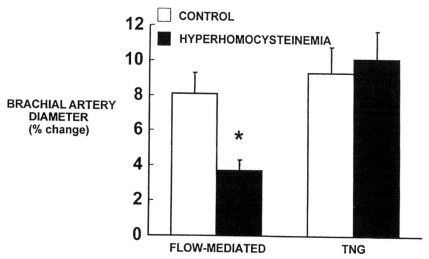

*Figure 3. The effect of homocysteine on brachial artery reactivity in humans. The vasodilator response of the brachial artery (expressed in % change in vessel diameter from baseline) to the endothelium-dependent stimuli of increased flow, resulting from reactive hyperemia, and the endothelium-independent agent nitroglycerin (TNG) was measured in 26 hyperhomocysteinemic subjects and 15 age- and gender-matched controls. The results represent the mean ± S.E.M. for all subjects (\*p=0.004). Reproduced with the permission of the American Heart Association from Tawakol et al; Circulation 1997;95:1119.*

homozygous and heterozygous homocystinuria, and an assessment of the effects of naturally occurring mild hyperhomocysteinemia. Chambers and colleagues evaluated flow-mediated dilation of the brachial artery in 13 healthy volunteers following an oral methionine load (of 100 mg/kg) [40]. The plasma homocysteine concentration rose from 9.3 ± 1.0 μM at baseline to 24.2 ± 3.6 μM and 30.5 ± 3.0 μM at 2 and 4 hours, respectively [40]. Mean flow-mediated dilation fell from 4.6 ± 0.8% at baseline to 0.7 ± 1.4% and −1.3 ± 0.8% at 2 and 4 hours, respectively [40]. Flow-mediated dilation strongly correlated with the plasma homocysteine concentration (p<0.001) [40]. In contrast, no significant difference was observed in vasodilation induced by nitroglycerin following the methionine load [40]. Thus, endothelium-dependent, but not endothelium-independent, vasodilation is impaired during the acute rise in plasma homocysteine concentrations following a methionine challenge.

In contrast to the acute rise in homocysteine following a methionine challenge, homozygous homocystinuria results in sustained elevations in the plasma homocystene levels. Impaired flow-mediated dilation, with preservation of nitroglycerin-mediated dilation, was demonstrated in 9 children with homozygous homocystinuria [41]. In contrast, in 14 of their obligate heterozygous parents, neither was the homocysteine level elevated nor flow-mediated dilation impaired [41]. More recently, mild hyperhomocysteinemia was found to be associated with impairment of endothelium-dependent vascular function [42, 43]. Tawakol and colleagues evaluated the effect of mild hyperhomocysteinemia (>16 μM) on endothelium-dependent vasodilation of the brachial artery in an elderly cohort (age 60 to 80 years) [43]. Flow-mediated, endothelium-dependent vasodilation was significantly impaired in the hyperhomocysteinemic subjects compared with control subjects (3.7 ± 0.6% versus 8.1 ± 1.2%; P=0.004) (Fig. 3) [43]. In contrast, endothelium-independent vasodilation induced by sublingual nitroglycerin was not different between the groups [43]. Similarly, Woo and colleagues found that a plasma homocysteine level above the 75$^{th}$ percentile in a cohort of middle-aged Chinese adults was associated with impaired endothelium-dependent, flow-mediated dilation of the brachial artery [42].

ENDOTHELIAL ANTITHROMBOTIC MECHANISMS

Despite marked platelet accumulation at the site of vascular injury and formation of platelet-rich thrombi, direct proaggregatory effects of hyperhomocysteinemia have not been uniformly demonstrated. It has been suggested that the propensity toward thrombosis seen in hyperhomocysteinemia is a consequence of effects on the platelet-vessel wall interaction. The vascular endothelium plays a dynamic role in preventing platelet adhesion and thrombosis. Normal antiaggregatory and antithrombotic actions of the endothelium include production of thrombomodulin, heparan sulfate, tPA, ecto-ADPase, and NO. Homocysteine may adversely effects vascular endothelial cell function to alter these antithrombotic mechanisms and create a milieu that strongly favors thrombus formation [44]. Thus, the thrombogenicity of hyperhomocysteinemia is a consequence of endothelial dysfunction that promotes the prothrombotic activity and impairs antithrombotic actions of the vascular endothelium.

Homocysteine alters the activity of factors within the coagulation cascade in a manner that promotes thrombosis. Exposure of cultured endothelial cells to homocysteine leads to increased conversion of endogenous factor V to activated factor V (or factor Va) [45]. This effect is explained by a decreased capacity of cultured endothelial cells to activate protein C as a consequence of diminished activity and surface expression of thrombomodulin, the thrombin cofactor responsible for protein C activation [46, 47]. Numerous in vitro studies support alterations in expression or activity of antithrombotic factors that can increase the propensity toward thrombosis; however, these studies typically use higher concentrations of homocysteine than encountered clinically. Diminished thrombomodulin-dependent activation of protein C has been demonstrated ex vivo with arterial segments from monkeys with diet-induced, moderate hyperhomocysteinemia [38].

Homocysteine may impair the activity of anticoagulant factors, stimulate the activity of procoagulants, and interfere with fibrinolytic activity of the endothelium, all of which facilitate thrombus formation. Homocysteine inhibits antithrombin III action by modulating the expression of anticoagulant heparan sulfate proteoglycans and, thus, altering its binding to endothelial cells [48]. Incubation of endothelial cells in culture with homocysteine increases tissue factor expression and activity [49]. In addition, homocysteine inhibits tissue-type plasminogen activator (t-PA) receptor function as preincubation of endothelial cells with homocysteine results in selective reduction in cellular binding sites for and activity of t-PA [50].

Through effects on the endothelium, homocysteine may indirectly promote platelet activation and aggregation, and, thus, increase the propensity toward thrombosis. Homocysteine reduces endothelial ecto-ADPase activity and depletes bioactive NO These actions serve to heighten the reactivity of circulating platelets. However, a similar degree of platelet activation *in vivo* has been demonstrated in diet-induced hyperhomocysteinemic monkeys [38]. Both hyperhomocysteinemic and control monkeys experienced a 30-40% decrease in venous platelet counts during intraarterial collagen infusion [38]. In contrast, heightened platelet response with a 3-fold increase in platelet consumption was observed in several homocystinuric patients as measured using [$^{51}$Cr]-labeled platelet turnover analysis [13].

## OTHER EFFECTS: CONTROL OF CELL GROWTH AND PROLIFERATION

Homocysteine alters the function of endothelial cells, in part, by modulating the expression of certain genes. Incubation of cultured human umbilical vein endothelial cells (HUVEC) with homocysteine induces the expression of multiple genes, including the upregulation of a stress protein, GRP78/BiP, and a bifunctional enzyme, methylenetetrahydrofolate dehydrogenase and methyltetrahydrofolate cyclohydrolase, involved in homocysteine metabolism [51]. In addition, homocysteine inhibits DNA synthesis in vascular endothelial cells and arrests their growth in the G1 phase of the cell cycle [52, 53]. This effect on cell growth appears to be mediated by decreased methylation and membrane association of a G1 regulator, p21$^{ras}$, with a reduction in mitogen-activated protein kinase activity [52]. These effects contrast with the observation of increased endothelial cell regeneration *in vivo* made by Harker and colleagues [14]. In contrast to the inhibitory effects seen on endothelial cell growth and proliferation, homocysteine has been shown to enhance vascular smooth muscle cell growth and proliferation in association with an increase in cyclin A1 and cyclin D expression [53]. In addition to the direct effects reported, homocysteine may facilitate vascular smooth muscle growth by impairing the inhibitory factors produced by the endothelium.


THERAPEUTIC INTERVENTIONS & EFFECTS ON ENDOTHELIAL FUNCTION

Therapies designed to lower plasma homocysteine levels or modify the antioxidant mechanisms in patients with hyperhomocysteinemia may influence the pathogenesis of arterial injury and dysfunction. Antioxidants may act as a sink for the reactive oxygen species generated during homocysteine oxidation. Supplementation with essential cofactors in methionine and homocysteine metabolism may lower plasma homocysteine levels. The reduction in oxidative stress, by direct action or through a reduction in homocysteine levels, may attenuate endothelial injury and dysfunction and possibly regulate the development and progression of atherosclerosis. Although studies have shown a benefit of vitamin supplementation with both folate and pyridoxine on homocysteine metabolism and levels, few studies have evaluated its consequences on endothelial function. Van den Berg and colleagues evaluated the effect of folic acid and pyridoxine supplementation on endothelial function in 48 young patients with peripheral arterial occlusive disease and mild hyperhomocysteinemia [54]. At baseline, homocysteine concentrations were abnormal in the fasting state in half of the subjects, and abnormal in all subjects following a methionine challenge [54]. Treatment with folic acid (5 mg) and pyridoxine (250 mg) for 12 weeks normalized the fasting and post-challenge homocysteine levels in 98% and 100% of patients, respectively [54]. Endothelial function was assessed in 18 of these subjects who completed therapy for 1 year by measuring von Willebrand factor (vWF) and thrombomodulin (TM) levels. An increased plasma level of vWF and TM were found at baseline and thought to reflect endothelial activation or injury. The increase in vWF level (by 235%) and TM level (by 57 ng/ml) observed at baseline decreased (to 170% and 49 ng/ml, respectively) with therapy [54]. Importantly, however, improvement in endothelium-dependent vasomotor function has not yet been demonstrated with treatment for hyperhomocysteinemia.

*Acknowledgement. We thank Ms. Stephanie Tribuna for her assistance in the preparation of this manuscript.*

## REFERENCES

1.  McCully KS. Vascular pathology of homocysteinemia: Implications for the pathogenesis of arteriosclerosis. Am J Pathol 1969;56:111-28.
2.  Clarke R, Daly L, Robinson K, et al. Hyperhomocysteinemia: an independent risk factor for vascular disease. N Engl J Med 1991;324:1149-55.
3.  Stampfer MJ, Malinow R, Willett WC, et al. A prospective study of plasma homocysteine and risk of myocardial infarction in US physicians. JAMA 1992;268:877-81.
4.  Selhub J, Jacques PF, Bostom AG, et al. Association between plasma homocysteine concentrations and extracranial carotid-stenosis. N Engl J Med 1995;332:286-91.
5.  Boers GH, Smals AG, Trijbels FJ, et al. Heterozygosity for homocystinuria in premature peripheral and cerebral occlusive arterial disease. N Engl J Med 1985;313:709-15.
6.  McCully KS, Ragsdale BD. Production of arteriosclerosis by homocysteinemia. Am J Pathol 1970;61:1-11.
7.  Donahue S, Struman JA, Gaull G. Arteriosclerosis due to homocysteinemia: Failure to reproduce the model in weanling rabbits. Am J Pathol 1974;77:167-73.
8.  Rinehart JF, Greenberg JD. Arteriosclerotic lesions in pyridoxine-deficient monkeys. Am J Pathol 1949;25:481-91.
9.  Reddy GS, Wilcken DE. Experimental homocysteinemia in pigs: comparison with studies in sixteen homocystinuric patients. Metabolism 1982;31:778-83.
10. Krishnaswamy K, Rao SB. Failure to produce atherosclerosis in *Macaca radiata* on a high-methionine, high-fat, pyridoxine-deficient diet. Atherosclerosis 1977;27:253-8.
11. Rolland PH, Friggi A, Barlatier A, et al. Hyperhomocysteinemia-induced vascular damage in the minipig. Captopril-hydrochlorothiazide combination prevents elastic alterations. Circulation 1995;91:1161-74.
12. Smolin LA, Crenshaw TD, Kurtycz D, Benevenga NJ. Homocysteine accumulation in pigs fed diets deficient in vitamin B-6: relationship to atherosclerosis. J Nutr 1983;113:2022-33.
13. Harker LA, Slichter SJ, Scott CR, Ross R. Homocysteinemia. Vascular injury and arterial thrombosis. N Engl J Med 1974;291:537-43.
14. Harker LA, Ross R, Slichter SJ, Scott CR. Homocysteine-induced arteriosclerosis. The role of endothelial cell injury and platelet response to its genesis. J Clin Invest 1976;58:731-41.
15. Harker LA, Harlan JM, Ross R. Effect of sulfinpyrazone on homocysteine-induced endothelial injury and arteriosclerosis in baboons. Circ Res 1983;53:731-9.
16. Wall RT, Harlan JM, Harker LA, Striker GE. Homocysteine-induced endothelial cell injury in vitro: a model for the study of vascular injury. Thromb Res 1980;18:113-21.
17. Welch GN, Upchurch G, Loscalzo J. Hyperhomocysteinemia and atherothrombosis. Ann NY Acad Sci 1997;811:48-58.
18. Loscalzo J. The oxidant stress of hyperhomocysteinemia. J Clin Invest 1996;98:5-7.

19. Starkebaum G, Harlan JM. Endothelial cell injury due to copper-catalyzed hydrogen peroxide generation from homocysteine. J Clin Invest 1986;77:1370-6.

20. Jones BG, Rose FA, Tudball N. Lipid peroxidation and homocysteine induced toxicity. Atherosclerosis 1994;105:165-70.

21. Dudman NP, Wilcken DE. Increased plasma copper in patients with homocystinuria due to cystathionine β-synthase deficiency. Clin Chim Acta 1983;127:105-13.

22. de Groot PG, Willems C, Boers GH, Gonsalves MD, van Aken WG, van Mourik JA. Endothelial cell dysfunction in homocystinuria. Eur J Clin Invest 1983;13:405-10.

23. Kirkland JB. Lipid peroxidation, protein thiol oxidation and DNA damage in hydrogen peroxide-induced injury to endothelial cells: role of activation of poly(ADP-ribose)polymerase. Biochim Biophys Acta 1991;1092:319-25.

24. Blundell G, Jones BG, Rose FA, Tudball N. Homocysteine mediated endothelial cell toxicity and its amelioration. Atherosclerosis 1996;122:163-72.

25. Jakubowski H. Metabolism of homocysteine thiolactone in human cell cultures. Possible mechanism for pathological consequences of elevated homocysteine levels. J Biol Chem 1997;272:1935-42.

26. Freedman J, Frei B, Welch GN, Loscalzo J. Glutathione peroxidase potentiates the inhibition of platelet function by S-nitrosothiols. J Clin Invest 1995;96:394-400.

27. Stamler JS, Osborne JA, Jaraki O, et al. Adverse vascular effects of homocysteine are modulated by endothelium-derived relaxing factor and related oxides of nitrogen. J Clin Invest 1993;91:308-18.

28. Upchurch GR Jr, Welch GN, Fabian AT, Pigazzi A, Keaney JF Jr, Loscalzo J. Stimulation of endothelial nitric oxide production by homocysteine. Atherosclerosis 1997;132:177-85.

29. Upchurch GR Jr, Welch GN, Fabian AJ, et al. Homocysteine decreases bioavailable nitric oxide by a mechanism involving glutathione peroxidase. J Biol Chem 1997;272:17012-7.

30. Upchurch GR Jr, Welch GN, Loscalzo J. Homocysteine, EDRF, and endothelial function. J Nutr 1996;126:1290S-4S.

31. Hultberg B, Anderson A, Isaksson A. The effects of homocysteine and copper ion on the concentration and redox status of thiols in cell line culture. Clin Chim Acta 1997;262:39-51.

32. Outinen PA, Sood SK, Liaw PC, et al. Characterization of the stress-inducing effects of homocysteine. Biochem J 1998;332:213-221.

33. Busse R, Mülsch A, Fleming I, Hecker M. Mechanisms of nitric oxide release from the vascular endothelium. Circulation 1993;87:V18-25.

34. Panganamala RV, Karpen CW, Merola AJ. Peroxide mediated effects of homocysteine on arterial prostacyclin synthesis. Prostaglandins Leukot Med 1986;22:349-56.

35. Wang J, Dudman NP, Wilcken DE. Effects of homocysteine and related compounds on prostacyclin production by cultured human vascular endothelial cells. Thromb Haemost 1993;70:1047-52.

36. Watanabe M, Osada J, Aratani Y, et al. Mice deficient in cystathionine β-synthase: animal model for mild and severe homocysteinemia. Proc Natl Acad Sci USA 1995;92:1585-9.

37. Quéré I, Hillaire-Buys D, Brunschwig C, et al. Effects of homocysteine on acetylcholine- and adenosine-induced vasodilation of pancreatic vascular bed in rats. Br J Pharmacol 1997;122:351-7.

38. Lentz SR, Sobey CG, Piegors DJ, et al. Vascular dysfunction in monkeys with diet-induced hyperhomocysteinemia. J Clin Invest 1996;98:24-9.

39. Eberhardt RT, Forgione M, Rudd MA, Trolliet MR, Cap A, Loscalzo J. Endothelial dysfunction in mice lacking the cystathionine β-synthase gene. Circulation 1998;in press.

40. Chambers JC, McGregor A, Jean-Marie J, Kooner JS. Acute hyperhomocysteinemia and endothelial dysfunction. Lancet 1998;351:36-7.

41. Celermajer DS, Sorensen K, Ryalls M, et al. Impaired endothelial function occurs in the systemic arteries of children with homozygous homocystinuria but not their heterozygous parents. J Am Coll Cardiol 1993;22:854-8.

42. Woo KS, Chook P, Lolin YI, et al. Hyperhomocysteinemia is a risk factor for arterial endothelial dysfunction in humans. Circulation 1997;96:2542-4.

43. Tawakol A, Omland T, Gerhard M, Wu JT, Creager MA. Hyperhomocysteinemia is associated with impaired endothelium-dependent vasodilation in humans. Circulation 1997;95:1119-21.

44. Harpel PC, Zhang X, Borth W. Homocysteine and hemostasis: pathogenetic mechanisms predisposing to thrombosis. J Nutr 1996;126:1285S-9S.

45. Rodgers GM, Kane WH. Activation of endogenous factor V by homocysteine-induced vascular endothelial cell activator. J Clin Invest 1986;77:1909-16.

46. Rodgers GM, Conn MT. Homocysteine, an atherogenic stimulus, reduces protein C activation by arterial and venous endothelial cells. Blood 1990;75:895-901.

47. Hayashi T, Honda G, Suzuki K. An atherogenic stimulus, homocysteine, inhibits cofactor activity of thrombomodulin and enhances thrombomodulin expression in human umbilical vein endothelial cells. Blood 1992;79:2930-6.

48. Nishinaga M, Ozawa T, Shimada K. Homocysteine, a thrombogenic agent, suppresses anticoagulant heparan sulfate expression in cultured porcine aortic endothelial cells. J Clin Invest 1993;92:1381-6.

49. Fryer RH, Wilson BD, Gubler DB, Fitzgerald LA, Rodgers GM. Homocysteine, a risk factor for premature vascular disease and thrombosis, induces tissue factor activity in endothelial cells. Arterioscler Thromb 1993;13:1327-33.

50. Hajjar KA. Homocysteine-induced modulation of tissue plasminogen activator binding to its endothelial cell membrane receptor. J Clin Invest 1993;91:2873-9.

51. Kokame K, Kato H, Miyata T. Homocysteine-respondent genes in vascular endothelial cells identified by differential display analysis. GRP78/BiP and novel genes. J Biol Chem 1996;271:29659-65.

52. Wang H, Yoshizumi M, Lai K, et al. Inhibition of growth and p21ras methylation in vascular endothelial cells by homocysteine but not cysteine. J Biol Chem 1997;272:25380-5.

53. Tsai JC, Perrella MA, Yoshizumi M, et al. Promotion of vascular smooth muscle cell growth by homocysteine: a link to atherosclerosis. Proc Natl Acad Sci USA 1994;91:6369-73.

54. Van den Berg M, Boers GH, Franken DG, et al. Hyperhomocysteinemia and endothelial dysfunction in the young patient with peripheral arterial occlusive disease. Eur J Clin Invest1995;25:176-81.

# 22. THE TREATMENT OF HIGH HOMOCYSTEINE CONCENTRATIONS IN HOMOCYSTINURIA: BIOCHEMICAL CONTROL IN PATIENTS AND THEIR VASCULAR OUTCOME

GODFRIED H.J. BOERS, SUFIN YAP, EILEEN NAUGHTEN AND
BRIDGET WILCKEN

SUMMARY

The natural history of individuals with homocystinuria due to cystathionine β-synthase deficiency was first documented in 1985 by Mudd et al [1]. Untreated, these individuals have severe hyperhomocysteinemia resulting in complications involving the eye (ectopia lentis), skeletal (osteoporosis, dolichostenomelia), vascular (thromboembolic events) and central nervous systems. Vascular complications are, however, the most striking cause of major morbidity and mortality in homocystinuric individuals. The aims of treatment must be to prevent or ameliorate particularly these life-endangering events by controlling or eliminating the severe hyperhomocysteinemia. There are currently three recognized modalities of treatment. For the pyridoxine responsive individual, pyridoxine in pharmacological doses in combination with folic acid and vitamin $B_{12}$ will correct the biochemical abnormalities. In pyridoxine-nonresponsive homocystinuria, a methionine restricted, cystine supplemented diet in combination with the use of pyridoxine, folic acid and vitamin $B_{12}$ is the treatment. However, good compliance with the diet may be difficult to obtain particularly in the late-detected individuals. Betaine, a methyl donor, may be useful in these individuals or as an adjunct to such a

K. Robinson (ed.), Homocysteine and Vascular Disease, 389-411.

diet. Additional medical measures that do not affect the biochemical abnormalities but aim at reducing or eliminating the thrombotic tendencies have also been used. These include dipyridamole, either alone or in combination with aspirin to normalise decreased platelet survival and minimise vascular intimal lesions, the avoidance of situations associated with an increased risk of thromboembolism and the use of high dose antithrombotic prophylaxis with heparin or warfarin in conditions with prolonged bedrest. From the data recently published by the centers treating a total of 84 homocystinuric individuals with 1314 patient-years of treatment in Australia [4], the Netherlands [5] and Ireland [6], 53 vascular events would have been expected if they had remained untreated according to the data of Mudd et al[1]. Instead only five have been recorded while on treatment (relative risk = 0.091 (95% CI 0.043 - 0.190); p<0.001). This clearly establishes that appropriate treatment of severe hyperhomocysteinemia significantly reduces the vascular risk in homocystinuria, albeit post-treatment homocysteine levels may still be several times higher than the cut-off point for homocysteine in the normal population. The present findings may have relevance to the current concept of mild hyperhomocysteinemia and its association with cardiovascular disease, in which the elevation of plasma homocysteine levels is considerably lower than the post-treatment levels reported by the three centers.

INTRODUCTION

In 1985, Mudd et al carried out a classic study documenting the natural history of 629 homocystinuric patients due to cystathionine β-synthase deficiency, the second most common treatable inherited disorder of amino acid metabolism[1]. The data obtained resulted in time-to-event graphs for each of the major recognized complications, namely ectopia lentis, radiographical osteoporosis, clinically detected thromboembolic events and mental retardation. These well-recognized time-to event graphs for the first time provided the clinician with a prognostic probability for the development of each stated complications when a patient remains untreated. More importantly, the result of this landmark study also establishes baselines for future evaluation of the effects of treatment in this disease.

The cardinal vascular sign in homocystinuria is thromboembolism, affecting both large and small arteries and veins[2]. It is also the most striking cause of major morbidity and mortality in homocystinuria [1,3]. Vascular occlusions may occur at any age and the natural history of clinically detected thromboembolic events have been documented in the abovementioned study by Mudd et al[1]: the probability of suffering from thromboembolism in an untreated patient before the age of 20 was 30% and it rose to 50% before the age of 30 years, with only minor differences in these probabilities between pyridoxine responsive and nonresponsive patients[1]. The study also disclosed that at the time of maximal risk (beyond the age of 10 years) there was 1 event per 25 years.

The purpose of this chapter is to outline the modalities of treatment available for severe hyperhomocysteinemia in patients with cystathionine β-synthase deficiency, to ascertain the biochemical control achieved and to discuss the effects of homocysteine-lowering on the vascular outcome of homocystinuria based on long-term data recently published by three centers in Australia, the Netherlands and Ireland [4-6, see Table 1].

## TREATMENT

### Clinical aims of treatment

The aims of treatment in homocystinuria vary according to the age of diagnosis. If cystathionine β-synthase deficiency is diagnosed in the newborn infant, as ideally it should be, the aim then must be to prevent the development of ocular, skeletal, intravascular thromboembolic complications and to ensure the development of normal intelligence. On the other hand, if the diagnosis is made late when some recognized complications have already occurred, then the clinician's goal must be to prevent life-endangering thromboembolic events and to prevent further escalation of the complications already suffered [7]. To achieve these clinical aims in treatment, one must try to control or eliminate the major biochemical abnormality characterized by cystathionine β-synthase deficiency, i.e. severe hyperhomocysteinemia.

### Strategies of treatment

There are currently three recognized modalities of homocysteine-lowering treatment:
1.  Pyridoxine (vitamin $B_6$), in combination with folic acid, vitamin $B_{12}$.
2.  Methionine restricted, cystine supplemented diet.
3.  Betaine.

*Table 1.* Demographics of HCU patients treated in Australia, The Netherlands and Ireland.[5,6,7]

| | Australia | The Netherlands | Ireland | Combined Data |
|---|---|---|---|---|
| Total no. of HCU patients | 40 | 30 | 25 | 95 |
| No. of pedigrees | 25 | 21 | 19 | 65 |
| Deaths before treatment | 8 | 1 | 0 | 9 |
| Total no. followed-up with treatment | 32 | 28 | 24 | 84 |
| No. of $B_6$ responders | 17 | 19 | 1 | 37 |
| No. of $B_6$ non-responders | 15 | 9 | 23 | 47 |
| Mean period of treatment (years) | | | | |
| $B_6$ responders | 16.6 | 13.2 | 11.7 | 13.8 |
| $B_6$ non-responders | 11.0 | 17.7 | 15.3 | 14.7 |
| Current mean (range) age-years | 30 (9-66) | 38.5(18-70) | 14.75(2.5-23.4) | 27.8(2.5-70) |

## Pyridoxine

Already in 1967, it had been demonstrated by Barber and Spaeth[8] that in some patients with homocystinuria high-dose pyridoxine treatment induces a complete or partial disappearance of their hyperhomocysteinemia, hypermethioninemia, and homocystinuria. This has been confirmed since then by many other authors[9-17]. Such a response was not due to overcoming of a depletion of vitamin $B_6$ in these patients. In Mudd's large survey on 629 patients, it was shown that at least 50% of the included patients did respond to pharmacological doses of pyridoxine[1]. Within sibships, pyridoxine responsiveness or nonresponsiveness was constant which suggested that there were at least two different genetic variant mutations in cystathionine β-synthase.

Pyridoxine is the precursor of cofactor pyridoxal phosphate upon which cystathionine β-synthase depends for its activity. Using sensitive enzyme assays in liver tissues or cultured skin fibroblasts it has been shown that pyridoxine responsive patients generally have at least traces of residual enzyme activity albeit as low as 1% to 2% of normal, and that nonresponsive patients did not[10,11,14,18-24]. Nevertheless, immunochemical studies on cultured fibroblasts by Skovby and coworkers[25,26], revealed the presence of immunoreactive enzyme antigen not only in patients with detectable activity but also in all but one of 6 studied patients with undetectable enzyme activity. Furthermore, they did not find a statistically significant correlation between the percentage of residual activity and the percentage of immunochemically detected enzyme antigen, indicating that other mechanisms apart from complete or partial gene deletion may account for deficient enzyme activity.

The correlation between *in vivo* responsiveness to pyridoxine and the in vitro presence of residual enzyme activity is not absolute as pyridoxine responsiveness has been reported in those homocystinuric patients without detectable residual activities[9,18,23,27,28] and, on the other hand, nonresponsive patients who did have such activity in their cultured fibroblasts[18,23,27]. The detection of no residual enzyme activity in the cultured fibroblasts of the former patients could have been the result of insufficiently sensitive enzyme assays and a residual activity may yet be measured in the liver of these patients because of the higher specific activity of the liver enzyme. Nevertheless, the finding of detectable enzyme activities in pyridoxine nonresponders indicates that the mere presence of residual enzyme activity is not the only prerequisite for clinical pyridoxine responsiveness.

The presence of some residual activity in responsive patients still enables them to convert about 1 gram methionine into inorganic sulphate per day, in contrast to nonresponders who lack this capacity[11]. Pyridoxine treatment enhances this capacity about twofold in responsive patients. However, normal

Table 2. Treatment regimens, biochemical criteria for B6 responsiveness, biochemical marker used in monitoring and its frequency in the Australian, Dutch and Irish centers treating HCU patients.

| | Australian | Dutch | Irish |
|---|---|---|---|
| Treatment regimens used: | | | |
| Dietary methionine restriction | General advice | Methionine 600mg[a] | Methionine 200-625mg |
| Pyridoxine (B6) mg/day | 100-200 | 750 (Adult) 200-500 (Child) | 100-800 (Adult) 150 (Neonate) |
| Folate (mg/day) | 5 | 5 | 5 |
| Vitamin B12 (IM) | Routine to B6 non-responsive patients | If deficient, given 1-2 monthly | Given if deficient |
| Betaine (grams/day) | 6-9 | 6 | 3-6 |
| Biochemical markers monitored | TfHcy[b] | TfHcy THcy[c] | fHcy[d] |
| Frequency of biochemical monitoring (per annum) | 1-2 | 1-2 | ≥8-10 |
| Criteria for B6 responsiveness | TfHcy <20μmol/L | TfHcy < 20μmol/L or THcy <50μmol/L | fHcy <5μmol/L |

[a] Dietary methionine restriction is used in only one Dutch HCU patient.
[b] TfHcy = total free homocysteine (protein-bound), taken as twice the fHcy plus mixed disulphides, homocysteine-cysteine.
[c] THcy (total homocysteine, both protein-bound and nonprotein-bound homocysteine) was used as a biochemical marker for monitoring since 1990 in the Dutch HCU patients. Prior to that, TfHcy was used.
[d] fHcy (free homocystine) is the free disulphide homocystine (homocysteine-homocysteine).

THcy: TfHcy: fHcy is approximately 5: 3-2:1.

*Table 3.* Patient-years of treatment, predicted and actual number of vascular events and biochemical control of HCU patients treated in Australia, The Netherlands and Ireland.

| | Australia | The Netherlands | Ireland | Combined Data |
|---|---|---|---|---|
| Total patient-years of treatment | | | | |
| $B_6$ responsive | 539 | 409 | 366 | 1314 |
| $B_6$ non-responsive | 281 | 250 | 12 | 543 |
| | 258 | 159 | 354 | 771 |
| Actual no. of vascular events while on treatment | 2 | 3 | 0 | 5 |
| Type[a] (no.) of events | PE (1) / MI (1) | AAA (2) / MI (1) | - | PE(1) / MI(2)/ AAA(2) |
| Predicted no. of vascular events if untreated 22 (after Mudd et al, 1985[1]) | 16 | 15 | 53 | |
| Relative risk | 0.088 | 0.181 | - | 0.091 |
| 95% Confidence Interval | 0.02-0.374 | 0.052-0.628 | - | 0.043-0.190 |
| p-values | p<0.001 | p=0.003 | p<0.001 | p<0.001 |
| Mean levels of homocysteine during long-term treatment (µmol/L) | | | | |
| $B_6$ responsive (no. of patients) | TfHcy[b] < 20 (17) | TfHcy = 7 (10)  THcy[b,c] = 30 (18) | fHcy[b] = 7.5 (1) | |
| $B_6$ nonresponsive (no. of patients) | TfHcy[c] = 33 (15) | TfHcy[c] = 34 (7)  THcy[c] = 88 (8) | fHcy[c] = 15.6 (23) | |

[a] PE = pulmonary embolism / MI = myocardial infarction / AAA = abdominal aortic aneurysm.

[b] Refer to Table 2, footnote b,c,d for explanation of the different homocysteine determinants used and their approximate equivalence.

[c] The Netherlands measured total homocysteine (THcy) from 1990.

humans are able to metabolise at least 12 grams of methionine per day. Therefore, complete restoration of the abnormal amino acid levels, as has been reported in many responsive patients while on treatment with pyridoxine[8,10-17,29], may be observed only in the fasting state or in case of moderate protein intake. Profiles of relevant amino acid levels in the fasting state and after a standardized methionine load off and on pyridoxine treatment are given by Boers et al[9]. From these data it is obvious that pyridoxine therapy leaves the capacity of pyridoxine responsive patients to handle a major methionine intake essentially unchanged.

The pyridoxine dose required to achieve successful biochemical control is titrated against plasma homocysteine levels. The optimal dose is reached when at a minimum dose of pyridoxine, the plasma homocysteine is at its lowest. Doses of pyridoxine required for a response varies markedly among pyridoxine responders. Barber and Spaeth achieved responses to doses of 250-500 mg/day [8] while Gaull utilized 800-1200 mg/day of pyridoxine for similar response[30]. However, a patient should not be considered unresponsive to pyridoxine until a dose of 500-1000 mg/day has been given for a period of several weeks [3]. In the neonates diagnosed by newborn screening programme, the Irish group has used a dose of 150 mg/day in three divided doses of pyridoxine to ascertain pyridoxine responsiveness while monitoring free homocystine[1], methionine and cystine[6, see Table 2]. The Dutch group has used a dose of 200-500 mg/day of pyridoxine in children and 750 mg/day in adults for six weeks, while monitoring total free homocysteine[2] and since 1990, total homocysteine[3] levels (free plus protein bound homocysteine)[5]. Using the same biochemical criteria for pyridoxine responsiveness, the Australian group has used a lower dose of 200 mg/day of pyridoxine[4].

Patient safety in the usage of these mega doses of pyridoxine has always featured in the minds of clinicians managing these individuals. Vitamin $B_6$ at doses from 200 mg to 6 gram has sporadically been considered as a cause of sensory neuropathy[31,32]. Remarkably, these side effects have never been observed in patients with homocystinuria who received long-term treatment (up to 24 years) with dosages up to 750 mg[33,34]. This is in line with the experience of the centers in this chapter reporting a total of 1314 patient-years of pyridoxine treatment in these patients[4-6, see Table 3].

It is important to remember that a biochemical response to pyridoxine may not occur in a potentially responsive patient if folate depletion is present [35]. Patients not given folic acid while on pyridoxine become folate-depleted

---

1 Free homocystine is the free disulfide homocystine (homocysteine-homocysteine)

2 The total free homocysteine (nonprotein-bound) is taken as twice the free homocystine plus mixed disulfides, homocysteine-cysteine.

3 Total homocysteine consists of both protein-bound and nonprotein-bound (total free) homocysteine.

unless supplemented, probably as a consequence of increased flux through the remethylation pathway. The dose of folic acid generally used has been 5 mg/day in adults. Furthermore, to avoid folate-refractoriness, it is mandatory to prevent deficiency of vitamin $B_{12}$, the cofactor in folate-mediated remethylation of homocysteine into methionine.

For those that are responsive to pyridoxine in combination with folic acid and vitamin $B_{12}$, it remains debatable as to whether long-term treatment with other measures such as methionine-restricted, cystine-supplemented diet or betaine supplementation provides the optimal biochemical control. Even the patients with maximal responsiveness to pyridoxine in the presence of adequate folate and $B_{12}$ have reduced tolerance to methionine during methionine loading tests and pyridoxine in these patients only corrects the biochemical abnormalities in the fasting state[36]. Such patients, in theory, may experience abnormal episodic surges in methionine or homocysteine following protein ingestion[3]. Hence, it follows that these patients may benefit from some methionine restriction or the use of small frequent feedings[36]. It is indeed the clinical practice to give general advice to these patients on reducing the intake of food containing methionine, at least distributing the methionine intake during the day.

**Methionine-restricted, cystine-supplemented diet**

A methionine-restricted, cystine-supplemented diet to correct the biochemical abnormalities is used in the treatment of pyridoxine nonresponsive homocystinuria. Such a diet was devised by Komrower et al [37] and Perry et al in 1966[38] . The diet was gelatine based with supplementation of essential amino acids except for methionine and with the addition of cystine, which becomes an essential amino acid in these patients[38]. Komrower treated a newborn sibling of two affected children allowing a daily methionine intake of 24 to 42 mg/kg body weight/day during the first year of life and about 15 to 25 mg/kg/day during the second year. The plasma methionine was titrated to normal or near normal values during treatment. The daily cystine intake was increased from 25 mg/kg to 73 mg/kg and then to 133 mg/kg of body weight, but the plasma cystine remained considerably less than normal [39]. After 2 years, a daily methionine intake of 10-15 mg/kg body weight reduced the plasma methionine and homocystine to normal or near normal. Despite poor dietary control at home, this child was judged to be clinically normal or near normal at 6.5 years old when last described[39].

Perry et al devised a similar diet initially as treatment for a newborn infants [38]. The diet entails reducing daily methionine intake to approximately 20-25 mg/kg body weight for infants, to 10-15 mg/kg body weight for growing children, and to 8-10 mg/kg for adults. L-cystine supplementation of 100-300 mg/kg body weight per day was instituted[7]. They found that with this diet, the patient's plasma methionine showed a dramatic reduction with continued presence of homocystine and continuously subnormal plasma cystine despite supplementation. However, the plasma cystine did approach normal on the occasions when the plasma homocystine had been unusually low[7]. This patient at 7.5 years old had normal growth and none of the recognized complications associated with the condition, a marked contrast to his two other affected siblings in whom severe clinical disease by age of 6 months had developed while not on diet[7]. These children were not pyridoxine responsive.

Amelioration of biochemical findings was also noted in those late detected cases in whom some clinical disease may be already present when a methionine-restricted, cystine-supplemented diet was commenced[7,39-42]. As expected, there was no reversal of the major abnormalities already present before the commencement of dietary treatment. However, further progression of complications seems to be halted or ameliorated[1]. Unfortunately, despite the amelioration of the biochemical abnormalities these dietary regimens have to be stopped regularly especially in adolescents due to lack of compliance[43,44]. Such a diet also would seem unpalatable to late-detected individuals as seen amongst the 15 Australian nonresponsive patients[4].

Of the 84 treated patients from the Australian, Dutch and Irish Centers, only 24 patients (1 from the Dutch group and 23 from the Irish group) are on a methionine-restricted, cystine-supplemented diet. These patients are all pyridoxine nonresponsive. The Australian group has not used the diet in their pyridoxine nonresponsive patients as they were late detected cases and found compliance with the diet unacceptable. The single Dutch homocystinuria patient, who was detected clinically and proved to be pyridoxine nonresponsive, is on a methionine restricted diet of 600mg daily and has persistent   by plasma total homocyteine > 100μmol/L despite betaine treatment[4]. Of the 23 Irish pyridoxine nonresponsive patients on diet, 21 were detected by the national newborn screening programme while the remaining two were missed on screening and detected late clinically, as both were breast-fed. Their current ages range from 2.5 -23.4 years and their methionine-restricted, cystine-supplemented diet has a methionine content ranging from 200-625mg daily. Breast milk, during infancy, or a registered infant formula was used as the source for methionine and the intake amount was titrated against the plasma methionine and free homocystine concentration. Frequent biochemical monitoring was necessary particularly during periods of growth spurts in order that a deficiency of methionine was not missed while keeping the plasma free homocystine as near normal as possible and corrected accordingly by increasing the intake. Two thirds of the total protein intake was derived from a synthetic methionine-free, cystine-supplemented mixture and the remaining third from the natural methionine-containing foods[6]. All remained on pyridoxine. Serum $B_{12}$ and folate were assayed regularly and if found to be deficient, the patient was supplemented. Perry et al in 1968 showed that plasma cystine and homocystine concentrations are inversely related[40]. They also demonstrated that tripling the dose of supplemental L-cystine from 1.5 to 4.5 g/day did not produce an increase in plasma cystine. Hence, despite the supplementation of L-cystine in patients on low methionine diets, it is important to point out here that normal plasma cystine concentrations cannot readily be achieved, particularly in the presence of raized plasma methionine and homocysteine, since a great proportion of the free cysteine in plasma becomes bound to homocysteine by disulfide linkage[45]. Currently, proprietary formulas based on a methionine-free synthetic mixture supplemented with cystine are virtually in exclusive use[49] replacing the early gelatine-based or soya diets. There is little in the published literature on the precise long-term experience of the use of methionine restricted, cystine supplemented diet as many centers managing patients with homocystinuria have not had the opportunity to commence dietary treatment in the neonatal period because only few countries have newborn screening for this disease.

## Betaine - a methyl donor

In pyridoxine nonresponsive patients, especially when treatment is started late, it is difficult to obtain good compliance with the methionine restricted diet [42,46-50]. Perry et al in 1968 first noted in a pyridoxine nonresponsive patient that the administration of choline, a precursor of the methyl donor betaine, decreased homocystine and increased methionine concentrations[40]. Since then, others workers have found similar effects in response to betaine in pyridoxine nonresponsive patients, namely a reduction in plasma homocysteine with a rise in plasma methionine in most cases [50-54] and plasma cysteine rises[39,51] usually in parallel with the reduction in homocysteine[55].

Betaine is presumed to produce its biochemical effects by increasing the rate of homocysteine remethylation by betaine-homocysteine methyltransferase as more substrate for this reaction is made available. The resultant hypermethioninemia does not appear to influence the pathophysiology of the disease and has so far not been reported to have any side effects. This finding has recently been confirmed by data from the Australian (n=15) and Dutch (n=10) group with a total of 226 patient-years of betaine treatment[4,5]. The Australian group reported on a further 74% decline in plasma total free homocysteine with the addition of betaine to a regimen consisting of pyridoxine, folate and vitamin $B_{12}$[4]. Similarly, the Dutch group reported on a further reduction of 47% and even 84%, with the addition of folate without and with betaine respectively, to a regimen of pyridoxine[5]. In three of the Australian patients treated with betaine, circulating methionine levels remained persistently above 1000μmol/L with no adverse effects noted. All the Dutch patients had methionine levels raized to their untreated levels while on betaine. Wilcken and Wilcken in 1997 concluded that betaine used as an additional therapy is safe and effective for at least 16 years[4]. Hence, betaine may also be useful in pyridoxine nonresponsive patients who will not tolerate methionine restriction or as an adjunct to such a diet[56]. Anhydrous betaine is usually prescribed at 3-9 g/day in two to three divided doses in adults[4,50,55].

## Additional therapeutic measures

The metabolism of vitamin $B_{12}$ interacts with the metabolism of methionine and folate where methylcobalamin acts as a cofactor of N5-methyl-tetrahydrofolate-homocysteine methyltransferase which remethylates homocysteine to methionine. Hence, it is important to monitor serum $B_{12}$ levels and supplement deficient patients. Wilcken and Wilcken recently reported on the regular use of hydroxycobalamin irrespective of $B_{12}$ levels in the Australian pyridoxine nonresponsive patients (n=15) which resulted in a further decline in homocysteine levels in some patients, but the efficacy in the absence of $B_{12}$ deficiency is not established[4]. Neither the Dutch and Irish groups have administered hydroxycobalamin routinely but, instead, have administered it in $B_{12}$ deficient patients[5,6]. Since foods of animal origin, the major dietary sources of vitamin $B_{12}$, are excluded from a low methionine diet, adequate $B_{12}$ intake is likely to be reduced[7].

Additional medical therapies aim at reducing or eliminating the thrombotic tendencies, but that do not affect the biochemical abnormalities have also been used in homocystinuria[45]. Harker et al reported that dipyridamole, a platelet aggregation inhibitor, either alone or in combination with aspirin normalized decreased platelet survival and showed a marked decrease in vascular intimal lesions [56-60]. They recommended a dose of dipyridamole 400 mg/day when used alone or dipyridamole 100 mg/day in combination with aspirin 1 g/day. Effectiveness of this regimen is debatable as Schulman et al reported on thromboembolic events suffered by 2 pyridoxine nonresponsive patients while on the regimen[60,61]. As the suggested dose of aspirin is potentially dangerous, Di Minno et al reported on the efficacy and safety of using low dose aspirin (50 mg/day) instead[62].

With respect to thromboembolic events which are the major cause of morbidity and mortality in patients with homocystinuria, it has been considered advisable to avoid activities associated with an increased risk of thromboembolism eg. the use of oral contraceptives and perhaps even pregnancy, surgery whenever possible and to correct any factors, eg. dehydration, that may lead to a hypercoagulable state. However, Wilcken reported on 19 major and 15 minor operations requiring an anaesthetic and there have been no thromboembolic complications[4]. At least 6 successful pregnancies, one in a patient treated with betaine have been recorded in women with homocystinuria[4,33,Boers unpublished data]. Nevertheless, in conditions with prolonged bedrest, high dose antithrombotic prophylaxis with heparin or warfarin preparations is indicated.

## RESULTS OF POOLED DATA

### Definition of the criteria for the determination of biochemical pyridoxine responsiveness

Both groups of patients with homocystinuria from Australia (n=40) and the Netherlands (n=30) consist of late detected cases who presented clinically (see Table 1). The biochemical status of pyridoxine responsiveness was assessed in each patient with a trial of oral pyridoxine while monitoring the total free homocysteine. The pyridoxine trial regimen used by the Australian group consisted of 100-200 mg of pyridoxine and 5 mg of folic acid daily. Their patients also received intermittent hydroxycobalamin injections if necessary, as dictated by serum $B_{12}$ levels[4]. The regimen used by the Dutch group consisted of 750 mg of pyridoxine (adults) and 200-500 mg of pyridoxine (children) daily for two weeks. Folic acid and vitamin $B_{12}$ were prescribed for those patients found to be deficient in these vitamins[5]. Both groups considered their patients pyridoxine responsive when the total free homocysteine was less than 20 μmol/L, while on the pyridoxine trial regimens[4,5,refer Table 2]. The cut-off point for the normal fasting total free homocysteine level in the Australian and Dutch population was defined as 6.0[51] and 5.6 μmol/L respectively[33]. Since 1990, the Dutch group has converted to using total homocysteine levels in their evaluation and levels less than 50 μmol/L are considered as the criterion for pyridoxine responsiveness[5; see Table 2]. The overall cut-off point for the Dutch normal total plasma homocysteine was 19 μmol/L with more specific cut-off points of 15,19 and 18 μmol/L for premenopausal women, postmenopausal women and for men respectively.

*Table 4.* Combined patient-years of treatment regimens in pyridoxine responsive and nonresponsive patients with homocystinuria treated in Austarlia, the Netherlands and Ireland.

| Regimen | $B_6$ responsive patients (n=37) | $B_6$ nonresponsive patients (n=47) | All patients (n=84) |
|---|---|---|---|
| $B_6$ + folate ± $B_{12}$ | 532 | 162 | 694 |
| Above + Betaine | 11 | 255 | 266 |
| All the above + diet | 0 | 13 | 13 |
| $B_6$ + folate + $B_{12}$ + diet | 0 | 354 | 354 |
| All treatment | 543 | 771 | 1314 |
| Mean years/patient | 14.7 | 16.4 | 15.6 |

The national newborn screening program for homocystinuria was implemented in 1971 in Ireland. Of the 24 patients from the Irish group, 21 were detected by newborn screening while the remaining three were detected late; two were breast-fed and only one is pyridoxine responsive. Upon diagnosis, all the neonates were given a trial of oral pyridoxine 150 mg in three divided doses per day[6]. Free homocystine and methionine were monitored every three days while on this daily regimen. Pyridoxine responsiveness was indicated by a rapidly falling methionine level and clearing of free homocystine from the plasma, while pyridoxine nonresponsiveness was indicated by persistently high or rising plasma methionine and free homocystine[6]. It is important to point out that the determination of pyridoxine responsiveness in a neonate can often be difficult in practice as a growth spurt, which utilises methionine thus lowering its conversion to homocysteine, could produce a biochemical response similar to that seen as a response to pyridoxine[Naughten unpublished data].

## Pooled biochemical data

In the past year, these three centers treating patients with homocystinuria have published their biochemical control and the long-term course, particularly the vascular outcome, for the first time since the use of the recognized treatment modalities. All groups commenced their patients (n=84) on treatment regimens (see Table 2) upon diagnosis[4-6]. The Australian and Dutch groups have targeted a level of total free homocysteine (nonprotein-bound) < 20 µmol/L and since 1990, the Dutch group has considered a total homocysteine level < 50 µmol/L as achieving good biochemical control[4,5]. The Irish group have used a target level of free homocystine < 5 µmol/L[6]. These three centers provide a total of 1314 patient-years of treatment on 84 patients[4-6, see Tables 1,3,4].

The biochemical data published from the three groups were analysed. Of the 32 Australian patients receiving effective treatment, the 17 who were pyridoxine responsive consistently maintained plasma total free homocysteine of < 20 µmol/L[4, see Table 3]. The remaining 15 pyridoxine nonresponsive patients had current mean total free homocysteine of 33 µmol/L[4, see Table 3]. Prior to 1990, the Dutch group (n=17) had a mean total free homocysteine of 18.2 µmol/L[see Table 3]. Since total homocysteine was measured from 1990, the Dutch group (n=26) showed a mean total homocysteine of 48 µ mol/L[see Table 3]. The Irish group (n=24) had results showing a mean free homocystine of 16 µmol/L [Naughten, unpublished data, see Table 3]. It is crucial to point out that the three centers have measured different fractions of homocysteine to monitor biochemical control ie. the Australian, Dutch and

Irish groups used total free homocysteine, total homocysteine and free homocystine respectively[see Table 2]. Hence, when considering the above biochemical control data, one has to remember that total homocysteine levels may be 2 to 3 times the total free homocysteine and as high as 5 times the free homocystine levels.

## Long-term actual versus expected vascular outcome

Vascular events were reported during the 1314 patient-years of treatment in the 84 patients treated in these three centers[4,5,6,see Table 3]. A total of five vascular events were recorded, two events occurred in two of the 32 treated Australian patients [4] and the remaining 3 events in three of the 28 treated Dutch patients [5], Boers unpublished data; see Tables 1,3]. All five events occurred in pyridoxine responsive patients at a mean (range) age of 48.8 (30-60) years. Two patients aged 56 and 60 years had abdominal aortic aneurysms, one aged 30 years had pulmonary embolism and two aged 43 and 55 years died from myocardial infarction[4,5]. The relatively younger Irish group (n=24) with a mean (range) age of 14.75 (2.5-23.4) years has remained free from vascular events [6, see Table 3].

The number of observed vascular events from these three centers were compared to the time-to-event graphs for untreated patients with homocystinuria, described by Mudd et al [1]. This study also disclosed that at the time of maximal risk ie. beyond the age of 10 years, there was 1 event per 25 years[1]. During 1314 patient-years of treatment in these 84 homocystinuria patients, 53 vascular events would have been expected if they remained untreated according to the data of Mudd et al[1]. Instead, only five vascular events have been recorded with treatment, relative risk = 0.091 (95% CI 0.043 - 0.190; p<0.001)[1] [ 1, see Table 3].

---

1   The Breslow-Day test for homogeneity of the odds ratio was also performed. This statistic tests the hypothesis that the odds ratios from the different countries are all equal. There was no evidence of unequality comparing the odds ratios of the different strata (countries) (Chi-Square = 2.663     DF = 2

Prob = 0.264). The number of actual events (as a proportion of the number of patient years) was compared to the expected number of events from Mudd et al[1], based on the same number of patient-years. The odds ratios from each of the 2x2 contingency tables for the different countries were combined using the Mantel-Haenzel procedure to give an estimate of the common odds ratio. The p-values quoted are based on the Chi-squared values from analysis of the individual contingency tables.

CONCLUSION

The aim of treatment in homocystinuria is to control and, if possible, normalize the severe hyperhomocysteinemia characteristically associated with the condition. In doing so, it is hoped that the clinical development of the recognized complications of untreated homocystinuria ie. ectopia lentis, thromboembolic events, osteoporosis and mental retardation, can be prevented or ameliorated, if already present at the start of treatment. Thromboembolic events, which may occur at any age, remain the most striking cause of morbidity and mortality in untreated patients. In 158 of the 629 patients studied by Mudd et al, a total of 253 thromboembolic events occurred, 51% in peripheral veins, 32% were cerebrovascular accidents, 11% affected peripheral arteries and only 4% led to myocardial infarctions [1]. The data recently published by the centers treating patients in Australia, the Netherlands and Ireland, which documents closely monitored long term biochemical control and vascular outcome during treatment, clearly establishes that effective treatment markedly reduces the vascular risk [4,5,6].

As thrombophilia can be a multigenic disorder, the presence of additional genetic risk factors for thrombosis may enhance the thrombotic tendency in homocystinuria. Resistance to activated protein C due to a single missense mutation, A506G (factor V Leiden), in the factor V gene is currently the single most common cause of inherited thrombophilia, accounting for 45% of cases [63]. Mandel et al in 1996 found that four out of four patients with homocystinuria and factor V Leiden had thrombosis while two other without factor V Leiden were free from thrombosis[64]. Since then, three other studies have contradicted this early report[65-67]. In the same year, Quere et al reported that factor V Leiden is not a necessary requirement for thrombosis to occur in homocystinuria patients [65]. This finding was also reported by Kluijtmans et al in the Dutch group of patients with homocystinuria where two of the three patients with homocysinuria and factor V Leiden had remained free from thrombosis[66]. A further five Dutch patients with homocystinuria and thrombosis did not carry factor V Leiden. Most recently, the Irish group reported on two homocystinuria patients with factor V Leiden treated from birth remaining free from thrombosis[67]. The data from these three studies would suggest that the presence of factor V Leiden in patients with homocystinuria is a significant confounding risk factor, but not a mandatory risk factor, for thrombosis to occur as has been earlier suggested by Mandel et al. It is interesting to note that three out of the six (50%) Dutch patients with homocystinuria and thrombosis carried the thermolabile methylene-tetrahydrofolate reductase mutation (C677T), making it a more relevant additional thrombotic risk factor than factor V Leiden[66].

The above studies have provided important data for the relevance of other genetic risk factors predisposing to thrombosis in patients with homocystinuria. Nevertheless, vascular outcome data presented by the Australian, Dutch and Irish centers has clearly established that treatment regimens used, producing marked reduction of the severe hyperhomocysteinemia, very significantly diminish vascular risk. The present findings may have relevance to the current concept of mild hyperhomocysteinemia, with elevated plasma homocysteine levels considerably lower than the post-treatment levels reported by the three above mentioned centers, as a risk factor for vascular disease[68-70]. It is important to note here that total homocysteine levels were usually reported in association with mild hyperhomocysteinemia as a risk factor for vascular events. Total homocysteine is at least 2 to 3 times that of total free homocysteine (as measured by the Australian group and the Dutch group prior to 1990) and may be as high as 5 times the free homocystine (measured by the Irish group). Since 1990, the Dutch group using total homocysteine to evaluate biochemical control, has recorded a mean total homocysteine level of 48 μmol/L in their patients. Despite this mean total homocysteine level being 2.5 times the Dutch cut-off point for normal total homocysteine of 19 μmol/L, there were only 3 vascular events recorded in 409 Dutch patient-years of treatment, compared with the expected 16 events if untreated[1].

All patients in this study, both the pyridoxine responsive and the non-responsive ones, were treated with vitamin $B_6$ in high doses. The clinically beneficial effect of homocysteine-lowering was clearly present in both groups despite the persistence for many years of follow-up of homocysteine blood levels several times higher than the cut-off point for what is considered an average concentration in normal population. Similar levels have been associated with very high risks of cardiovascular events in numerous case-control and also prospective studies. Even the rise of homocysteine of one standard deviation above the mean in the normal population leads to an increase of relative risk of coronary disease of 60%[70]. In our patients, however, vascular events became rare after start of treatment. This could be due, at least partially, to some protective antithrombotic effects of high vitamin $B_6$ blood levels. Recent epidemiological studies on the association between mild or moderate hyperhomocysteinemia and cardiovascular disease indeed confirmed an inverse correlation between vitamin $B_6$ levels and cardiovascular risk, independently of their homocysteine-lowering effect[71-73]. Vitamin $B_6$ has been shown to inhibit platelet aggregation and prolong clotting time[74,75]. Also an increase of antithrombin III activity[76] and even a cholesterol-lowering effect[74] have been reported. Some of the ongoing clinical trials on the effect of homocysteine-lowering intervention on cardiovascular risk include the study of the separate effects of folic acid and of vitamin $B_6$ supplementation[77]. If a positive outcome of high vitamin $B_6$ blood levels unrelated with their eventual homocysteine-lowering effect will be confirmed, much more efforts should be put into elucidating the antithrombotic mechanisms of high vitamin $B_6$ levels. The findings could have relevance to the current concept of mild hyperhomocysteinemia and its association with cardiovascular disease, in which the causal role of a mildly elevated homocysteine level is not definitively proven yet.

In conclusion, appropriate treatment of severe hyperhomocysteinemia significantly reduces the vascular risk in patients with homocystinuria, albeit post-treatment homocysteine levels may still be several times higher than the cut-off point for values in the normal population.

*Acknowledgement. The authors wish to acknowledge Pamela Howard, National Center for Inherited Metabolic Disorders, The Children's Hospital, Temple Street, Dublin 1, Ireland, for statistical analysis of the data.*

## REFERENCES

1. Mudd SH, Skovby F, Levy HL et al. The natural history of homocystinuria due to cystathionine β-synthase deficiency. Am J Hum Genet 1985; 37: 1-31.

2. Carson NAJ. Homocystinuria: Clinical and biochemical heterogeneity. In: Cockburn F, Gitzelmann R, eds. Inborn errors of metabolism in humans. Lancaster, England: MTP Press Limited, 1982: 53-67.

3. Ubbink JB, Becker PJ, Vermaak WJ, Delport R. Results of B-vitamin supplementation study used in a prediction model to define a reference range for plasma homocysteine. Clin Chem 1995a; 41: 1033-7.

4. Wilcken DEL, Wilcken B. The natural history of vascular disease in homocystinuria and the effects of treatment. J Inher Metab Dis 1997; 20: 295-300.

5. Kluijtmans LAJ, Boers GHJ, Kraus JP et al. The molecular basis of homocystinuria due to cystathionine β-synthase deficiency in Dutch homocystinuria patients. Effects of CYSTATHIONINE -SYNTHASE genotype on biochemical and clinical phenotype, and on response upon treatment. Am J Hum Genet - In Press.

6. Yap S, Naughten E. Homocystinuria due to cystathionine β-synthase deficiency in Ireland: 25 years' experience of a newborn screened and treated population with reference to clinical outcome and biochemical control. J Inher Metab Dis 1998; 21: 738-47.

7. Perry TL. Homocystinuria. In: Nyan WL, ed. Heritable disorders of amino acid metabolism. New York: John Wiley & Sons, Inc, 1974: 395-428.

8. Barber GW, Spaeth GL. Pyridoxine therapy in homocystinuria. Lancet 1967; 1: 337.

9. Boers GHJ, Smals AGH, Drayer JIM, Trijbels FJM, Leermakers AI, Kloppenborg PWC. Pyridoxine does not prevent homocystinuria after methionine loading in adult homocystinuria patients. Metabolism 1983; 32: 390-7.

10. Seashore MR, Durant JL, Rosenberg LE. Studies of the mechanism of pyridoxine responsive homocystinuria. Pediatr Res 1972; 6: 187-96.

11. Mudd SH, Edwards WA, Loeb PM, Brown MS, Laster I. Homocystinuria due to cystathionine synthase deficiency: the effect of pyridoxine. J Clin Invest 1970; 49: 1762-73.

12. Barber GW, Spaeth GL. The successful treatment of homocystinuria with pyridoxine. J Pediatr 1969; 75: 463-78.

13. Hollowell JG, Coryell ME, Hall WK, Findley JK, Thevaos TG. Homocystinuria as affected by pyridoxine, folic acid, and vitamin $B_{12}$. Proc Soc Exper Biol Med 1968; 129: 327-33.

14. Yoshida T, Tada K, Yokoyama Y, arakawa T. Homocystinuria of vitamin B6 dependent type. Tokohu J Exp Med 1968; 96: 235-42.

15. Gaull GE, Rassin DK, Sturman JA. Enzymatic and metabolic studies of homocystinuria: effects of pyridoxine. Neuropaediatrie 1969; 1: 199-226.

16. Hooft C, Carton D, Samyn W. Pyridoxine treatment in homocystinuria. Lancet 1967; 1: 1384.

17. Carson NA, Carré IJ. Treatment of homocystinuria with pyridoxine. Arch Dis Child 1969; 44: 387-92.

18. Uhlendorf BW, Conerly EB, Mudd SH. Homocystinuria: studies in tissue culture. Pediatr Res 1973; 7: 645-8.

19. Mudd SH, Laster L, Finkelstein JD, Irreverre F. Studies on homocystinuria. In: Himwich HE, Kety SS, Smythies JR, eds. Amines and schizophrenia. New York: Pergamon Press, 1965: 246-56.

20. Gaull GE, Sturman JA, Schaffer F. Homocystinuria due to cystathionine synthase deficiency: enzymatic and ultrastructural studies. J pediatr 1974; 84: 381-90.

21. Porter PN, Grishaver MS, Jones OW. Characterization of human cystathionine β-synthase. Evidence for the identity of human L-serine dehydratase and cystathionine β-synthase. Biochim Biophys Acta 1974; 364: 128-39.

22. Poole JR, Mudd SH, Conerly EB, Edwards WA. Homocystinuria due to cystathionine synthase deficiency. Studies on nitrogen balance and sulfur excretion. J Clin Invest 1975; 55: 1033-48.

23. Bittles AH, Carson NAJ. Homocystinuria: studies on cystathionine β-synthase, S-adenosylmethionine synthetase and cystathionase activities in skin fibroblasts. J Inher Metab Dis 1981; 4: 3-6.

24. Kim Y, Rosenberg LE. On the mechanism of pyridoxine responsive homocystinuria. II. Properties of normal and mutant cystathionine β-synthase from cultured fibroblasts. Proc Natl Acad Sci U.S.A. 1974; 71: 4821-5.

25. Skovby F, Kraus J, Redlich C, Rosenberg LE. Immunochemical studies on cultured fibroblasts from patients with homocystinuria due to cystathionine β-synthase deficiency. Am J Hum Genet 1982; 34: 73-83.

26. Skovby F, Kraus JP, Rosenberg LE. Homocystinuria: Biogenesis of cystathionine β-synthase subunits in cultured fibroblasts and in an in vitro translation system programmed with fibroblast messenger RNA. Am J Hum Genet 1984; 36: 452-9.

27. Fowler B, Kraus J, Packman S, Rosenberg LE. Homocystinuria. Evidence of 3 distinct classes of cystathionine β-synthase mutants in cultured fibroblasts. J Clin Invest 1978; 61: 645-53.

28. Fowler B, Sardharwalla IB. Homocystinuria: cystathionine synthase activity in cultured skin fibroblasts: In: International Symposium on inborn errors of metabolism in humans, Switzerland 1980: 20.

29. Brenton DP, Cusworth DC. The response of patients with cystathionine synthase deficiency to pyridoxine. In: Carson NAJ, Raine DN, eds. Inherited disorders of sulfur metabolism. Edinburgh: Churchill Livingston, 1971: 264-74.

30. Gaull GE, Rassin DK, Struman JA. Pyridoxine-dependency in homocystinuria. Lancet 1968; 2: 1302.

31. Parry GJ, Bredensen DE,. Sensory neuropathy with low dose pyridoxine. Neurology 1985; 53: 1466-8.

32. Schaumberg H, Kaplan J, Windebanke A, Vick N, Rasmus S, Pleasure D, Brown MJ. Sensory neuropathy from pyridoxine abuse. N Engl J Med 1983; 309: 445-8.

33. Boers GHJ. Homocystinuria, a risk factor of premature vascular disease. Clinical Research Series no 3. Dordrecht-Holland/Riverton-USA, Foris Publications, 1986.

34. Mpofu C, Alani SM, Whitehouse C, Fowler B, Wraith JE. No sensory neuropathy during pyridoxine treatment in homocystinuria. Arch Dis Child 1991; 6: 1081-2.

35. Morrow G III, Barnes LA. Combined vitamin responsiveness in homocystinuria. J Pediatr 1972; 81: 946-54.

36. Refsum H, Helland S, Ueland PM. Radioenzymic determination of homocysteine in palsma and urine. Clin Chem 1985; 31: 624-8.

37. Komrower GM, Lambert AM, Cusworth DC, Westfall RG. Dietary treatment of homocystinuria. Arch Dis Child 1966; 41: 666-71.

38. Perry TL, Dunn HG, Hansen S, MacDougall L, Warrington PD. Early diagnosis and treatment of homocystinuria. Pediatrics 1966; 37: 502-5.

39. Komrower GM, Sardharwalla IB. The dietary treatment of homocystinuria. In: Carson NAJ, Raine DN, eds. Inherited disorders of sulfur metabolism. Edinburgh. Churchill-Livingston, 1971: 254-63.

40. Perry TL, Hansen S, Love DL, Crawford LE, Tischler B. Treatment of homocystinuria with a low-methionine diet, supplemental cystine, and a methyl donor. Lancet 1968; 2: 474-8.

41. Carson NAJ. Homocystinuria: Treatment of a 5-year old retarded child with a natural diet low in methionine. Am J Dis Child 1967; 113: 95.

42. van Sprang FJ, Wadman SK. Treatment of homocystinuria. In: Inherited disorders of sulfur metabolism, edited by Carson NAJ and Raine DN. Churchill Livingston, Edinburgh 1971: 275.

43. Brenton DP, Cusworth DC, Dent CE, Jones EE. Homocystinuria, clinical and dietary studies. Q J Med 1966; 35: 325-46.

44. Parkinson MS. Therapeutic problems of adolescent homocystinuria. Proc R Soc Med 1969; 62: 909-10.

45. Mudd SH, Levy HL, Skovby F. Disorders of transsulfuration. In Scriver CR, Beaudet AL, Sly WS, Valle D, eds. The metabolic and molecular bases of inherited disease, 7th. edn. New York: McGraw-Hill, 1995: 1279-327.

46. Andria G, Sebastio G. Homocystinuria due to cystathionine β-synthase deficiency and related disorders. In: Fernandes J, Saudubray JM, van den Berghe G,eds.: Inborn

metabolic diseases-diagnosis and treatment, (2nd. Edn.), Springer-Verlag Berlin Heidelberg, New York, 1996: 177-82.

47. Brenton DP, Cusworth DC, Dent CE, Jones EE. Homocystinuria. Proc R Soc Med 1963; 56: 996-7.

48. Parkinson MS. Therapeutic problems of adolescent homocystinuria. Proc R Soc Med 1969; 62: 909-10.

49. Smolin LA, Benevenga NJ. The use of cyst(e)ine in the removal of protein-bound homocysteine. Am J Clin Nutr 1984; 39: 730.

50. Berlow S, Bachman RP, Berry GT, Donnell GN, Grix A, Levitsky LL, Hoganson G, Levy HL. Betaine therapy in homocystinuria. Brain Dysfunction 1989; 2: 10.

51. Wiley VC, Dudman NPB, Wilcken DEL. Interrelations between plasma free and protein-bound homocysteine and cysteine in homocystinuria. Metabolism 1988;37:191-5.

52. Wilcken DEL, Dudman NPB, Tyrrell PA. Homocystinuria due to cystathionine β-synthase deficiancy - The effects of betaine treatment in pyridoxine-responsive patients. Metabolism 1985; 34: 1115-21.

53. Wiley VC, Dudman NPB, Wilcken DEL. Free and protein-bound homocysteine and cysteine in cystathionine β-synthase deficiency: Interrelations during short- and long-term changes in plasma concentrations. Metabolism 1989; 38: 734-9.

54. Smolin LA, Benevenga J, Berlow S. The use of betaine for the treatment of homocystinuria. J Pediatr 1981; 99: 467-72.

55. Wilcken DEL, Wilcken B, Dudman NPB, Tyrrell PA. Homocystinuria - The effects of betaine in the treatment of patients not responsive to pyridoxine. N Engl J Med 1983; 309: 448-53.

56. Harker LA, Ross R, Slighter SJ, Scott CR. Homocysteine-induced arteriosclerosis. The role of endothelial cell injury and platelet response in its genesis. J Clin Invest 1976; 58: 731-41.

57. Harker LA, Ross R. Prevention of homocysteine induced arteriosclerosis: sulphinpyrazone endothelial protection. In: Abe T, Sherry S, eds. A new approach to reduction of cardiac death. Bern-Stuttgart-Vienna: Hans Huber Publishers, 1979: 59-72.

58. Harker LA, Scott CR. Platelets in homocystinuria. N Engl J Med 1977; 296: 818.

59. Harker LA, Ross R. Sulphydryl-mediated vascular disease. Eur J Clin Invest 1978; 8: 199.

60. Schulman JD, Agarwal B, Mudd SH, Shulman NR. Pulmonary embolism in a homocystinuric patient during treatment with dipyridamole and acetylsalicylic acid. N Engl J Med 1978; 299: 661.

61. Schulman JD, Mudd SH, Shulman NR, Landvater L. Pregnancy and thrombophlebitis in homocystinuria. Blood 1980; 56: 326.

62. Di Minno G, Davi G, Margaglione M, Cirillo F, et al. Abnormal high thromboxane biosynthesis in homozygous homocystinuria. Evidence for platelet involvement and probucol-sensitive mechanism. J Clin Invest 1993; 92: 1400-6.

63. Bertina RM, Koelman BPC, Koster T et al. Mutation in blood coagulation factor V associated with resistance to activated protein C. Nature 1994; 369: 64-67.

64. Mandel H, Brenner B, Berant M et al. Coexistence of hereditary homocystinuria and factor V Leiden - Effects on thrombosis. N Engl J Med 1996; 334: 763-8.

65. Quere I, Lamarti H, Chadefaux-Vekemans B. Thrombophilia, homocystinuria and mutation of the factor V gene. N Engl J Med 1996; 335: 289.

66. Kluijtmans LAJ, Boers GHJ, Verbruggen B, Trijbels FJM, Novakova IRO, Blom HJ. Homozygous cystathionine β-synthase deficiency, combined with factor V Leiden or thermolabile methylenetetrahydrofolate reductase in the risk of venous thrombosis. Blood 1998; 91: 2015-8.

67. Yap S, O'Donnell KA, O'Neill C, Mayne PD, Thornton P, Naughten E. Factor V Leiden (Arg506Gln), a confounding genetic risk factor but not mandatory for the occurrence of venous thromboembolism in homozygotes and obligate heterozygotes for cystathionine β-synthase deficiency. Thromb Haemost 1999;81:502-5.

68. Mayer EL, Jacobsen DW, Robinson K. Homocysteine and coronary atherosclerosis. J Am Coll Cardiol 1996; 27: 517-27.

69. Motulsky AG. Nutritional ecogenetics: homocysteine-related arteriosclerotic vascular disease, neural tube defects, and folic acid. Am J Hum Genet 1996; 58: 17-20.

70. Boushey CJ, Beresford SAA, Omenn GS, Motulsky AG. A quantitative assessment of plasma homocysteine as a risk factor for vascular disease: probable benefits of increasing folic acid intakes. JAMA 1995; 274: 1049-57.

71. Robinson K, Arheart K, Refsum H et al. Low circulating folate and vitamin B$_6$ concentrations. Risk factors for stroke, peripheral vascular disease, and coronary artery disease. Circulation 1998; 97: 437-43.

72. Rimm EB, Willet WC, Hu FB et al. Folate and vitamin B$_6$ from diet and supplements in relation to risk of coronary heart disease among women. JAMA 1998; 279: 359-64.

73. Folsom AR, Nieto J, McGovern PG et al. Prospective study of coronary heart disease incidence in relation to fasting total homocysteine, related genetic polymorphisms, and B vitamins. Circulation 1998; 98: 204-10.

74. Brattstrom L, Stavenow L, Galvard H et al. Pyridoxine reduces cholesterol and low-density lipoprotein and increases antithrombin III activity in 80-year old man with low plasma pyridoxal 5'-phosphate. Scand J Clin Lab Invest 1990; 50: 873-7.

75. Turner RC, Matthews DR, Lang DA et al. Is vitamin B$_6$ an antithrombotic agent? Lancet 1981; 317: 1299-1301.

76. Subbarao K, Kuchibhotla J, Kakkar VV. Pyridoxal 5'-phosphate: a new physiological inhibitor of blood coagulation and platelet function. Biochem Pharmacol 1979; 28: 531-4.

77. Clarke R. An overview of the homocysteine lowering clinical trials. In: Robinson K, editor. Homocysteine and vascular disease. Dordrecht, The Netherlands: Kluwer Academic Publishers,1999: 413-429.

# 23.  AN OVERVIEW OF THE HOMOCYSTEINE LOWERING CLINICAL TRIALS

ROBERT CLARKE

## SUMMARY

Epidemiological studies have shown that cases with coronary, cerebral, or peripheral vascular disease have higher homocysteine levels than controls, but substantial uncertainty exists about the strength of any risk associations in age and sex-specific groups and in those with and without prior vascular disease. Folic acid and other B-vitamins are highly effective in delaying the vascular complications in patients with homocystinuria, who have markedly elevated levels. However, the effect on vascular risk of homocysteine reduction among those with lower levels is unknown, which has prompted calls for large-scale clinical trials to test this hypothesis. There was substantial uncertainty about the optimal regimen for lowering homocysteine levels. But many of these issues have recently been clarified by a meta-analysis of 12 randomized trials of vitamin supplements to lower homocysteine levels. The meta-analysis showed that the proportional and absolute reductions in homocysteine varied according to pre-treatment homocysteine levels, from 16% (95% CI: 11% to 20%) among those in the bottom fifth to 39% (95% CI: 36% to 43%) among those in the top fifth. After standardizing for a pretreatment homocysteine of 12 $\mu$mol/l and folate level of 12 nmol/l, there was no longer any heterogeneity in the proportional reductions in homocysteine achieved in the individual trials. Under these circumstances, the meta-analysis estimated that dietary folic acid reduced homocysteine levels by 25% (95% CI: 23 to 28%) with similar effects in a daily dosage range of 0.5 mg to 5 mg. Vitamin $B_{12}$ (mean 0.5 mg) produced an additional

*K. Robinson (ed.), Homocysteine and Vascular Disease,* 413-429.

reduction in blood homocysteine of 7%, whereas vitamin $B_6$ had no additional effects on homocysteine levels. Vitamin $B_6$ is effective at lowering homocysteine levels after methionine loading, which appears to have an independent effect on vascular risk. In view of the independent effects of folic acid and vitamin $B_6$, clinical trials with factorial designs (where participants are randomly assigned to receive to receive folic acid or placebo, and individuals in each group are subsequently randomly assigned to receive either vitamin $B_6$ or placebo) would allow assessment of the separate and combined effects of both vitamins without materially increasing the number of patients. Current and planned large-scale clinical trials to assess the effects of vitamin supplements on risk of vascular disease should provide reliable evidence for this hypothesis in almost 40000 patients with prior heart disease and several thousand patients with a prior stroke or TIA. Collaborative analysis of the post-publication follow-up of individual participants in the separate trials should provide reliable evidence of the importance of folic acid and vitamin $B_6$ in age-specific groups, and different disease categories, and across a wide range of pre-treatment homocysteine levels. The results of these trials are required before advocating widespread screening for elevated homocysteine levels or advocating the use of vitamin supplements in high-risk individuals or changing population mean levels of folate (by fortification of flour) for the prevention of cardiovascular diseases.


INTRODUCTION


Moderately elevated concentrations of blood total homocysteine have been identified as a promising area of research for the prevention of cardiovascular disease [1]. Many studies, conducted in various settings, and in different populations have reported that cases with coronary disease [2-23], stroke [24-30] or peripheral vascular disease [31-36], have higher homocysteine levels than controls. The initial studies were mainly "case-control" (or "retrospective") studies, which compared homocysteine levels in blood samples collected after the onset of disease in cases with those in controls. Weaker associations have been reported in some prospective studies in which blood was taken some years before vascular disease was diagnosed [2,3,6], with no association reported in others [4,5]. In addition, elevated homocysteine levels have been associated with an increased risk of mortality among patients with established coronary disease [37]. It is unclear the extent to which the discrepant results of different study designs are due to random error, bias (due to the effects of illness on blood homocysteine levels) or incomplete adjustment for confounding factors (such as smoking, blood pressure, and cholesterol). Furthermore, substantial uncertainty persists about the strength of the relationship of homocysteine with vascular disease in age and sex-specific groups and about the graded nature of increasing risk with increasing homocysteine levels across the distribution found in the general population, which have prompted a meta-analysis of individual participant data from all the observational studies to address these issues.

While folic acid and other B-vitamin supplements are highly effective in delaying the vascular complications in patients with homocystinuria, who have markedly elevated homocysteine levels [38,39], the effect on risk of vascular disease of homocysteine reductions among those with moderately elevated levels is unknown, which has prompted calls for large-scale clinical trials to test this hypothesis [40,41]. However, even moderate reductions in the risk of vascular diseases associated with dietary supplementation with folic acid and other B-vitamins would be of substantial public health importance, if these could be reliably demonstrated. But, detection of reductions in the risk of vascular disease of about 10 to 15% associated with the use of folic acid supplements would require that large-scale clinical trials be conducted in high-risk populations and adopt regimens and procedures that will maximise the difference between the treatment groups for an adequate duration. Until recently, there was substantial uncertainty about the optimal regimen for lowering homocysteine levels, but many of these issues have been clarified by a meta-analysis of the randomized trials of vitamin supplements to lower homocysteine levels [42]. This review examines the available evidence for the proportional and absolute reductions in homocysteine levels that might be expected from dietary supplementation with folic acid, vitamin $B_{12}$ and vitamin $B_6$ from the meta-analysis of the Homocysteine Lowering Trialist's Collaboration [42], and considers the issues involved in the design of large-scale clinical trials to assess the effect on vascular risk of lowering blood homocysteine levels.

## FOLIC ACID

Folate, in the form of 5-methyltetrahydrofolate is a co-substrate for methionine synthase, the enzyme required for the remethylation of homocysteine to methionine. This folate derivative donates its methyl group to a cobalamin attached to methionine synthase which enables remethylation of homocysteine to methionine. Blood folate levels increase in a graded manner with increasing intake of dietary folate, and are inversely correlated with homocysteine levels [43]. Data from the Framingham study indicated that mean plasma homocysteine levels declined progressively with increasing folate intake until the mean folate intake exceeded about 400 to 600 µg/day, but about two thirds of the Framingham study population had folate intakes below about 400 µg/day [43]. The average intake of folate has increased substantially in recent years in some popula

**Table1: Blood concentrations of homocysteine in the individual trials**

| Author of primary report (& reference) | Treatment comparisons with doses of vitamins (mg)[†] | N | Mean homocysteine (µmol/l) | | | |
|---|---|---|---|---|---|---|
| | | | Pre-treat. | Post-treat. | Difference (& SD) | Ratio (& SD) of Post : Pre homocysteine |
| Brattstrom[53] | C | 20 | 14.5 | 15.1 | 0.6 (1.2) | 1.0 (0.1) |
| | 2.5F | 16 | 16.9 | 12.0 | -4.9 (3.9) | 0.7 (0.2) |
| | 10F | 17 | 15.8 | 11.3 | -4.5 (3.5) | 0.7 (0.1) |
| den Heijer I[54] | P | 27 | 18.9 | 17.8 | -1.1 (5.6) | 1.0 (0.2) |
| | 5F, 0.4B12, 50B6 | 25 | 18.7 | 11.3 | -7.0 (7.0) | 0.7 (0.2) |
| den Heijer II[54] | P | 36 | 11.9 | 11.4 | -0.6 (2.7) | 1.0 (0.2) |
| | 0.5F | 36 | 12.4 | 9.7 | -2.8 (2.4) | 0.8 (0.2) |
| | 5F | 35 | 12.1 | 8.9 | -3.2 (2.2) | 0.8 (0.1) |
| | 0.4B12 | 36 | 12.6 | 11.3 | -1.3 (2.0) | 0.9 (0.2) |
| | 5F, 0.4B12, 50B6 | 35 | 12.1 | 8.3 | -3.8 (3.9) | 0.7 (0.2) |
| den Heijer III[54] | P | 46 | 14.0 | 14.5 | 0.5 (5.6) | 1.0 (0.4) |
| | 5F, 0.4B12, 50B6 | 46 | 15.9 | 10.3 | -5.7 (9.7) | 0.7 (0.2) |
| Ubbink I[55] | P | 17 | 30.0 | 30.7 | -0.7 (9.1) | 1.0 (0.3) |
| | 0.6F | 19 | 28.4 | 16.8 | -11.6 (6.2) | 0.6 (0.2) |
| | 10B6 | 17 | 28.2 | 27.9 | -0.3 (9.6) | 1.0 (0.4) |
| | 0.4B12 | 18 | 30.6 | 26.0 | -4.6 (9.1) | 0.9 (0.3) |
| | 0.6F, 0.4B12,10B6 | 20 | 26.9 | 13.6 | -13.3 (7.3) | 0.5 (0.2) |
| Ubbink II[56] | P | 13 | 23.5 | 22.1 | -1.4 (4.8) | 1.0 (0.2) |
| | 1F, 0.4B12, 10B6 | 13 | 29.3 | 11.5 | -17.8 (13.8) | 0.5 (0.2) |
| Naurath[57] | P | 142 | 13.9 | 13.4 | -0.5 (2.7) | 1.0 (0.2) |
| | 1.1F, 1B12, 5B6 | 143 | 12.7 | 8.4 | -4.4 (3.5) | 0.7 (0.2) |
| Pietrzik I[58] | P | 37 | 8.1 | 8.7 | 0.6 (1.2) | 1.1 (0.1) |
| | 0.4F, 0.1B12, 2B6 | 33 | 7.2 | 5.8 | -1.4 (1.3) | 0.8 (0.2) |
| Pietrzik II[58] | P | 86 | 8.1 | 8.2 | 0.2 (1.4) | 1.0 (0.2) |
| | 0.4F, 2B6 | 42 | 7.8 | 6.6 | -1.2 (1.2) | 0.9 (0.1) |
| Woodside[59] | P | 55 | 9.9 | 9.0 | -0.9 (1.8) | 0.9 (0.2) |
| | 1F, 0.02B12, 7.2B6 | 57 | 11.9 | 7.8 | -4.3 (3.4) | 0.7 (0.1) |
| Cuskelly[60] | C | 8 | 7.0 | 6.7 | -0.2 (0.7) | 1.1 (0.1) |
| | 0.4F | 9 | 5.8 | 5.0 | -0.8 (1.0) | 0.9 (0.2) |
| Saltzman[61] | P | 5 | 11.5 | 12.2 | 0.7 (1.5) | 1.1 (0.1) |
| | 2F | 5 | 19.6 | 15.0 | -4.6 (3.5) | 0.8 (0.1) |

[†]F represents folic acid, B12 represents vitamin $B_{12}$, B6 represents vitamin $B_6$, C represents an untreated open control and P represents a placebo control group.

tions, such as the United States, due to greater use of multivitamin supplements containing folic acid and the introduction of fortification of grain products with folic acid in 1998. Nevertheless, a substantial proportion of the US population still have intakes of folate that are sub-optimal for homocysteine levels. A UK dietary survey of the elderly in the mid-1990's, suggested that the average folate intake was about 200 to 250 µg/day [44]. Folic acid is a synthetic chemical form of folate, which is used in fortified food or supplements and has about twice the bioavailability of food folate [45]. This must be taken into account when comparing the dietary intake data with that of the effect of vitamin supplements.

## VITAMIN $B_{12}$

Vitamin $B_{12}$, as methylcobalamin, is also required for the remethylation of homocysteine to methionine as coenzyme for methionine synthase. Blood vitamin $B_{12}$ levels are inversely correlated with blood homocysteine levels. Individuals with cobalamin deficiency have particularly high levels of homocysteine. But, in contrast with folic acid, most diets contain adequate vitamin $B_{12}$ with a median intake of about 5 ug/day. While the prevalence of pernicious anemia increases with increasing age, as many as 20 to 30% of the elderly are unable to absorb dietary vitamin $B_{12}$ because of gastric achlorhydria [46]. Administering folic acid supplements to patients who are vitamin $B_{12}$ deficient may "mask" the diagnosis by correcting the anemia and allowing the neurological dysfunction to progress to irreversible neuropathy [47-49]. The concern that folic acid may cause hematological changes to improve or disappear, but fail to correct or prevent the neurological complications can be addressed by screening for vitamin $B_{12}$ deficiency before starting therapy, or by adding sufficient vitamin $B_{12}$ to supplements containing folic acid.

## VITAMIN $B_6$

Vitamin $B_6$ in the active form as pyridoxal 5'-phosphate, is a cofactor for cystathionine β-synthase, one of the two enzymes required for the metabolism of homocysteine to cysteine. Some, but not all, studies show that blood homocysteine levels are inversely related to blood levels of vitamin $B_6$ [43,50]. While supplementation with folic acid is very effective at lowering basal total homocysteine levels, vitamin $B_6$ is more effective at lowering homocysteine levels after a methionine load (where vitamin $B_6$ is a co-factor for the key enzyme involved in the transsulfuration pathway) [51]. Some epidemiological studies suggest that low $B_6$ levels are related to risk of vascular disease independent of

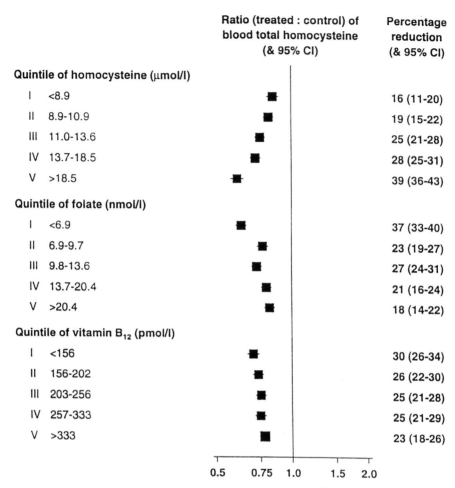

*Figure 1: Reductions in blood homocysteine concentrations with folic acid supplements according to pretreatment blood concentrations of homocysteine, folate and vitamin $B_{12}$. Squares indicate the ratios of post-treatment blood homocysteine concentrations among subjects allocated folic acid to those of controls. The size of each square is proportional to the number of individuals studied, and the horizontal line through the square indicates the 95% CI for the ratio (Reproduced with permission).*

their effect on either fasting or post-methionine load homocysteine levels [50,52]. Supplementation with vitamin $B_6$ in particular is highly effective in delaying the vascular and other complications of homocystinuria [38,39].

## META-ANALYSIS OF THE VITAMIN TRIALS TO LOWER HOMOCYS-TEINE LEVELS

Substantial uncertainty persisted about the proportional and absolute reductions in blood total homocysteine levels that could be achieved by varying doses of folic acid or other B-vitamins, partly because the non-randomized studies were unreliable and partly because the previous randomized trials of vitamin supplements were either too small or were carried out in unrepresentative populations. Hence, a meta-analysis of 12 randomized trials [53-61], involving individual data from 1114 participants was carried out to address these issues. There was substantial heterogeneity in the blood concentrations of homocysteine and the reductions in absolute levels achieved in the individual trials (Table 1). The proportional and absolute reductions in blood homocysteine produced by folic acid supplements were greater at higher pre-treatment blood homocysteine levels and at lower pre-treatment blood folate levels. Even after adjustment for differences in the folic acid regimen, the homocysteine lowering effect of folic acid ranged from a proportional reduction of 16% (11% to 20%) in subjects in the bottom fifth of the homocysteine concentration to a 39% (36% to 43%) reduction among subjects in the top fifth (Figure 1). After standardizing pre-treatment blood levels of homocysteine to 12 µmol/l and folate levels to 12 nmol/l (i.e. approximate average levels for Western populations), there was no longer any heterogeneity in the proportional reductions in homocysteine levels achieved in the individual trials (Figure 2). Under these circumstances, the meta-analysis estimated that dietary supplementation with folic acid reduced blood homocysteine levels by 25% (95% CI: 23 to 28%), with similar effects in the range of 0.5 to 5 mg folic acid daily (Figure 1). Vitamin $B_{12}$ (mean: 0.5 mg daily) produced an additional 7% (95% CI: 3 to 10%) reduction in blood homocysteine, whereas vitamin $B_6$ (mean: 16.5 mg daily) had no additional effects. Hence, the meta-analysis suggested that in typical western populations, daily supplementation with both 0.5 to 5 mg folic acid and about 0.5 mg vitamin $B_{12}$ would be expected to reduce blood homocysteine levels by about one-quarter to one-third. Studies in most western populations indicate that the average concentration of blood homocysteine is about 12 µmol/l, and so a reduction of about one quarter to one third might correspond to an absolute reduction of about 3 to 4 µmol/l (e.g. from about 12 µmol/l to about 8 to 9 µmol/l).

## FOLIC ACID ALONE OR ADDED VITAMIN $B_{12}$ AND VITAMIN $B_6$

Among the vitamins studied, folic acid had the dominant homocysteine-lowering effect.

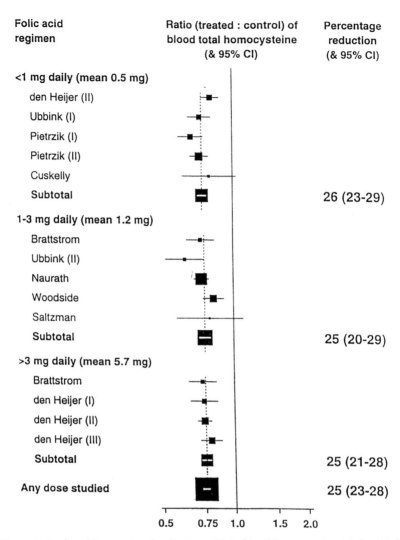

*Figure 2:Predicted Proportional reductions (%) in blood homocysteine levels with folic acid supplementation (0.5 to 5mg daily) after standardization for a pre-treatment folate level of 12µmol/L and a homocysteine level of 12µmol/L.The squares indicate the ratios of post-treatment blood homocysteine among individuals allocated folic acid supplements to those of those of individuals allocated controls. The size of each square is proportional to the number of individuals studied, and the horizontal line through the square indicates the 95% CI for the ratio (Reproduced with permission).*

Addition of vitamin $B_{12}$ to folic acid had a small additional homocysteine-lowering effect. However, vitamin $B_{12}$ would be added primarily to avoid the theoretical risk of neuropathy due to unopposed folic acid therapy in vitamin $B_{12}$ deficient patients, even those with intrinsic factor deficiency or malabsorption states. The addition of vitamin $B_{12}$ to folic acid would simplify treatment regimens since vitamin $B_{12}$ deficiency is common in the elderly and the standard screening tests for vitamin $B_{12}$ deficiency may not always detect it. By contrast, vitamin $B_6$ did not appear to have any significant effect on homocysteine levels, but these trials did not assess the effects of homocysteine lowering after methionine loading, which are influenced by vitamin $B_6$. Since vitamin $B_6$ levels are associated with cardiovascular risk, independent of their association with homocysteine levels, maximum reduction in risk may be achieved with the optimum intake of both vitamins. In view of the independent effects of folic acid and vitamin $B_6$, clinical trials with factorial designs (where participants are randomly allocated to receive either folic acid or placebo, and individuals in each group are subsequently randomized to receive either vitamin $B_6$ or placebo), would allow assessment of the separate and combined effects of both vitamins without materially increasing the required number of patients.


## CHOICE OF TARGET POPULATION AND SAMPLE SIZE

The meta-analysis of the published epidemiological studies of homocysteine and coronary heart disease suggests that a prolonged absolute difference of 3 to 5 µmol/l in blood total homocysteine levels may be associated with about 30% less coronary heart disease. Consequently, if half of the epidemiologically predicted reduction is achieved within a few years, (as seems to be the case with total cholesterol [62-64]), an absolute difference of 3-5 µmol/l in blood homocysteine levels may be associated with 15% less coronary heart disease. The sensitivity of a clinical trial to detect a difference, if one exists, depends not so much on the number randomized, but on the number of "events", such as death or non-fatal cardiovascular events that would be expected before the end of the trial. Hence clinical trials should be conducted in high risk populations (e.g., prior vascular disease), and adopt regimens and procedures that will maximise a difference that can be sustained between the treatment groups for an adequate duration.


## ONGOING OR PLANNED TRIALS OF HOMOCYSTEINE LOWERING THERAPY

The current and planned large-scale clinical trials to assess the effects of vitamin supplements on risk of vascular disease, if successful, should provide reliable

**Table 2: Current and planned clinical trials to assess the effect of homocysteine lowering on risk of cardiovascular disease**

| Study title & coordinating centre | Projected sample size | Homocysteine lowering regimen |
| --- | --- | --- |
| Vitamin Intervention for Stroke Prevention (VISP); Wake Forest University, USA | 3600 | Folic acid (2.5 mg)+ B-6 (25 mg)+ B-12 (0.4 mg) v Folic acid (0.02 mg)+ B-6 (0.2 mg) + B-12 (0.06 mg) |
| Women's Antioxidant and Cardiovascular Disease Study (WACS), Harvard Medical School, USA | 6-8000 | Folic acid (2.5mg)+ B-6 (50 mg) + B-12 (1 mg) v placebo |
| Study of the Effectiveness of Additional Reductions in Cholesterol and Homocysteine (SEARCH) University of Oxford, England | 12000 | Folic acid (2 mg) + B-12 (1mg) v placebo in a 2 x 2 factorial design with Simvastatin (80 mg v 20 mg) |
| Cambridge Heart Antioxidant Study (CHAOS-2) University of Cambridge, England | 4000 | Folic acid (5mg) v placebo |
| Norwegian Study of Homocysteine Lowering with B-vitamins in Myocardial Infarction. (NORVIT). University of Tromso, Norway | 3000 | Folic acid (5 mg x 2 weeks + 0.8 mg) + B-12 (0.4 mg) v placebo in a 2 x 2 factorial design with B-6 (40 mg) v placebo |
| Bergen Vitamin study University of Bergen, Norway | 2000 | Folic acid (5 mg x 2 weeks + 0.8 mg) + B-12 (0.4 mg) v placebo in a 2 x 2 factorial design trial with B-6 (40 mg) v placebo. |
| Prevention with A Combined Inhibitor and Folate In Coronary heart disease (PACIFIC) University of Sydney, Australia. | 10000 | Folic acid (0.2 mg or 2 mg) v placebo in a 2 x 2 factorial design with Omapatrilat.(Doses to be chosen after results of the pilot study) |

evidence for the effects of these vitamins on risk of vascular disease in almost 40,0000 patients with prior coronary heart disease and a lesser number with a prior stroke. The target populations, sample size and treatment regimens to be adopted in the current clinical trials to test the homocysteine hypothesis are shown in Table 2. All trials will examine the effects of folic acid or placebo in populations at high risk of vascular disease, but some will also receive vitamins $B_{12}$ and $B_6$ or placebo (Table 2).

Combined therapy of folic acid and vitamin $B_6$ vs placebo might be expected to produce a greater reduction in vascular risk than a trial testing folic acid alone vs placebo, but such trials would be unable to distinguish the relative importance of either vitamin. The two US trials have included vitamin $B_6$ in combination with folic acid and vitamin $B_{12}$. The Vitamin in Stroke Prevention (VISP) trial plans to randomize 3600 patients with a prior stroke or transient ischemic attack to either folic acid (2.5 mg) and $B_6$ (25mg) and $B_{12}$ (400 μg ) or very low dose folic acid (20 μg) and $B_6$ (200 μg) and $B_{12}$ (6 μg). The Women's Antioxidant Cardiovascular Study (WACS) has a 2x2x2 factorial design trial of vitamin E (600 IU every other day), vitamin C (500 mg every day), and beta-carotene (50 mg every other day), in over 8000 women with a history of prior vascular disease or other high risk, and this trial was recently modified to include additional random allocation to either folic acid (2.5 mg), and vitamin $B_6$ (50 mg) and vitamin $B_{12}$ (1mg) vs placebo. The two Norwegian trials, using identical treatment regimens in different clinical settings will assess the independent effects on cardiovascular risk of folic acid and vitamin $B_6$ separately using 2 x 2 factorial designs. Two large-scale homocysteine lowering trials will be carried out in the UK. The Study of the Effectiveness of Additional Reductions in Cholesterol and Homocysteine (SEARCH) is a 2 x 2 factorial design trial which will assess the effects on coronary heart disease of blood homocysteine reductions with folic acid (2 mg) and vitamin $B_{12}$ (1mg) vs placebo, and of standard versus larger cholesterol reductions with "statin" therapy (80mg vs 20mg daily Simvastatin). The SEARCH trial plans to randomise 12000 patients with a history of a prior myocardial infarction over a period of 2 years, with minimum follow-up of at least 4 years. The Cambridge Heart and Antioxidant Study (CHAOS-2) will assess the effects of folic acid (5 mg) or placebo in 4000 patients with a prior myocardial infarction or unstable angina. In Australia, a pilot trial is currently underway for the Prevention with a Combined Inhibitor and Folate In Coronary heart disease (PACIFIC) trial that will assess the effects on blood homocysteine of folic acid (0.2 mg vs 2 mg vs placebo) in conjunction with blood pressure reduction in 800 patients with a prior myocardial infarction, unstable angina or a risk factor profile predictive of a higher than average subsequent risk of coronary events. The results of this pilot trial should be particularly informative as the lower dose of folic acid (0.2 mg) approximates to about the upper limit of what could be achieved through dietary folate or food fortification. If the magnitude of the homocysteine reduction achieved with the lower dose is equivalent to the higher dose, the organizers plan to adopt this regimen in a trial of 10000 such patients. In addition to the VISP trial, further trials of homocysteine lowering therapy are currently being planned for patients with prior stroke or transient ischemic attack.

CONCLUSION

Epidemiological studies suggest that patients with vascular disease have higher homocysteine levels than healthy controls, although the true strength of association appears substantially less than that which was previously estimated [1]. Since homocysteine levels are easily reduced by folic acid and other B-vitamins may have additional benefits on cardiovascular risk, it is of substantial public health interest to determine whether supplementation one or other such vitamins may reduce the risk of cardiovascular disease. Observational studies cannot exclude the influence of confounding due to other dietary or non-dietary factors which may explain much of the moderate relative differences observed in such studies. Long-term large-scale clinical trials of such vitamins are required to address these questions. The design of the ongoing and planned large-scale trials of homocysteine lowering therapy, should provide randomized evidence for the effects of homocysteine lowering therapy on cardiovascular risk over the next decade. All of these large-scale trials will be carried out in high risk populations of patients with prior vascular disease or other high risk of such events. Individual trials differ somewhat in the choice of vitamin regimen adopted for lowering blood homocysteine levels. All trials have adopted similar end-points such as fatal and non-fatal coronary heart disease (and some include coronary revascularization procedures, such as coronary artery grafts or angioplasty), hemorrhagic and other strokes, total and site-specific cancers etc, which should enable the principal investigators in each trial to collate the individual participant data from their studies in a systematic overview of the post-publication follow-up of their separate results. A systematic overview of all trials of folic acid-based therapy would provide randomized evidence of any benefits (or hazards) of lowering homocysteine levels in about forty thousand patients with coronary heart disease and several thousand patients with prior cerebrovascular disease. Such an overview could compare the relative importance of folic acid and vitamin $B_6$ on vascular risk, and provide reliable evidence of the effects on mortality risks of these vitamins in age-specific subgroups, and in different disease categories, and across a wide range of blood homocysteine levels. Until these large-scale trials of homocysteine lowering therapy are completed, definitive recommendations about widespread screening of patients for elevated homocysteine levels cannot be justified. Furthermore, the results of these trials are required before advocating the use of vitamin supplements in high-risk individuals or changing the population mean levels of folate (by fortification of flour) for the prevention of cardiovascular diseases. Introduction of fortified flour for the prevention of neural tube defects before the trials of vascular disease are conducted could, however, complicate the assessment of any benefits or risks of lowering homocysteine concentrations in this way.

## REFERENCES

1. Boushey C, Beresford SAA, Omenn GS, Motulsky AG. A quantitative assessment of plasma homocysteine as a risk factor for vascular disease: probable benefits of increasing folic acid intakes. JAMA 1995;274.1049-57.

2. Stampfer MJ, Malinow MR, Willett WC, Newcomer LM, Upson B, Ullmann D, et al. A prospective study of plasma homocyst(e)ine and risk of myocardial infarction in US physicians. JAMA 1992;268:877-81.

3. Wald NJ, Watt HC, Law MR, Weir DG, McPartlin J, Scott J. Homocysteine and ischaemic heart disease: results of a prospective study with implications regarding prevention. Arch Int Med 1988;158:862-7.

4. Evans RW, Shaten BJ, Hempel JD, Cutler JA, Kuller LH. Homocyst(e)ine and risk of cardiovascular disease in the Multiple Risk Factor Intervention Trial. Arterioscler Thromb Vasc Biol 1997;17:1947-53.

5. Alfthan G, Pekkanen J, Jauhiainen M, Pitkaniemi J, Karvonen M, Tuomilehto J, et al. Relation of serum homocysteine and lipoprotein(a) concentrations to atherosclerotic disease in a prospective Finnish population based study. Atherosclerosis 1994;106:9-19.

6. Arnesen E, Refsum H, Bonaa KH, Ueland PM, Forde OH, Nordrehaug JE. Serum total homocysteine and coronary heart disease. Int J Epidemiol 1995;24:704-9.

7. Malinow MR, Ducimetiere P, Luc G, Evans AE, Arvelier D, Cambien F, Upson BM. Plasma homocyst(e)ine levels and graded risk for myocardial infarction: findings in two populations at contrasting risk for coronary heart disease. Atherosclerosis 1996;126:27-34.

8. Graham IM, Daly LE, Refsum HM, Robinson K, Brattström LE, Ueland PM et al. Plasma homocysteine as a risk factor for vascular disease: The European Concerted Action Project. JAMA 1997;277:1775-81.

9. Verhoef P, Kok FJ, Kruyssen DA, Schouten EG, Witteman JC, Grobbee DE, et al. Plasma total homocysteine, B vitamins, and risk of coronary atherosclerosis. Arterioscler Thromb Vasc Biol 1997;17:989-95.

10. Schwartz SM, Siscovick DS, Malinow MR, Rosendaal FR, Beverly RK, Hess DL, et al. Myocardial infarction in young women in relation to plasma total homocysteine, folate, and a common variant in the methylenetetrahydrofolate reductase gene. Circulation 1997;96:412-7.

11. Loehrer FM, Angst CP, Haefeli WE, Jordan PP, Ritz R, Fowler B. Low whole-blood S-adenosylmethionine and correlation between 5-methyltetrahydrofolate and homocysteine in coronary artery disease. Arterioscler Thromb Vasc Biol 1996;16:727-33.

12. Verhoef P, Stampfer MJ, Buring JE, Gaziano JM, Allen RH, Stabler SP et al. Homocysteine metabolism and risk of myocardial infarction: relation with vitamins $B_6$, $B_{12}$ and folate. Am J Epidemiol 1996; 143;845-59.

13. von Eckardstein A, Malinow MR, Upson B, Heinrich J, Schulte H, Schonfeld R, et al. Effects of age, lipoproteins, and hemostatic parameters on the role of homocyst(e)inemia as a cardiovascular risk factor in men. Arterioscler Thromb 1994;14:460-4.

14. Genest JJ Jr, McNamara JR, Salem DN, Wilson PW, Schaefer EJ, Malinow MR, et al. Plasma homocyst(e)ine levels in men with premature coronary artery disease. Impaired homocysteine metabolism in early-onset cerebral and peripheral occlusive arterial disease. J Am Coll Cardiol 1990;16:1114-9.

15. Hopkins PN, Wu LL, Wu J, Hunt SC, James BC, Vincent GM, et al. Higher plasma homocyst(e)ine and increased susceptibility to adverse effects of low folate in early familial coronary artery disease. Arterioscler Thromb Vasc Biol 1995;15:1314-20.

16. Pancharuniti N, Lewis CA, Sauberlich HE, Perkins LL, Go RC, Alvarez JO, et al. Plasma homocyst(e)ine, folate, and vitamin $B_{12}$ concentrations and risk for early-onset coronary artery disease. Am J Clin Nutr 1994 Apr;59(4):940-8.

17. Robinson K, Mayer EL, Miller DP, Green R, van Lente F, Gupta A, et al. Hyperhomocysteinemia and low pyridoxal phosphate. Common and independent reversible risk factors for coronary artery disease. Circulation 1995;92:2825-30.

18. Dalery K, Lussier Cacan S, Selhub J, Davignon J, Latour Y, Genest J Jr. Homocysteine and coronary artery disease in French Canadian subjects: relation with vitamins B12, B6, pyridoxal phosphate, and folate. Am J Cardiol 1995;75:1107-11.

19. Ubbink JB, Vermaak WJH, Bennett PJ, van Staden DA, Bisbort S. The prevalence of hyperhomocysteinemia and hypercholesterolemia in angiographically defined coronary heart disease. Klin Wochenschr 1991;69:527-34.

20. Blacher J, Montalescot G, Ankri A, Chadefaux Vekemans B, Benzidia R, Grosgogeat Y, et al. [Hyperhomocysteinemia in coronary artery diseases. Apropos of a study on 102 patients]. Arch Mal Coeur Vaiss 1996;89:1241-6.

21. Malinow MR, Sexton G, Auerbach M, Grossman M, Wilson D, Upson B. Homocyst(e)inemia in daily practice. Coronary Artery Dis 1990;1:215-220.

22. Lolin YI, Sanderson JE, Cheng SK, Chan CF, Pang CP, Woo KS, et al. Hyperhomocysteinemia and premature coronary artery disease in the Chinese. Heart 1996;76:117-22.

23. Israelsson B, Brattström LE, Hultberg BL. Homocysteine and myocardial infarction. Atherosclerosis 1988;71:227-33.

24. Brattström L, Israelsson B, Norrving B, Bergquist D, Thorne J, Hultberg B, Hamfelt A. Impaired homocysteine metabolism in early-onset cerebral and peripheral occlusive arterial disease. Effects of pyridoxine and folic acid treatment. Atherosclerosis 1990; 81:51-60.

25. Coull BM, Malinow MR, Beamer N, Sexton G, Nordt F, deGarmo P. Elevated plasma homocyst(e)ine concentration as a possible independent risk factor for stroke. Stroke 1990;21:572-6.

26. Verhoef P, Hennekens CH, Malinow MR, Kok FJ, Willett WC, Stampfer MJ. A prospective study of plasma homocyst(e)ine and risk of ischemic stroke. Stroke 1994;10:1924-30.

27. Lindgren A, Brattström L, Norrving B, Hultberg B, Andersson A, Johansson BB. Plasma homocysteine in the acute and convalescent phases after stroke. Stroke 1995;26:795-800.

28. Petri M, Roubenoff R, Dallal GE, Nadeau MR, Selhub J, Rosenberg IH. Plasma homocysteine as a risk factor for atherothrombotic events in systemic lupus erythematosis. Lancet 1996; 348:1120-4.

29. Perry IJ, Refsum H, Morris RW, Ebrahim SB, Ueland PM, Shaper AG. Prospective study of serum total homocysteine and risk of stroke in middle-aged British men. Lancet 1995;346:1395-8.

30. Evers S, Koch H,G, Grotemeyer KH, Lange B, Deufel T, Ringelstein EB. Features, symptoms, and neurophysiological findings in stroke associated with hyperhomocysteinemia. Arch Neurol 1997;54:1276-1282.

31. Molgaard J, Malinow MR, Lassvik C, Holm A, Upson B, Olsson AG. Hyperhomocyst(e)inemia: an independent risk factor for intermittent claudication. J Int Med 1992:231:273-9.

32. Bergmark C, Mansoor MA, Swedenborg J, deFaire U, Svardal AM. Ueland PM. Hyperhomocyst(e)inemia in patients operated for lower extremity ischemia below the age of 50 – effect of smoking and extent of disease. Eur J Vasc Surg 1993;7:391-6.

33. Valentine RJ, Kaplan HS, Green R, Jacobsen DW, Myers SI, Clagett GP. Lipoprotein(a), homocysteine and hypercoagulable states in young men with premature peripheral atherosclerosis: a prospective controlled analysis. J Vasc Surg 1996;23:53-61.

34. Malinow MR, Kang SS, Taylor LM, Coull B, Inahara T, Mukerjee D, Sexton G, Upson B. Prevalence of hyperhomocyst(e)inemia in patients with peripheral occlusive disease. Circulation 1989:79:1180-8.

35. Taylor LM, DeFrang RD, Harris EJ, Porter JM. The association of elevated plasma homocysteine with progression of peripheral vascular disease. J Vasc Surg 1991;13:129-36.

36. Cheng SW, Ting AC, Wong J. Fasting total plasma homocysteine and atherosclerotic peripheral vascular disease. Ann Vasc Surg 1997; 11:217-23.

37. Nygård O, Nordrehaug JE, Refsum H, Ueland PM, Farstad M, Vollset SE. Plasma homocysteine levels and mortality in patients with coronary artery disease. N Engl J Med 1997;337:230-36.

38. Mudd SH, Skovby F, Levy HL, Pettigrew KD, Wilcken B, Pyeritz RE et al. The natural history of homocystinuria due to cystathionine beta-synthase deficiency. Am J Hum Genet 1985;37: 1-31.

39. Wilcken DE, Wilcken B. The natural history of vascular disease in homocystinuria and the effects of treatment. J Inherit Metab Dis. 1997; 20: 295-300.

40. Stampfer MJ, Malinow MR. Can homocysteine lowering reduce cardiovascular risk? Engl J Med 1995;332:328-9.

41. Graham I, Meleady R. Heart attacks and homocysteine. Br Med J 1996;313:1419-20

42. Homocysteine Lowering Trialist's Collaboration. Lowering blood homocysteine with folic acid based supplements: meta-analysis of randomized trials. Br Med J 1998;316:894-98.

43. Selhub J, Jacques PF, Wilson PW, Rush D, Rosenberg IH. Vitamin status and intake as primary determinants of homocysteinemia in an elderly population. JAMA 1993,270:2693-8.

44. Bates CJ, Mansoor MA, van der Pols J, Prentice A, Cole TJ, Finch S. Plasma total homocysteine in a representative sample of 972 British men and women aged 65 and over. EurJ Clin Nutr 1997; 51: 691-7.

45. Daly S, Mills JL, Molloy A, Conley M, Lee YJ, Kirke PN et al. Minimum effective dose of folic acid for food fortification to prevent neural tube defects. Lancet 1997;350:1666-1669.

46. Stabler SP, Allen RH, Savage DG, Lindenbaum J. Clinical spectrum and diagnosis of co-balamin deficiency. Blood 1990;76:871-81.

47. Savage DG, Lindenbaum J. Folate-cobalamin interactions: In Folate in Health and Dis-ease. Ed LB Bailey. New York: Marcel Dekker Inc, 1995: 237-285.

48. Lindenbaum J, Healton EB, Savage DG, Brust JCM, Garrett TJ, Podell ER et al. Neurop-sychiatric disorders caused by cobalamin deficiency in the absence of anemia or macrocy-tosis. N Engl J Med 1988;31 8:1720-8.

49. Cambell NRC. How safe are folic acid supplements? Arch Int Med 1996;156: 1638-44.

50. Robinson K, Arheart K, Refsum H, Brattstrom L, Boers G, Ueland P et al. Low circulating folate and vitamin B6 concentrations: risk factors for stroke, peripheral vascular disease, and coronary artery disease. Circulation. 1998; 97: 437-43.

51. Bostom AG, Jacques PF, Nadeau MR, Williams RR, Elliston RC, Selhub J. Postme-thionine load hyperhomocysteinemia in persons with normal fasting total plasma homo-cysteine:initial results from the NHLBI Family Heart Study. Atherosclerosis 1995;116:147-51.

52. Rimm EB, Willett WC, Hu FB, Sampson L, Colditz G, Manson JA et al. Folate and vita-min $B_6$ from diet and supplements in relation to risk of coronary heart disease among women. JAMA 1998;279:359-364.

53. Landgren F, Israelsson B, Lindgren A, Hultberg B, Andersson A, Brattstrom L. Plasma homocysteine in acute myocardial infarction: homocysteine-lowering effect of folic acid. J Int Med 1995;237:381-8.

54. den Heijer M, Brouwer IA, Bos GMJ, Blom HJ, Spaans AP, Rosendaal FR et al. Vitamin supplementation reduces blood homocysteine levels: a controlled trial in patients with ve-nous thrombosis and healthy volunteers. Arterioscl Thromb Vasc Biol 1998;18(3):356-61.

55. Ubbink JB, Vermaak WJH, van der Merwe A, Becker PJ, Delport R. Potgieter HC. Vita-min requirements for the treatment of hyperhomocysteinemia in humans. J Nutr 1994,124:1927-33.

56. Ubbink JB, van der Merwe A, Vermaak WJH, Delport R. Hyperhomocysteinemia and the response to vitamin supplementation. Clinical Invest 1993;71:993-8.

57. Naurath HJ, Joosten E, Riezler R, Stabler SP, Allen RH, Lindenbaum J. Effects of vitamin $B_{12}$, folate, and vitamin $B_6$ supplements in elderly people with normal serum vitamin con-centrations. Lancet 1995;346:85-89.

58. Dierkes J. Vitamin requirements for the reduction of homocysteine blood levels in healthy young women. PhD thesis, University of Bonn,1995.

59. Woodside JV, Yarnell JWG, Young IS, McCrum EE, Patterson CC, Gey F, et al. The ef-fects of oral vitamin supplementation on cardiovascular risk factors. Proc Nutr Soc 1997;56:149 A.

60. Cuskelly G, McNulty W, McPartlin J, Strain JJ, Scott JM. Plasma homocysteine response to folate intervention in young women. Ir J Med Sci 1995;164:3.

61. Saltzman E, Mason JB, Jacques PF, Selhub J, Salem D, Schaefer EJ et al. B vitamin sup-plementation lowers homocysteine levels in heart disease. Clin Res 1994; 42:172A.

62. Scandinavian Simvastatin Survival Study Group. Randomized trial of cholesterol lowering in 4444 patients with coronary heart disease: the Scandinavian Simvastatin Study (4S). Lancet 1994;344:1383-1389.

63. Sacks FM, Pfeffer MA, Moye LA, Rouleau JL, Rutherford JD, Cole TG et al. The effects of pravastatin on coronary events after myocardial infarction in patients with average cholesterol levels. N Engl J Med 1996;335:1001-9.

64. Shepherd J, Cobbe SM, Ford I, Isles CG, Lorimer AR, Macfarlane PW et al. For the West of Scotland Coronary Prevention Study Group. Prevention of coronary heart disease with pravastatin in men with hypercholesterolemia. N Engl J Med 1995;333:1301-7.

# 24. SUMMARY AND FUTURE DIRECTIONS FOR EPIDEMIOLOGICAL, PREVENTIVE AND BASIC RESEARCH

STEPHEN P. FORTMANN, BARRY SHANE AND
ARNO G. MOTULSKY

Future research on the epidemiology of homocysteine as a risk factor for cardiovascular disease must be understood in the general context of research on epidemiology and prevention. The major causes of cardiovascular disease are well understood, particularly as they contribute to epidemic cardiovascular disease, and include mass exposure to high levels of dietary saturated fat, physical inactivity, obesity, hypertension and cigarette smoking. While it is frequently stated that these "classical" risk factors account for only 50% of the cardiovascular disease incidence, this statement is based on the imprecision of multivariate risk models and ignores the significant limitations to the predictive power of these models from measurement error (1). From a population perspective, the classical risk factors are likely to account for 70 to 85 percent of cardiovascular disease incidence (2). Thus, one of the principal challenges to cardiovascular disease prevention is to apply current knowledge to a much higher proportion of the population at risk by improving clinical prevention efforts and by finding effective ways of changing health-related behavior at the community level (3). This will be a particularly great challenge in the developing world, where the majority of cardiovascular disease events already occurs (4-6).

The search for new risk factors, including homocysteine, nevertheless remains important. In developed countries, the best plans for controlling cardiovascular disease include both population-wide components and interventions directed at high risk subgroups. Since the prediction of cardiovascular disease risk at the individual level is imprecise, the discovery of

*K. Robinson (ed.), Homocysteine and Vascular Disease*, 431-436.

new risk factors may improve the cost-effectiveness of interventions for high-risk subgroups by increasing the precision of risk prediction. In addition, identification of new risk factors stimulates further investigation on the etiology of cardiovascular disease, advancing both general knowledge and identifying additional potential for prevention and treatment. Newer risk factors may also uncover subgroups that are at high risk that cannot now be identified. Homocysteine appears to be fulfilling most of these areas for potential advancement.

The epidemiological relationship of homocysteine to cardiovascular disease is presented in several of the chapters in this book. As reviewed in those chapters, numerous cross-sectional, case-series, and case-control studies document that patients with arteriosclerotic diseases have higher levels of homocysteine than patients without such diseases. Such cross-sectional designs are subject to several forms of bias, including the distinct possibility that elevated homocysteine levels are a result, rather than a cause, of the cardiovascular disease. There is growing evidence that inflammation plays a role in cardiovascular disease the pathogenesis of which provides a possible mechanism by which extensive atherosclerotic disease might result in higher homocysteine levels (7). In addition, controlling for confounding factors, including dietary folate, other B vitamin intake, and cigarette smoking, has not always been adequate. Fewer prospective studies have been reported and these have produced mixed results. Some have failed to find an association (8) and in others the association is weaker than in cross-sectional studies, or is eliminated by controlling for potential confounding variables (9). The strength of an association is one of the principal criteria for assessing the likelihood that the association is causal, so the weakened or absent risk in studies with prospective designs is troublesome. Likewise, the failure to find an association between coronary disease and the TT polymorphism of the methylenetetrahydrofolate reductase gene is puzzling, since carriers of this genotype have higher levels of homocysteine, particularly with suboptimal folate nutrition. These findings would seem to make it more likely that the association between homocysteine and cardiovascular disease is confounded by some other factor. Additional prospective studies do not warrant a high priority since clinical trials are already in progress to test whether lowering homocysteine levels prevents cardiovascular disease. Such intervention trials will provide much stronger evidence concerning the causal hypothesis than any observational study. Unfortunately, studies in the United States, where folate fortification of foods started in 1998, may be difficult to interpret since the control groups will also now have lower homocysteine levels. Whenever possible, large prospective studies ought to evaluate homocysteine as a risk factor, particularly in more heterogeneous populations (e.g., including more ethnic subgroups). The suggestion that homocysteine may be a more potent risk factor in women (see chapter by Verhoef) should also be evaluated more extensively in prospective studies, since some of the reported studies were limited to men.

As noted above, the strongest evidence for a cause and effect relationship between a risk factor and a disease is obtained in clinical trials where the risk factor is manipulated and disease incidence is compared in treatment and control groups. However, the results of clinical trials cannot always be generalized, since the various inclusion and exclusion criteria and dosage used may not apply to the general population. All these factors need to be carefully analyzed in evaluating overall trial results. For example, the influence of pretreatment homocysteine level is likely to be critical, since patients with homocystinuria have extremely marked increases in the level of homocysteine and appear to benefit from treatment to lower it (see chapter by Rubba, Di Minno, and Andria). Thus, the benefit to patients with only modest increases of homocysteine (12 and 20 µmol/L) may be limited to those at the higher levels. The possibility that other correlates of homocysteine level, such as age, smoking, and diet, might modify the effect of the treatment also will need to be examined.

Much of the interest in homocysteine as a risk factor results from the potential for treatment with a simple, inexpensive, and probably innocuous intervention, folic acid supplementation. As noted in the chapter by Ueland, Refsum, and Schneede, several lifestyle factors that lower homocysteine levels are also of proven benefit through other mechanisms. In addition, folic acid fortification of food introduced to prevent neural tube defects in newborns is already established in the United States and may be initiated elsewhere. Even the current degree of folic acid fortification (estimated to provide an average of 100µg additional folic acid per day) will result in population-wide lowering of homocysteine that would be expected to have an impact on the incidence of cardiovascular disease if elevated homocysteine is causally related (see chapter by Wilson and Jacques). Thus the potential for future prevention of cardiovascular disease through homocysteine lowering is very great indeed (10). The optimum level of fortification with folic acid alone or with other vitamins (pyridoxine and vitamin $B_{12}$) will need to be determined if cardiovascular disease benefits can be demonstrated.

A number of major mechanistic questions, however, remain to be answered. The beneficial effects of folate and betaine on disease progression in patients with severe $B_6$-nonresponsive cystathionine β-synthase deficiency is the strongest evidence that elevated homocysteine is the primary cause of the vascular complications in these patients. These treatments cannot rescue the metabolic defect but they can divert homocysteine into methionine. A plethora of mechanisms have been suggested to explain the adverse effects of elevated homocysteine. Some of these may be correct but none have been unequivocally established. If it is a cause, rather than an effect of vascular complications, the adverse mechanisms operative in chronic mild hyperhomocysteinemia may be different from that in severe hyperhomocysteinemia.

Establishing the role of a chronic mild elevation of a metabolite in the cause of a condition is always difficult. Do effects seen at high levels of a metabolite reflect chronic exposure to lower levels? Even if effects are noted, any potential mechanism explaining the role of homocysteine in the development of vascular complications has to address the question: why homocysteine, what is special about this compound that makes the effect specific for homocysteine? Several chapters in this book discuss mechanisms involving oxidative stress or effects on nitric oxide production and utilization. Some of these attractive mechanisms attribute specificity to the chemical properties of homocysteine. Homocysteine is a stronger nucleophile than other plasma and cellular thiols and is more prone to oxidation than cysteine. However, much of this chemical difference would be negated under physiological conditions because of the higher concentration of cysteine. Although specificity for homocysteine versus cysteine has been demonstrated in some of these studies, the actual mechanism by which homocysteine causes the specific change remains to be elucidated. Similarly, very interesting effects on the growth of epithelial and smooth muscle cells have been reported together with homocysteine-specific effects on expression of genes regulating cell growth. Again, why homocysteine elicits these effects remains to be clarified. Another suggested mechanism involves binding of homocysteine to specific receptors. This type of mechanism, although not well developed at the moment, would be attractive as an explanation for specificity. Finally, one specific effect of homocysteine compared to other sulfhydryl compounds that has been known for many years is its metabolism to adenosylhomocysteine. Adenosylhomocysteine is an inhibitor and regulator of many methyltransferase reactions that are involved in the regulation of multiple processes in growth, development and metabolism. It is somewhat surprising that relatively few studies have addressed whether paradigms that cause changes in plasma homocysteine also influence the levels of other metabolites such as adenosylhomocysteine in tissues, and this should be an area of further study in the future. The recent development of animal models in which key enzymes of homocysteine metabolism have been genetically altered should provide interesting experimental systems to explore chronic effects of hyperhomocysteinemia. These models will also facilitate studies on whether changes in other metabolites distinct from homocysteine are the causative agents directly linked to chronic disease.

Homocysteine is just one player in a complex series of metabolic interconversions that are required for the supply of methionine and cysteine. Methionine is an essential amino acid and is one of the more limiting amino acids in the food supply. It is somewhat unusual compared to other amino acids in the degree that it is utilized for anabolic reactions distinct from protein synthesis, providing the methyl group for most biological methylations and the sulfur for cysteine synthesis. The large flux of the methyl group of methionine into methyl group metabolism has necessitated a process for the re-synthesis of methionine from homocysteine. The regulation of these processes, which are described in several chapters, is complex and is designed to maintain methionine and methyl group status in the face of differences in dietary intakes of methionine and also differences in vitamin status (11,12). Failure of these regulatory balances may be reflected by elevated levels of homocysteine. Chronic changes in methyl group status are more likely to adversely affect health than small changes in plasma homocysteine levels. Various interventions such as increased vitamin intakes have been proposed to reduce circulating homocysteine. Increased vitamin intake is attractive because it appears innocuous. However, more attention should be placed in the future on the potential effect of such treatments on other indicators of methyl group homeostasis and status.

## REFERENCES

1.  MacMahon S, Peto R, Cutler J, et al. Blood pressure, stroke, and coronary heart disease. Part 1, Prolonged differences in blood pressure: prospective observational studies corrected for the regression dilution bias. Lancet 1990;335:765-74.
2.  Negri E, La Vecchia C, Franzosi MG, Tognoni G. Attributable risks for nonfatal myocardial infarction in Italy. Preventive Medicine 1995;24:603-609.
3.  Stone EJ, Pearson TA. Community trials for cardiopulmonary health: Directions for public health practice, policy, and research. Ann Epidemiol 1997;S7:S1 - S124.
4.  Reddy K, Yusuf S. Emerging epidemic of cardiovascular disease in developing countries. Circulation 1998;97:596-601.
5.  Murray C, Lopez A. Alternative projections of mortality and disability by cause 1990-2020: Global Burden of Disease Study. Lancet 1997;349:1498-1504.
6.  Mackay J. The global tobacco epidemic: The next 25 years. Public Health Reports 1998;113:14-21.
7.  Ross R. Atherosclerosis--an inflammatory disease. N Engl J Med 1999;340:115-26.
8.  Evans R, Shaten B, Hempel J, Cutler J, Kuller L. Homocyst(e)ine and risk of cardiovascular disease in the Multiple Risk Factor Intervention Trial. Arterioscler Thromb Vasc Biol 1997;17:1947-1953.
9.  Folsom AR, Nieto FJ, McGovern PG, et al. Prospective study of coronary heart disease incidence in relation to fasting total homocysteine, related genetic polymorphisms, and B vitamins: the Atherosclerosis Risk in Communities (ARIC) study. Circulation 1998;98:204-210.

10. Boushey CJ, Beresford SAA, Omenn GS, Motulsky AG. A quantitative assessment of plasma homocysteine as a risk factor for vascular disease: probable benefits of increasing folic acid intakes. JAMA 1995;274:1049-1057.

11. Selhub J, Miller JW. The pathogenesis of homocysteinemia: interruption of the coordinate regulation by S-adenosylmethionine of the remethylation and transsulfuration of homocysteine. Am J Clin Nutr 1992;55:131-138.

12. Finkelstein JD, Martin JJ. Methionine metabolism in mammals. Distribution of homocysteine between competing pathways. J Biol Chem 1984;259:9508-13.

# INDEX